Current Topics in Intensive Care Number 2

CURRENT TOPICS IN INTENSIVE CARE

Current Topics in Intensive Care Number 2

edited by

J.F. Bion
Senior Lecturer in Intensive Care Medicine
University Department Anaesthesia and Intensive Care
Queen Elizabeth Hospital,
Birmingham, UK

W.B. SAUNDERS COMPANY LTD
London · Philadelphia · Toronto
Sydney · Tokyo

W.B. Saunders Company Ltd 24–28 Oval Road
London NW1 7DX

The Curtis Center
Independence Square West
Philadelphia, PA 19106–3399, USA

Harcourt Brace & Company
55 Horner Avenue
Toronto, Ontario, M8Z 4X6, Canada

Harcourt Brace & Company, Australia
30–52 Smidmore Street
Marrickville
NSW 2204, Australia

Harcourt Brace & Company, Japan
Ichibancho Central Building
22–1 Ichibancho
Chiyoda-ku, Tokyo 102, Japan

This book is printed on acid-free paper

A catalogue record for this book is available from the British Library

ISBN 0–7020–1871–6

Typeset by J&L Composition Ltd, Filey, North Yorkshire
Printed by WBC Book Manufacturers Ltd, Bridgend, Mid Glamorgan

Contents

Contributors *vii*
Contents of Number 1 *ix*
Preface *x*

1i Advances in American Prehospital Emergency Medical Services 1
Paul E. Pepe

1ii Advances in Prehospital Care 21
Thomas Kerz and Wolfgang F. Dick

2 Pulmonary Vasomotor Dysfunction in Acute Lung Injury 41
Marc Leeman and Robert Naeije

3 Serious Illness in Pregnancy and Childbirth 55
Barry N.J. Walters

4 Initial Management of the Poisoned or Overdosed Patient 82
Francis J. De Roos and Lewis R. Goldfrank

5 Treatment Limitation Decisions 102
J.F. Bion

6 Modern Techniques for Measuring Body Composition in Patients who are Critically Ill 125
Lindsay D. Plank and Graham L. Hill

7 New Developments in Specialized Nutrition Support 144
Thomas R. Ziegler

8 Antioxidant Therapy 175
C. Deby, G. Hartstein, G. Deby-Dupont and M. Lamy

9 Growth Factors in Tissue Healing 206
Malcolm R. Alison

10 Muscle Dysfunction in Critical Illness 238
John Coakley and Richard Ross

11 Surfactant Physiology and Therapy in Acute Lung Injury 256
Peter D. Macnaughton and Timothy W. Evans

Contributors

Dr M.R. Alison, Senior Lecturer in Experimental Pathology, Department of Histopathology, Royal Postgraduate Medical School, Hammersmith Hospital, Du Cane Road, London W12 0NN, UK.

Dr J.F. Bion, Senior Lecturer in Intensive Care Medicine, University Department of Anaesthesia and Intensive Care, North 5, Queen Elizabeth Hospital, Birmingham B15 2TH, UK.

Dr John Coakley, Department of Intensive Care, St Bartholomew's Hospital, West Smithfield, London EC1A 7BE, UK.

Dr Carol Deby, Centre for Biochemistry of Oxygen, Department of Anesthesia and Intensive Care Medicine, CHU Sart Tilman-Bât B35, 4000 Liège, Belgium.

Dr Deby-Dupont, Department of Anaesthesia, Centre Hospitalier Université de Liège, Sart Tilman, B35–400 Liège, Belgium.

Professor Dr med W. Dick, Head of Department, Klinik für Anaesthesiologie, Klinikum der Johannes Gutenberg-Universitat Mainz, Langenbeckstrasse 1, Postfach 3960, 6500 Mainz, Germany.

Dr T.W. Evans, Reader in Critical Care, National Heart & Lung Institute, Consultant in Intensive Care & Thoracic Medicine, Royal Brompton National Heart & Lung Hospital, London SW3 6NP, UK.

Professor Lewis Goldfrank, Medical Director, New York City Poison Control Center, Department of Health, 455 First Avenue #123, New York 10012, USA.

Dr Gary Hartstein, Department of Anesthesia and Intensive Care Medicine, CHU Sart Tilman-Bât B35, 4000 Liège, Belgium.

Professor Graham Hill, University Department of Surgery, Fifth Floor, Auckland Hospital, Auckland 3, New Zealand.

Dr Thomas Kerz, Klinik für Anaesthesiologie, Klinikum der Johannes Gutenberg-Universitat Mainz, Langenbeckstrasse 1, Postfach 3960, 6500 Mainz, Germany.

Professor Maurice Lamy, Department of Anaesthesia, Centre Hospitalier Université de Liège, Sart Tilman, B35-400 Liège, Belgium.

Dr Marc Leeman, Department of Intensive Care & Laboratory of Cardiovascular & Respiratory Physiology, Erasme Hospital, Free University of Brussels, B-1070 Brussels, Belgium.

Dr P.D. Macnaughton, Senior Registrar in Intensive Care, Westmead Hospital, Westmead, NSW 2145, Australia.

Dr Robert Naeije, Department of Intensive Care & Laboratory of Cardiovascular & Respiratory Physiology, Erasme Hospital, Free University of Brussels, B-1070 Brussels, Belgium.

Professor Paul Pepe, Department of Medicine, Surgery and Pediatrics, Baylor College of Medicine; Director, City of Houston Emergency Medical Services, Center for Resuscitation and Emergency Medical Services, 410 Bagby, Suite 300, Houston TX 77002, USA.

Dr L.D. Plank, University Department of Surgery, Fifth Floor, Auckland Hospital, Auckland 3, New Zealand.

Dr Francis De Roos, Fellow in Medical Toxicology, New York City Poison Control Center, Department of Health, 455 First Avenue #123, New York 10012, USA.

Dr Richard Ross, Department of Endocrinology, St Bartholomew's Hospital, West Smithfield, London EC1A 7BE, UK.

Dr B.N.J. Walters, Clinical Senior Lecturer in Obstetric Medicine, King Edward Memorial Hospital for Women, Bagot Road, Subiaco, Western Australia 6008, Australia.

Dr Thomas Ziegler, 818 Guinevere Way, Lilburn, Georgia 30247, USA.

Current Topics in Intensive Care: No 1
Contents

1 Developments in Intracranial Pressure Monitoring and Investigation of Head Injured Patients
Stephen B. Lewis, Peter L. Reilly and John A. Myburgh

2 Nitric Oxide: its Role and Application in the Critically Ill
Rolf Rossaint and Konrad J. Falke

3 Applications of Monoclonal Antibody Technology in the Critically Ill
Janice L. Zimmerman

4 Monitoring of Ventilation and Respiration in Acute Lung Injury
Tom Clutton-Brock and B. Venkatesh

5 New Ventilatory Strategies in Severe Respiratory Failure
Hilmar Burchardi, Michael Sydow and Carl-Peter Criee

6 Regional or Organ Blood Flow and Oxygen Consumption: Observations in Septic Shock
L.G. Thijs

7 Splanchnic Ischaemia
Ulf Haglund and Agneta Montgomery

8 Management of the Patient Resuscitated from Sudden Cardiac Death
Challon J. Murdock and Michael J.E. Davis

9 Acute Renal Replacement Therapy
Rinaldo Bellomo

10 Neurological Changes During Severe Sepsis
Charles F. Bolton, G. Bryan Young and Douglas W. Zochodne

11 Audit and Quality Assurance in Critical Care
J.F. Bion

Preface

In this second edition of *Current Topics in Intensive Care*, I and my co-authors have chosen aspects of clinical medicine and applied physiology that are of current interest to clinicians and for which there is new information. Our contributors have examined aspects of: pre-hospital emergency care; acute lung injury; obstetric critical illness; poisoning; the ethics of treatment limitation; and new techniques for measuring the changes in body composition, which accompany the metabolic derangements of multiple organ failure. We have also devoted several chapters to techniques of preventing tissue damage and enhancing tissue repair. While it is not our purpose in this series to produce specific themes, the underlying principle of Volume 2 is the need to improve our ability to identify and treat patients at risk of critical illness much earlier on, with the intention of preventing subsequent organ system failures. Of course, this is not always possible, and in those patients with established organ system failures, strategies for restoring tissue repair may offer some hope for the future in that group of patients for whom intensive care at present defers, but cannot prevent, their subsequent death. We hope that this volume will provide illumination and stimulation to our colleagues in intensive care.

I would like to acknowledge with thanks the contributors to this volume who have provided high quality scientific papers of clinical relevance. I also appreciate the assistance of my co-editors and the help of Margaret Macdonald and her colleagues at W.B. Saunders.

J.F. Bion

1i

Advances in American Prehospital Emergency Medical Services

Paul E. Pepe

OVERVIEW

In the late 1960s and early 1970s, critical care medicine came of age as a recognized discipline. Simultaneously, in Europe, the United States (US) and other countries, certain critical care physicians took their knowledge and intensive care talents out of the hospital setting (Pepe et al., 1990). They had come to appreciate that the earlier key interventions were provided for patients with life-threatening manifestations of coronary artery disease, the better the results. As a result, in those communities where such out-of-hospital critical care services were established effectively, many lives were saved (Pepe et al., 1990).

Likewise, delivery of sophisticated prehospital care for severe injury became an important offshoot of such out-of-hospital intensive care programmes. With the evolution of trauma centres, prehospital care and transport became an integral component of injury management.

Eventually, in the US and other venues, most of the prehospital care services, both for trauma care and coronary artery disease, were delegated to specially-trained personnel, the forerunners of today's paramedics (Pepe et al., 1990). In addition, these prehospital care providers took on additional responsibilities such as the care of patients with the sequelae of diabetes, congestive heart failure, stroke, and other acute illnesses. As a result, formal programmes of out-of-hospital emergency care soon became a routine part of each municipalities' public safety obligations to its citizens.

Emergency medical services (EMS), as a formal system of public safety, has now been in existence for more than a quarter century. Citizens worldwide expect EMS as a basic function of government and society, just as much as public schools and police protection. Across the US alone, a response to an EMS incident occurs every two seconds. The terms 'paramedic' and '9–1–1' (or their equivalents) have become household words in North America and, likewise EMS systems have also begun to proliferate, in some form or fashion, around the world.

Similarly, in the world of intensive care medicine, EMS has maintained a relatively high profile, particularly because many critical care physicians supervise or regularly interact with EMS programmes. More importantly, most of today's clinical data regarding resuscitation medicine have been derived from EMS systems. Therefore, a detailed review of developments in specific EMS therapeutics might be less than novel. None the less, even for the most sophisticated of EMS experts, it would still be worthwhile to step back and summarize some of the more global controversies that have evolved in out-of-hospital emergency medical care delivery during the past few years in North America.

CURRENT CONTROVERSIES IN AMERICAN PREHOSPITAL CRITICAL CARE

From the joint perspective of leading EMS specialists (see Acknowledgements), some of the most compelling issues to address would be those revolving around the following headings:

The Value of Advanced Life Support Interventions – do they make a difference?

The Value of Responses with Warning Lights and Sirens – are they always necessary?

EMS Management and Deployment Strategies – cost versus care.

The Ethics of Research, Futility and Cost Containment in the Prehospital Setting.

EMS as the Practice of Medicine – the evolving role of the physician.

The Value of Advanced Life Support Interventions

Approximately 25 years ago, a certain breed of critical care physicians took to the streets of North America and Europe to challenge the notion that many of those dying out in the community from heart disease and injury were unsalvageable (Pepe et al., 1990). Bringing with them many of their intensive care tools such as defibrillators, endotracheal tubes, intravenous cannulation and a host of pharmacological interventions, they delivered *advanced life support* in the streets as well as in people's homes and workplaces. In some places, particularly North America, the skills and procedures of these pioneers were passed on to *paramedics* (non-physician, specially-trained personnel). In many communities in the US, for example, firefighters went through intensive training under expert physician tutelage and were extremely successful in saving lives, particularly of those with *Sudden Death Syndrome* (cardiac arrest associated with ventricular fibrillation). It was apparent that using these advanced skills and procedures, paramedics provided a way to deliver life-saving care in a cost-effective manner.

In some venues, lesser skilled basic *emergency medical technicians* (EMTs) were also trained to provide and assist with the basic (non-invasive) skills such as spinal immobilization and basic CPR. However, in those communities where only EMTs provided care, or where advanced care was delayed significantly, survival rates were not as good. It was assumed, therefore, that physician-level advanced life support (or at least paramedic-level skills) were required to effect a good EMS system. In fact, the concept eventually was extrapolated in most of the US toward a philosphy that, the more paramedics one could train, the better the life-saving effect.

But perhaps this presumption was premature. In the mid-1980s, trauma surgeons in the US began to debate the value of a 'scoop and run' versus a 'stay and play' approach to prehospital trauma care, inferring that advanced life support (ALS) procedures provided by paramedics (e.g., intravenous access at the scene) delayed definitive care (Border et al., 1983; Smith et al., 1985; Pepe et al., 1990; Bourn, 1992). A spill-over effect soon occurred and others began to question the prehospital use of other invasive interventions provided by prehospital care personnel (paramedics), such as furosemide and even endotracheal intubation.

In fact, by the last 1980s, it was beginning to be appreciated that most of the standard procedures used in EMS are empiric and of unproven efficacy in the prehospital setting (Bourn, 1992). For example, to date, only two interventions seem to have sound support for cases of sudden death associated with ventricular fibrillation (VF) (Cummins et al., 1991; Bourn, 1992; Pepe et al., 1994); *early basic CPR* by bystanders and *early defibrillation*. Most recently, it has become recognized, more and more, that clinical research findings supporting the use of time-honoured pharmacological interventions, such as adrenaline (epinephrine) and lignocaine (lidocaine), were not as strong as one would like (Wesley et al., 1991; Pepe et al., 1994). This realization has become particularly relevant considering their endorsement as national and international standards of care for cardiac arrest management (Cummins et al., 1991; Emergency Cardiac Care Committee, 1992). In fact, some would even suggest that, under certain circumstances, their use may be very detrimental (Wesley et al., 1991; Pepe et al., 1994).

In addition, in the area of trauma care, growing evidence has suggested that the use of traditional interventions such as the pneumatic anti-shock garment (PASG) and even intravenous (IV) fluid infusions may be detrimental under certain circumstances (Mattox et al., 1989; Honigman et al., 1991; Bickell et al., 1992, 1994; Pepe and Maio, 1993). Similarly, despite the recent enthusiasm for bolstering EMS for children (EMS-C), including the prolific training of EMS personnel in paediatric intubation and intra-osseous injection, few data are available to prove the absolute efficacy of any of these interventions. Furthermore, because paediatric resuscitations are comparatively infrequent, proper statistical analysis is nearly impossible.

The resulting inference is that the absolute need for prehospital ALS providers (i.e. paramedics, nurses or physicians) may be quite limited, if at all necessary. Today, with the advent of automated defibrillators, defibrillation can be delivered earlier than ever before by basic life support (BLS) providers (Weaver et al., 1988; Cummins et al., 1991; Becker and Pepe, 1993). In addition, many are now advocating the use of alternative invasive airways (e.g., the Combitube® or PTL®) by BLS providers (Atherton and Johnson, 1993; Pepe et al., 1993a). Thus the distinctions betwen ALS and BLS may be fading quickly and the absolute need for traditional ALS providers is being questioned (Pepe et al., 1994). For example, such approaches actually have been proposed recently to help to establish more cost-effective EMS staffing strategies for certain Provinces in Canada, particularly in those venues where physicians have traditionally provided prehospital ALS services. In an era of medical cost-containment and shrinking governmental budgets, the alternative of using lesser-trained personnel for presumably equivalent efficacy is growing attractive. In addition, the US Department of Transportation (DOT) has recently developed a new 'Blueprint' training curriculum package for emergency medical technicians (EMTs). This 'blueprint' outlines a new approach to training standards that focuses on certain skills and less so on titles such as EMT-basic or EMT-paramedic. Therefore, the traditional lines have now been blurred even further with this latest initiative from a time-honoured bastion of classifications and standards for EMS providers.

But perhaps paramedics and other ALS providers can serve another role. It is well-accepted that appropriate patients with evolving myocardial infarction are benefited by the earliest possible treatment with thrombolytics (Eisenberg et al., 1993). This has prompted the notion of prehospital administration of this therapy to improve patient outcome (European Myocardial Infarction Project Group, 1993; Weaver et al., 1993). In recent trials of prehospital versus in-hospital thrombolytics, however, there were no demonstrable differences in survival rates (Weaver et al., 1993). On the other hand, part of the explanation was a 'study effect', with the early prehospital detection of S–T elevations on the prehospital 12-lead electrocardiograph (ECG), a larger percentage of patients were treated in-hospital within a 'golden hour' following the onset of their myocardial ischaemia symptoms. In these cases, mortality rates were negligible and infarct size was less than 1% in nearly half of the cases (Weaver et al., 1993). Thus the use, by ALS providers, of a prehospital 12-lead ECG, which uses a computerized algorithm capable of identifying 75% of infarcts in evolution, was the most likely key to success. Still, this may only imply a benefit of the special ECG and not necessarily the use of ALS skills themselves. Conceptually, the growing technology of computers and automation may cause the eventual extinction of the traditional 'eyes, ears and hands of the doctor'. It may also herald the extinction of prehospital care physicians as primary care givers where they still exist (such as in parts of Europe and Canada).

So should we reconsider the need for paramedics and other prehospital ALS providers? Maybe not. While there is a growing scepticism toward the value of prehospital ALS procedures, objective evidence still supports their value (Pepe et al., 1994). For example, studies have shown that many out-of-hospital cardiac arrest patients presenting with asystole or rhythms other than VF (and therefore not requiring defibrillation) have been successfully resuscitated following significant periods of basic CPR (Pepe et al., 1993). In fact, as many as 20% of out-of-hospital cardiac arrest survivors never receive defibrillation – only the other ALS procedures (Pepe et al., 1993b). In turn, without such on-scene ALS, very few survive (Bonnin et al., 1993; Kellerman, 1993).

The implication is that some aspect of ALS (other than defibrillation) must be of value (Pepe et al., 1994). We do not yet understand how it works, but some component of ALS seems to be effective. Likewise, tolerance of prehospital circulatory arrest associated with severe injury appears to be significantly prolonged by endotracheal intubation (Durham et al., 1992). In such critical situations, the ET tube, placed by ALS providers in the prehospital setting, has been shown to provide moribund victims of penetrating injuries with the ability to withstand circulatory arrest for a slightly longer period of time, thus improving their chances for survival (Copass et al., 1984;

Durham et al., 1992). Additionally, the provision of simple ALS therapies that can quickly relieve a patient from hypoglycaemic coma or active seizures, is of obvious value, even if they have not been studied in formal scientific trials.

In a recent cost-effectiveness study of pharmacological interventions provided by a large urban EMS system, only 5% of all patients attended required drug therapy. However, the use of these drugs were all indicated, safe and appropriate in almost all cases (Zachariah et al., 1994a). It is also intuitive that, despite overall results in studies of prehospital thrombolytic therapy (Weaver et al., 1993), certain patients with prolonged myocardial ischaemia may not fare as well if they do not receive thrombolytics as soon as possible (i.e., in the prehospital setting). Whether because of patient stoicism or because of geographical distances, response and transport intervals after the onset of myocardial ischaemia symptoms may be significantly prolonged. In turn, further and significant myocardial damage may be avoided in certain cases where the time for hospital transport would place the patient far beyond the 'golden hour' of early reperfusion. Here, experience, judgement and advanced skills are all of value.

In conclusion, while the majority of patients calling for EMS do not require ALS care, a significant number will benefit from ALS under certain circumstances. Future research efforts will be needed to delineate those subgroups which will achieve such benefit and, in turn, how best to train and deploy appropriate personnel to maximum effect. Along the same lines, the classic role of paramedics and prehospital care physicians may be evolving even further. Recently, some health care systems have considered the use of paramedics as 'Barefoot doctors' who, like visiting health nurses, would be sent out to do home 'check-ups' and immunizations. In this case, however, the 'Barefoot paramedic' can provide and receive direct feedback to and from the 'on-line' physician at the base station. Such a non-emergency role for the paramedic will certainly be a major image change if this concept takes root.

For now, however, the majority of EMS researchers would support the provision of ALS, but with caution. Continued research, scrutiny and cost-effective deployment strategies (see below) should become future goals of EMS systems.

Warning Lights and Sirens

In the past, ambulances were seen as a vehicle to rush patients quickly to the hospital for emergency care. Today, much of the life and death care takes place at the scene. In addition, however, much of EMS does not involve *immediate* life-threatening emergencies. Like ALS procedures, the true value of EMS responses that utilize warning lights and sirens (WL&S) has not been well-documented. Although the use of WL&S is a traditional approach in public safety, some special interests and academicians alike have begun to challenge the time-honoured notion that *every* emergency call deserves a 'fast as possible' response facilitated by WL&S. Although studies examining comparable actuarial data for the average driver (collisions per miles driven) have been lacking, proponents of a limited use of WL&S believe that a large number of collisions and vehicular mishaps are associated with the use (or abuse) of WL&S. These collisions are not only those involving the emergency vehicles but also those involving a 'wake-effect' in which other vehicles collide when other drivers in traffic are distracted or brake fast in response to the WL&S.

The National Association of EMS Physicians (NAEMSP) recently developed a position statement which outlines the need for better discretion in WL&S use as well as better guidelines for their activation. Hopefully, future guidelines will be based on sound medical criteria. For example, while an out-of-hospital cardiac arrest case may be an appropriate circumstance for responses using WL&S, abdominal pain in a 20-year-old male may not warrant such a response. Likewise, criteria for the use of WL&S during transport from the scene back to hospitals are in need of medical scrutiny. For example, a person with a gunshot wound (GSW) to the lower abdomen should probably be transported using WL&S despite a 'stable' appearance (e.g. because of possible iliac artery injury) whereas another person with a serious GSW to the lower leg may not necessarily need WL&S. If bleeding is controlled and intravenous fluids are being infused, a patient can be transported in due time, despite an initial tachycardia and a 'cool and clammy appearance'. Likewise, once a patient is resuscitated from cardiac arrest, a rapid transport to the hospital is usually not warranted.

Recently, several investigations have attempted to see if WL&S use actually improves response time significantly (not to mention patient outcomes). Interestingly, the preliminary data suggest only a one or two minute saving in the average response intervals for the urban and suburban setting (Zachariah et al., 1994b). However, these results are also skewed and the range of time differentials may be significant (e.g. 5 min). In some cases, such as sudden cardiac arrest or a GSW to the chest accompanied by difficulty in breathing, these differentials would very likely affect outcome (Copass et al., 1984;

Cummins et al., 1991; Durham et al., 1992; Pepe and Maio, 1993). However, in the majority of cases to which EMS crews respond, the absence of WL&S may have very little effect except perhaps for an increased number of complaints stemming from the traditional public expectations of a WL&S response.

Nevertheless, the data are sparse and academic medical input, until recently, has been even sparser. Again, future studies delineating the efficacy of WL&S, should be undertaken, not only in terms of response time, but patient outcome as well. However, the more appropriate target for study may not simply be the WL&S response, it must also include a closer examination of the emergency vehicle operator's safety training and his or her subsequent compliance with that training. Intuitively, it is more likely that an overzealous driver causes the traffic mishap by misuse of WL&S and not the WL&S themselves. In fact, it may be found that when safety is used, proper use of WL&S may even decrease the collision rate, including those resulting from the 'wake-effect'.

EMS Management and Deployment Strategies

Perhaps the greatest controversy in EMS revolves around the issue of how best to manage EMS and how to deploy EMS responders. There are probably more opinions than there are different types of EMS systems. The debates regarding the necessity and limitations of ALS and even the use of WL&S have fuelled this controversy even further. While some promote an all-ALS ambulance system (Ornato, 1990), others would even put paramedics on neighbourhood firetrucks as ALS first-responders. On the other hand, given the previous discussion, there are those who would use only a basic life support (BLS) ambulance service where the BLS providers provide automated defibrillation and alternative airway skills (Weaver et al., 1988; Cummins et al., 1991; Pepe et al., 1993a).

Some would base their EMS systems in the municipal/county Fire Department, some at a hospital, some in a 'third service' (i.e. police, fire and 'EMS'), and some in the local health department. Some would favour a private ambulance service, others a municipal service, a 'public utility model', or police or even military services.

Beyond these considerations are hybrid configurations where private or third service ambulance crews serve as back-up to fire service rescue squads or firetruck first-responders. These configurations are further compounded by the differences in access and dispatch systems and the differences in urban and non-urban areas or the potential for using police as first-responders or military for rescue work. For each of these potential alternatives, there are dozens more. Even if one were to believe in the superiority of one configuration over the others, political, social, and economic factors usually prohibit its implementation (or even its testing in a demonstration project).

As stated previously, the use of an all ALS ambulance system has been proposed by many as a way to ensure the timely response of the highest level of care to all patients (Ornato, 1990; Wilson et al., 1992). Such systems are often amplified by the use of vehicular tracking systems and system status management techniques where deployment is tethered to the predicted temporal demand for service (Marshall, 1987). On the other hand, others have argued in favour of a tiered ALS/BLS ambulance response, citing better utilization of paramedics by sparing them for the very small percentage of cases that truly need their services (Cobb et al., 1976; McManus et al., 1977; Curka et al., 1993). Interestingly, the traditional EMS systems that have documented a true life-saving effect in their communities have utilized such a strategy coupled with an aggressive fire engine first-responder programme (Cobb et al., 1976; McManus et al., 1977; Pepe et al., 1991; Curka et al., 1993). Although intuitively it seems that an all ALS system would be better, proponents of the tiered ALS/BLS systems cite better retention of an experienced cadre of paramedics who are highly skilled by virtue of concentrated skills as well as closer medical supervision and focused training (Cobb et al., 1976; McManus et al., 1977; Curka et al., 1993).

In many parts of the United Kingdom, the US, and other countries, government health departments manage the EMS system. In the US, however, fire departments run the majority of local EMS programmes. None the less, in recent years, private ambulance services have begun to assert that they can provide better management and cheaper costs. In turn, fire-based systems argue with this position claiming certain operational advantages (longevity, cross-training, diminished bureaucracy for the EMS system). These issues have been the topics of mushrooming seminars on EMS management in the US. Many of these educational offerings have begun to feature computer-modelling and even business practices to market EMS as a health care consumer product. In addition, more and more automation and the extraordinary evolution of computerized data collection technologies have resulted in blossoming quality improvement techniques which may either awe or intimidate traditional EMS managers. Unfortunately, the end-points of such products often feature indirect measurements of patient care (e.g. more precise documentation of response intervals and optimization of unit-hour utilization) and not necessarily patient outcomes.

A related area of controversy has been the use of helicopters for EMS, particularly in the urban areas of US. Though some well-controlled systems have established clear, workable guidelines for air medical triage and response, several problems still exist in many venues. Even when protocols are followed, local first-responding units often have competitive interactions with air medical agencies, engendering interpersonal and inter-agency confrontation. In addition, proprietary interests and competition have obstructed appropriate and even safe utilization of this expensive resource. Furthermore, explicit scientific data supporting the specific value of air medical systems have not always been convincing. This issue has grown more and more pressing in an era of health reform and cost-containment. None the less, there is intuitive value to providing a transportational system for those in outlying areas and distant venues who truly could benefit from more immediate access to a higher level of comprehensive medical care. The future challenge to the EMS community is to try to achieve this idealistic goal in a virtual sea of public misperceptions, overutilization, ego-politics and proprietary interests.

Whatever the claims may be for air or ground services, few EMS leaders are willing to agree to a consensus except for the metaphor of a multi-component 'chain of survival' which provides early access, early first aid (e.g. CPR) by bystanders, early first response (with airway and defibrillation capabilities) and early ALS (Cummins et al., 1991; Becker and Pepe, 1993). In fact, in the evolving era of automated defibrillation, the use of minimally-trained first-responders (i.e. police or firefighters) has finally attracted some broad-based appeal (Weaver et al., 1988; Pepe et al., 1991; Becker and Pepe, 1993; Hoekstra et al., 1993). In many places, both political resistance and a false perception of a dramatic fiscal impact have both continued to hamper the use of such existing resources (e.g. firetrucks) to facilitate early defibrillation (Pepe et al., 1991). None the less, the use of firefighter crews as first-responders who provide automated defibrillation (as well as other BLS skills) comes the closest to the universal acceptance among all of the EMS deployment strategies currently promulgated in the United States (and several other European countries as well). Recent research now has documented that the cost and resource utilization of such a service is almost negligible (Pepe et al., 1991). In fact, in many venues, the first-responder firetruck is considered to be the backbone of the EMS programme and fire crews routinely accompany paramedic responses for the majority of ALS responses (Cobb et al., 1976; McManus et al., 1977; Pepe et al., 1991; Curka et al., 1993; Hoekstra et al., 1993).

Regardless of philosophy, further research is encouraged to delineate the most effective training level and response schedule for this particular deployment strategy. Likewise, in areas where volunteer fire services are utilized and response may be somewhat delayed, the routine use of on-duty police and other security officers for early defibrillation response also deserves further study. Eventually, proper data gathering will provide us with facts that may evenually overcome traditional training boundaries, as well as the political barriers that can often obstruct better patient care.

The Ethics of Research, Futility and Cost-Containment in the Prehospital Setting

Since the 1970s, only a few individual systems had been routinely involved in EMS research and scientific evaluation. But by the 1990s, research and scientific publication had become widely accepted as a standard function of EMS systems. Between 1989 and 1994, the number of EMS-related papers submitted and presented at scientific meetings had increased exponentially and journals even began to have special EMS and resuscitation issues. EMS paper submissions have recently dominated academic emergency medicine meetings.

None the less, with the blossoming of such widespread research has come questions of ethics. As described above, the proper application and use of ALS, WL&S, and EMS deployment schemes have not been well-documented. In turn, this has stimulated the need for well-designed scientific study and, specifically, prospective controlled clinical trials (Pepe, 1990, 1993a, 1993b). But when such studies have been proposed or implemented, certain 'red flags' have been raised as well. Among those banners were the issues of cost, additional workload on prehospital care providers and concerns over informed consent (Davis and Maio, 1993). The problems stem from the clear inability of sick and injured patients (or even their families) to give truly informed consent, particularly under the duress of an emergency situation. In some communities, superb research initiatives have been scuttled by this concern. In others, the consent to research interventions is considered to be a form of prospective community-wide 'implied consent' to provide either the standard of care (or something that is potentially better) when the emergency number is dialled (Pepe, 1993b). These issues have been the focus of many recent (and forthcoming) publications and conferences. It is also a major issue undergoing discussion at the National Institute of Health, the major US governmental funding agency for medical research. Ironically, although the intent of controlled studies is to determine both efficacy and complications, the US Food and Drug Administration has taken strong exception to waiver of consent except for known benign procedures.

Indeed, other ethical issues have come to the forefront of EMS discussions. For example, the problems of 'whom to resuscitate' and when to terminate resuscitation efforts became a major focus of the American Heart Association's most recent National Standards Conference on Emergency Cardiac Care (McIntyre et al., 1992). Although guidelines have been proposed for years, more recently, improved and more practical protocols have begun to surface (Bonnin et al., 1993; Kellerman, 1993; Pepe et al., 1993c). Several recent prospective studies have confirmed that, unless patients are resuscitated successfully with the return of spontaneous circulation at the scene, continued efforts at the hospital are futile. With the exception of those with persistent ventricular fibrillation, all survivors will achieve spontaneous pulses within 20–25 minutes after the initiation of standard Advanced Cardiac Life Support (ACLS) procedures (Bonnin, et al., 1993). Accordingly, resuscitation efforts can be terminated on-scene if pulses cannot be restored in that time period.

As termination criteria have now been improved, so have criteria for waiving the initiation of efforts. To date, rigor mortis, lividity or confirmed terminal illness have been used as objective criteria for waiving efforts. Recent studies now suggest that those with unwitnessed arrests who do not receive bystander CPR and present to paramedics with asystole, have no chance of surviving, and resuscitation efforts can be waived.

While the motivating factor for developing these criteria has been medical futility, other driving forces include cost-containment and cost-effective utilization of available resources. In turn, the concern exists that such practices to waive or terminate therapeutic efforts must not be abused. Also, it must be kept in mind that those guidelines may need to be modified once new therapeutic modalities become available to researchers and practitioners. There is no worse place for self-fulfilled prophecies than in the practice of resuscitology (Durham et al., 1992; Bonnin et al., 1993; Kellerman, 1993; Pepe et al., 1993b).

Another evolving area of ethics combines all of these previous factors of research and cost-containment, namely the interaction with industry-sponsored research. Conflict of interest may become an issue when the EMS researcher attempts to study new interventions, particularly when desperately-needed financial support is provided by the manufacturer or developer. Also, by the mere fact that

EMS physicians are often public figures who have the public trust at stake, even a *perception* of conflict of interest should be avoided 'at all costs'. EMS physicians and researchers must not only be pillars of integrity, they must never give anyone the excuse to claim they are not!

EMS as the Practice of Medicine

The original North American EMS programmes were soundly rooted with physician leadership; subsequent programmes evolved in the 1970s without this integral element (Pepe and Stewart, 1986; Pepe et al., 1990; Falk, 1993). In most communities, medical direction for EMS was provided by committees or physician 'advisers'. By the mid-1980s, the failure of most EMS systems to meet engendered expectations of life-saving was being recognized by a growing number of physicians (Smith et al., 1985; Becker et al., 1991; Pepe et al., 1993d; Lombardi et al., 1994). In some cases, trauma surgeons criticized unacceptable delays in the prehospital setting caused by paramedics who were attempting to provide 'stabilizing' procedures for the critically injured (Smith et al., 1985). In other situations, it was a recognition of very low survival rates for sudden death in many of our nation's major EMS systems (Braun et al., 1990; Becker et al., 1991; Cummins et al., 1991; Becker and Pepe, 1993).

It soon became appreciated that the reason for many EMS system inadequacies was a profound lack of expert physician involvement and credibility (Pepe and Stewart, 1986; Pepe et al., 1990). Few US physicians responsible for EMS systems had ever practised prehospital clinical care. Therefore most were very detached from the actual mechanics of EMS operations and clinical practice demands. As a result, medical protocols and training for paramedics were hospital-oriented. Worse yet, 'cookbook' protocols had replaced the elemental apprenticeship and day-to-day mentorship of physicians who were expert in the actual delivery of prehospital care (Pepe et al., 1990). Such mentorship had been the rule in the original US EMS systems some 20–25 years ago (Pepe et al., 1986, 1990). However, by the 1980s, this key element had become rare nationwide (Falk, 1993). Renewed recognition of this key element of expert physician leadership has now led to the rapid development of full-time EMS physician positions in many US EMS systems (Falk, 1993; Pepe et al., 1993d).

In some large cities, several physicians are now dedicated to EMS medical direction on a full-time basis. Likewise, on-scene participation, training and supervision are now becoming well-accepted, if not commonplace, practices of North American EMS physicians (Stewart et al., 1987; ACGME, 1990; Pepe and Curka, 1991). In fact, the components of full-time medical direction and expert quality assurance have even become the keystone feature of many private ambulance services bidding for city or county contracts to provide EMS.

But while the key element of physician supervision has become well-accepted, the exact hierarchical role of the EMS physician is still debated. Should the EMS physician be the EMS system manager as well (e.g. the public health director model)? There exists strong sentiment that physicians unfamiliar with good EMS system management practices can make things worse by simplistic application of medical practices. Also, good managers may not be good physicians . . . and vice versa. Management means responsibility and, 90% of the time, responsibility means headaches, such as budget battles, personnel and disciplinary controversies, as well as primeval political choreography!

Taking it a step further, should EMS physicians continue to practise medicine or should they evolve into vestigial practioners who now develop health care business plans? It is not uncommon today for EMS medical directors to go back to school for Masters of Business Administration or Master of Public Health (MBA or MPH) degrees. Should that be standard fare? More and more EMS physicians have begun to envision EMS in terms of public health care delivery. In turn, their perspectives and concerns have evolved far beyond the more pedestrian pros and cons of anti-shock garments or the use of certain pharmacological interventions. Their growing concern is the ultimate survival of the emergency health care system as a whole. The answers to these questions are not easy and, in this case, they will probably be long in coming.

Still, what has definitely become an established consensus over the past decade, is that EMS, whether it involves basic or advanced skills, is a unique practice of medicine. In this practice, the resources are not only blood pressure cuffs and defibrillators, but also the various elements effecting the medical care, such as dispatch procedures, emergency medical technicians (EMTs), and transportation vehicles. Therefore, in most venues today, the EMS physician is no longer seen as a medical adviser alone. He or she must not only have final approval over the use of all of these medical resources but also must be at (or near) the helm of the decision-making process. Because the EMS physician must have credibility, this means that the EMS physician must have a grass-roots command of these various entities and functions, including routine hands-on experience in the actual patient care (prehospital) setting. But, the development of such attributes are not created in a void. Eventually, the proper grooming of future EMS physicians will also need to be institutionalized in the form of an expert apprenticeship under expert EMS physician mentors (Pepe and Stewart, 1986; Stewart et al., 1987; ACGME, 1990; Pepe and Curka, 1991; Falk, 1993). In turn the American Board of Emergency Medicine is exploring the potential for subspecialty boards. Likewise, the Society for Academic Emergency Medicine and the National Association of EMS physicians have developed formal fellowship curricula (Krohmer et al., 1994).

In contrast to the US, where greater involvement of specialized physicians is now being sought, physicians at the roadside have been the rule in many European countries. Ironically, there now exist various movements in many of those countries to reduce physician involvement and develop paramedic programmes (i.e. where specially-trained non-physician personnel can deliver advanced life support procedures in the field). In Eastern Canada, it has been debated to what extent non-physician EMS personnel should be trained. Economically, if advanced techniques have minimal proven value, the need for paramedics has no longer been considered a necessity by some. Instead, training basic emergency medical technicians (EMTs) who provide automated defibrillation and some 'intermediate' airway techniques (e.g. the Combitube®), has been the goal. Nevertheless, the need for physicians or paramedics is still argued by others. Currently, some Canadians and Europeans are closely studying the relative value of these services.

Regardless of staffing configurations, however, there appears to be a trend to have both physicians and paramedical personnel (trained to some advanced degree or another) in EMS systems. In both the North American and European situations (as well as many Australian and Asian settings), the overall trend appears to be moving toward a system of care where non-physician, specially-trained EMS personnel provide the majority of basic and even the advanced medical skills in out-of-hospital settings. However, in all circumstances, there is a clear role for expert physician supervisors who *routinely* participate in field care (sometimes to deliver primary care in the most serious cases), or, more often, who supervise the care delivered at all levels, both basic and advanced. Regardless of practise philosophy, expert physician leadership is the universal constant. Moreover, it has become widely-recognized that the level of clinical and educational involvement of an EMS physician correlates with EMS system success. Therefore, the proper tutelage of future EMS physicians must be a priority.

Miscellaneous Issues

Although many of the issues discussed above appear to be the major areas of discussion in EMS, there are many more topics of concern of physicians involved in this evolving area of emergency public health care. Polls of leading EMS physicians also cite issues such as: rural EMS; funding for EMS systems and medical director positions; advocacy for EMS personnel and prevention of EMS personnel 'burn-out' syndrome; communicable disease procedures; and multiple other day-to-day problems in the delivery of prehospital care. Interestingly, topics which were very important to EMS physicians a few years ago, such as the development and exchange of patient care protocols or issues of liability for EMS activities, have seemed to be placed on the back burner for now. Other topics that have taken a back seat in recent years are issues of dealing with firefighter or EMS unions as well as the problems of due process and discipline of EMS personnel. None the less, in some EMS systems, some of these issues are still of paramount concern for EMS physicians and administrators alike. Thus, the focus of this text is simply an assimilation of the thoughts of certain leading individuals in EMS and should not underestimate the importance of other issues for the many EMS practitioners trying to improve emergency health care delivery for their patients throughout the world.

RESOLUTION OF CURRENT ISSUES

The future of EMS and the current issues, as previously discussed, all involve unresolved areas of controversy or development that will require scientific evaluation or, at the very best, expert judgement. The common denominator to achieve their eventual resolution will most likely be found by addressing the last issue, namely a focus on a proper evaluation of the practice of prehospital medicine. With the evolving and expanding role of physicians who specialize full-time in EMS and prehospital medical care, all of these issues should receive a more sophisticated and academic approach, (Pepe et al., 1990, 1993d; Krohmer et al., 1994), particularly if we are successful in training and properly moulding future EMS physicians (Stewart et al., 1987; ACGME, 1990; Pepe and Curka, 1991; Krohmer et al., 1994). Today, some of the most respected leaders in academic EMS were the 'apprentices' of the EMS physician role models from places like Seattle and Pittsburgh (Pepe and Stewart, 1986; Stewart et al., 1987; Pepe et al., 1990, 1993d). Experience has also shown, however, that

EMS physicians, even when involved full-time, may actually obstruct or reverse progress because of their lack of proper mentorship. Therefore, a focused future goal for academic emergency and critical care medicine should be the proper development of EMS fellowships and subspeciality training under academically-oriented mentors who have achieved excellence in EMS, both clinically and scholastically. The generation and eventual proliferation of such expert specialists will constitute the best common demoninators for proper resolution of the key issues under discussion, not to mention the entire future development of EMS.

ACKNOWLEDGEMENTS

The author thanks Drs Norman Dinerman, Raymond Fowler, Leonard Cobb, Herbert Garrison, Don Yealy and David Persse (this year's SAEM Physio Control EMS Fellow) for their gracious input and enthusiasm for emergency health care delivery as well as Nina Meher-Homji for preparation of the manuscript.

REFERENCES

Accreditation Council for Graduate Medical Education (1990) *Special Requirement for Residency Training in Emergency Medicine*. ACGME, Chicago, IL, p. 11.

Atherton, G.L., Johnson, J.C. (1993) Ability of paramedics to use the Combitube^{TM} in prehospital cardiac arrest. *Annals of Emergency Medicine* **22**: 1263–1268.

Becker, L.B., Pepe, P.E. (1993) Ensuring the effectiveness of community-wide emergency cardiac care. *Annals of Emergency Medicine* **22** (part II): 354–365.

Becker, L., Ostrander, M., Barrett, J. et al. (1991) Outcome of CPR in a large metropolitan area: Where are the survivors? *Annals of Emergency Medicine* **20**: 355–361.

Bickell, W.H., Bruttig, S.P., Millnamow, G.A., O'Benar, J., Wade, C.E. (1992) Use of hypertonic saline/dextran versus lactated Ringer's solution as a resuscitation fluid after uncontrolled aortic haemorrhage in anesthetized swine. *Annals of Emergency Medicine* **21**: 1077–1085.

Bickell, W.H., Wall, M.J., Pepe, P.E. et al. (1994) A comparison of immediate versus delayed fluid resuscitation for hypotensive patients with penetrating torso injury. *New England Journal of Medicine* **331**: 1105–1109.

Bonnin, M.J., Pepe, P.E., Clark P.S., Kimball K.T. (1993) Distinct criteria for termination of resuscitation in the out-of-hospital setting. *Journal of the American Medical Association* **270**: 1457–1462.

Border, J.R., Lewis, F.R., Aprahamian, C. et al. (1983) Prehospital trauma care – stabilization or scoop and run. *Journal of Trauma* **23**: 708.

Bourn, S. (1992) Give me proof – is EMS really worth it? *Journal of Emergency Medical Services* **17**: 83–85.

Braun, O., McCallion R., Fazackerly, J. (1990) Characteristics of midsized urban EMS systems. *Annals of Emergency Medicine* **19**: 536–546.

Cobb, L.A., Alvarez, H., Copass M.K. (1976) A rapid response system for out-of-hospital cardiac emergencies. *Medical Clinics of North America* **60**: 283–290.

Copass, M.K., Oreskovich, M.R., Bladergroen, M.R., et al. (1984) Prehospital cardiopulmonary resuscitation of the critically injured patient. *American Journal of Surgery* **148**: 20.

Cummins, R.O., Ornato, J.P., Thies, W., Pepe, P.E. (1991) The American Heart Association Emergency Cardiac Care Committee's Subcommittee on Advanced Cardiac Life Support. Improving survival from sudden cardiac arrest: the 'chain of survival concept'. *Circulation* **83**: 1832–1847.

Curka, P.A., Pepe, P.E., Ginger V.F., et al. (1993) Emergency medical services priority dispatch: *Annals of Emergency Medicine* **22**: 1688–1695.

Davis, E., Maio, R.F. Ethical issues in prehospital research. (1993) *Prehospital and Disaster Medicine* **8**(suppl.): S11–S14.

Durham, L.A., Richardson, R.J., Wall, M.J., Pepe, P.E., Mattox, K.L. (1992) Emergency centre thoracotomy: impact of prehospital resuscitation. *Journal of Trauma* **32**: 775–779.

Eisenberg, M.S., Aghababian, R.V., Bossaert, L. et al. (1993) Thrombolytic therapy. *Annals of Emergency Medicine* **22**: 417–427.

Emergency Cardiac Care Committee, Subcommittee on Advanced Cardiac Life Support (ACLS), (1992) American Heart Association. Adult advanced cardiac life support. Part III, Guidelines for cardiopulmonary resuscitation and emergency cardiac care. *Journal of the American Medical Association* **268**: 2199–2241.

European Myocardial Infarction Project Group. (1993) Prehospital thrombolytic therapy in patients with suspected acute myocardial infarction. *New England Journal of Medicine* **329**: 383–389.

Falk, J.L. (1993) Medical direction of emergency medical service systems: A full-time commitment whose time has come. *Critical Care Medicine* **21**: 1259–1260.

Hoekstra, J.W., Banks, J., Martin, D., et al. (1993) The effect of first responder automated defibrillation on time to therapeutic interventions during out-of-hospital cardiac arrest. *Annals of Emergency Medicine* **22**: 1247–1253.

Honigman, B., Lowenstein, S.R., Moore, E.E., et al. (1991) The role of the pneumatic antishock garment in penetrating cardiac wounds. *Journal of the American Medical Association* **266**: 2398–2401.

Krohmer, J.R., Swor, R.A., Benson, N.H., et al. (1994) Prototype curriculum for a fellowship in EMS. *Prehospital and Disaster Medicine* **9**: 73–77.

Kellerman, A.L. (1993) Criteria for dead-on-arrivals, prehospital termination of CPR and do-not-resuscitate orders. *Annals of Emergency Medicine* **22**: 47–51.

Lombardi, G., Gallagher, E.J., Gennis, P. (1994) Outcome of out-of-hospital cardiac arrest in New York City: The pre-hospital arrest survival evaluation (Phase) study. *Journal of the American Medical Association* **271**: 678–683.

McIntyre, K.M., Crimmins, T.J., Safar, P., Lo B., Weir, R.F., Pepe, P.E. (1992) Ethical considerations in resuscitation; Part VIII. Emergency Cardiac Care Committee and Subcommittees, American Heart Association. Guidelines for cardiopulmonary resuscitation and emergency cardiac care. *Journal of the American Medical Association* **268**: 2282–2288.

McManus, W.F., Tresch, D.D., Darin, J.C. (1977) An effective prehospital emergency system. *Journal of Trauma* **17**: 304–310.

Marshall, L. Tracking the wild ambulance fleet. (1987) *Journal of Emergency Medical Services* **12**: 32–38.

Mattox, K.L., Pepe, P.E., Bickell, W.H., et al. (1989) The MAST controversy: Analysis of 911 hypotensive patients prospectively randomized. *Journal of Trauma* **29**: 1104–1112.

Ornato, J.P. (1990) The need for ALS in urban and suburban EMS systems (editorial). *Annals of Emergency Medicine* **12**: 1469–1470.

Pepe, P.E. (1990) Controlled studies in the prehospital setting: a viable, important venue for clinical research. *Prehospital and Disaster Medicine* **5**: 285–288.

Pepe, P.E. (1992) Anti-shock garments: more harm than good. *Journal of Critical Illness* **7**: 166–168.

Pepe, P.E. (1993a) Out-of-hospital research in the urban environment. *Prehospital and Disaster Medicine* **8** S20–24.

Pepe, P.E. (1993b) Out-of-hospital resuscitation research: Rationale and strategies for controlled clinical trials. *Annals of Emergency Medicine* **22**: 17–23.

Pepe, P.E., Curka, P.A. (1991). Scene supervision of EMS. In Swor, R. (ed.) *Quality Management in Prehospital Care*, Chap. 7, pp 203–211. St Louis: C.V. Mosby & Co.

Pepe, P.E., Maio, R.F. (1993) Evolving challenges in prehospital trauma services – current issues and suggested evaluation tools. *Prehospital and Disaster Medicine* **8** (suppl. 1): S25–S34.

Pepe, P.E., Stewart, R.D. (1986) The role of the physician in the prehospital setting. *Annals of Emergency Medicine* **15**: 1480–1483.

Pepe, P.E., Bonnin, M.J., Mattox, K.L. (1990) Regulating the scope of EMS services. *Prehospital and Disaster Medicine* **5**: 59–63.

Pepe, P.E., Kelly, J.E., Ivy, M.V., et al. (1991) Resource utilization and impact of using fire apparatus for a fully-integrated EMS first-responder program (abstract). *Annals of Emergency Medicine* **20**: 488.

Pepe, P.E., Zachariah, B.S., Chandra, N. (1993a) Invasive airway techniques in resuscitation. *Annals of Emergency Medicine* **22** (part II): 393–403.

Pepe, P.E., Levine, R.L., Fromm, R.E., Curka, P.A., Clark, P.S. (1993b)

Cardiac arrest presenting with rhythms other than ventricular fibrillation: Contribution of resuscitation efforts toward total survivorship. *Critical Care Medicine* **21**: 1838–1843.

Pepe, P.E., Brown, C.G., Bonnin, M.J., et al. (1993c) Prospective validation of criteria for on-scene termination of resuscitation efforts after out-of-hospital cardiac arrest (abstract). *Annals of Emergency Medicine* **22**: 884–885.

Pepe, P.E., Mattox, K.L., Duke, J.H., Fisher, P.B., Prentice, F.D. (1993d) The effect of fulltime specialized physician supervision on the success of a large urban emergency medical services system. *Critical Care Medicine* **21**: 1279–1286.

Pepe, P.E., Abramson, N.J., Brown, C.G. (1994) Advanced cardiac life support – does it really work? *Annals of Emergency Medicine* **23**: 1037–1041.

Smith, J.P., Bodai, B.I., Hill, A.S. et al. (1985) Prehospital stabilization of critically injured patients: A failed concept. *Journal of Trauma* **25**: 65.

Stewart, R.D., Paris, P.M., Heller, M. (1987) Design of a resident in-field experience for an emergency medicine residency curriculum. *Annals of Emergency Medicine* **16**: 175–179.

Weaver, W.D., Hill, D., Fahrenbruch, C.E., et al. (1988) Use of the automatic external defibrillator in the management of out-of-hospital cardiac arrest. *New England Journal of Medicine* **319**: 661–666.

Weaver, W.D., Cergueira, M., Hallstrom, A.P., et al. (1993) The Myocardial Infarction, Triage, and Intervention trial of prehospital versus hospital initiated thrombolytic therapy. *Journal of the American Medical Association* **270**: 1211–1216.

Wesley, R.C., Resh, W., Zimmerman, D. (1991) Reconsideration of the routine and preferential use of lidocaine in emergent treatment of ventricular arrhythmias. *Critical Care Medicine* **19**: 1439–1444.

Wilson, B, Gratton, M.C., Overton, J., Watson, W.A. (1992) Unexpected ALS procedures on non-emergency ambulance calls: the value of a single-tier system. *Prehospital and Disaster Medicine* **7**: 380–382.

Zachariah, B.S., Pepe, P.E., Curka, P.A. (1994a) Analysis of medication usage in an urban EMS system (abstract). *Academy of Emergency Medicine* **1**: 315.

Zachariah, B.S., Pepe, P.E., Persse, D.E., Curka, P.A. (1994b) The effect of warning lights and sirens on EMS response intervals (abstract). *Annals of Emergency Medicine* **23**: 637.

1ii

Advances in Prehospital Care

Thomas Kerz, Wolfgang F. Dick

INTRODUCTION

New treatment strategies and technical devices have been developed for the care of the critically ill. Only very rarely has their usefulness in prehospital medicine been determined in the field; instead, prehospital medicine mostly transferred in-hospital management strategies to patients who had to be treated in completely different surroundings. This article examines the main innovations and controversies critically, from the perspective of the standpoint of the pre-hospital care provider.

AIRWAY MANAGEMENT

American Heart Association (AHA) guidelines recommend endotracheal intubation as the gold standard for emergency airway care (AHA, 1992). However, because of insufficient training of paramedical personnel, other devices such as masks, oro- or nasopharyngeal airways or the (o)esophageal obturator airway (EOA) are commonly used by this group of emergency care providers. There are several problems associated with all types of device; Hankins et al. (1993) describe an unacceptably high complication rate when emergency medical service EMS personnel tried to insert EOAs or endotracheal tubes. These problems are mainly due to the infrequent use and consequent insufficient practice of EMS staff. Therefore, there is an urgent need for new developments to improve airway management when skilled personnel are not on the scene.

Pharyngo-Tracheal-Lumen Airways (PTLA)

These are inserted blindly and will thus generally be placed oesophageally. Multiple apertures at pharyngeal level allow insufflation of the lungs while the oesophagus and oropharynx are blocked by inflatable balloons. A similar device is the Combitube® which has a modified pharyngeal balloon. If the PTLA/Combitube® occasionally is placed into the trachea, ventilation is performed as with a genuine endotracheal tube. Animal and human data indicate effectiveness of this method, and case reports support its value when endotracheal intubation is not possible (Eichinger et al., 1992; Klauser et al., 1992). When ICU nurses performed emergency intubation with either the Combitube® or the endotracheal tube, insertion of the first was quicker, and blood gases showed comparable results for each device (Staudinger et al., 1993). Evaluation in a prehospital CPR setting demonstrated the effectiveness of the Combitube® as a primary airway as well as back-up to the endotracheal tube, but the authors considered the latter as the preferred method (Atherton and Johnson, 1993). Bartlett et al. (1992) compared a pharyngotracheal lumen airway (PTL, similar to the Combitube®) with endotracheal intubation (ET) in 111 pre-hospital cardiac arrest patients. No differences were found between the two devices in blood gas analysis on arrival at the hospital, but ventilation with the PTL was achieved significantly quicker than with the ET tube.

The Laryngeal Mask Airway (LMA)

This consists of a tube which ends in an inflatable wall forming a seal around the laryngeal inlet. LMA insertion technique is relatively easy. At least in adult patients it has been shown to be easier to learn than the handling of the Guedel airway, bag and face mask (Alexander et al., 1993). Davies et al. (1990) also pointed out the ease and high rate of success of the method compared to endotracheal intubation when used by inexperienced personnel. However, a minimal period of formal training is mandatory in order to achieve high success rates (Tolley et al., 1992). In 8–33% of reported LMA placements, more than one attempt is needed (Maltby et al., 1990; Smith and White, 1992). Applicability of the LMA to children is more difficult and still under discussion. Case reports demonstrate the LMAs usefulness when conventional intubation is not possible (Calder et al., 1990; Greene et al., 1992). The mask has been used sucessfully during CPR by junior anaesthesia staff with no previous experience (Kokkinis, 1994). In patients with cervical spine injuries the LMA has been described as preventing secondary trauma to the spinal cord (Pennant et al., 1992).

Neither the LMA or the PTLA/Combitube® provide protection against aspiration (Koehli, 1991). As all patients treated by the

EMS system are at a specific risk for this complication, the airway should be secured by endotracheal intubation whenever possible. Nevertheless, when endotracheal intubation fails or is possibly harmful, trained personnel may find either the PTLA/Combitube® or the LMA invaluable tools for artificial ventilation. However, successful artificial ventilation can be provided by many means (e.g. Bag–valve–mask), and emphasis should be laid more on the importance of securing some ventilation of the lungs, rather than placing too much reliance on specific devices.

Oximetry

Portable pulse oximeters allow the quick, on-line, non-invasive, continuous determination of arterial oxygen saturation in emergency care patients. They have been recommended to detect patients at risk of serious desaturation, and to guide oxygen therapy (Ellinger et al., 1988; McGuire et al., 1988). In a closed-claims analysis from 17 insurance companies relevant to claims filed between 1974 and 1988, oximetry (together with capnometry) was considered potentially preventive in 93% of the anaesthetic-related mishaps (Tinker et al., 1989).

Several shortcomings of the technique must be taken into account: In a moving ambulance, pulse oximetry (and capnometry) were found less accurate as the severity of shock progressed (Low, 1993, data presented at the 1993 meeting of the World Association for Emergency and Disaster Medicine, Stockholm). Depending on the type of oximeter, only partial O_2 saturation (SpO_2) is measured (ratio between oxyhaemoglobin and reduced haemoglobin). Therefore, if there is a considerable amount of dyshaemoglobinaemia (e.g. in smoking, smoke poisoning, suicide attempt with car exhaust gases, ingestion of nitrates), oxygen transport is grossly overestimated (Mertzlufft, 1990; Reinhard and Luxem, 1992). Patients with severe anaemia will have normal values for O_2 saturation, but will have significant reduction in O_2 content. These patients might consequently experience severe tissue damage with normal SpO_2 values. In preterm infants and newborns, hyperoxia (PaO_2 > 150 mmHg) is not detected and may lead to irreparable retrolental fibroplasia. For this paediatric subgroup, an SpO_2 of 90–95% is recommended (Vogel et al., 1988). Correct measurements may be rendered impossible by hypothermia, vasoconstriction, low blood pressure, hyperbilirubinaemia, patient movements and the use of nail enamel.

Capnometry

As with oximetry, capnometry is a routine form of monitoring during anaesthesia. Portable capnometers give the opportunity to measure end-tidal E_tCO_2 concentration during prehospital care of emergency patients (Jantzen and Hennes, 1991). Qualitative and semi-quantitative (colorimetric; Strunin and Williams, 1989) determination of carbon dioxide is easy (Ornato et al., 1992), but quantitative capnometry has outstanding advantages and should be used whenever possible. As the first generation of these capnometers was far too heavy and had insufficient battery working times, new monitoring systems have been developed. Not only E_tCO_2, but also ECG, blood pressure (invasive and non-invasive), and SpO_2 can now be recorded on a single monitor of low weight and satisfactory mains-independency.

End-tidal CO_2 concentration depends on ventilation, circulation, and metabolism. Thus, monitoring of E_tCO_2 may help to clarify several problems. Correct endotracheal intubation can be verified, and dislocation or kinking of the tube during transport can be recognized immediately. Inadvertent hyper- or hypocapnia can be avoided. Though difficult to distinguish from each other, deterioration of cardiac output (CO) or reduction of pulmonary perfusion (pulmonary embolism) can be detected. Because of the correlation of E_tCO_2 with CO and coronary perfusion pressure, many authors have correlated E_tCO_2 values with the adequate performance of CPR and the chances of successful resuscitation (Barton and Callaham, 1988; Sanders et al., 1989; Callaham and Barton, 1990). However, when adrenaline is given during resuscitation, this correlation is lost and cannot be used to predict outcome (Martin et al., 1990; Paradis et al., 1990; Trillo et al., 1994). Finally, in hypo- or hyperthermic patients, ventilation patterns can be adjusted to changing metabolic demands.

CARDIOPULMONARY RESUSCITATION

Active Compression–Decompression (ACD)

This method of thoracic compression–decompression was found to be effective when a San Francisco housewife sucessfully resuscitated her husband by means of a toilet plunger. She thought of this method when her husband collapsed in the confines of a small toilet room. On a second occasion 6 months later, the husband again was successfully resuscitated with the plunger, this time by his son (Lurie et al., 1990).

The ACD-device which was constructed after these initial experiences permits active decompression of the chest, thereby increasing venous return (Tucker et al., 1993b). Cohen et al. (1991, 1992) investigated the ACD device in dogs and in humans in cardiac arrest. In the 1992 study, patients in cardiac arrest received standard advanced cardiac life support (ACLS) while intra-arterial pressure devices, transoesophageal echocardiography, and capnometry were installed. Then, either 2 minutes of standard CPR followed by 2 minutes of ACD CPR or vice versa was performed. Mean E_tCO_2 was 4.3 vs. 9.0 mmHg (standard vs. ACD), systolic arterial pressure 52.5 vs. 88.9 mmHg, and the velocity time integral (an index of forward flow) was 7.3 cm vs. 17.5 cm. Three of the ten patients studied regained a stable pulse after 2 minutes of ACD CPR, after more then one hour had been spent with standard CPR.

Cerebral, myocardial, and renal perfusion have been found increased when compared with standard CPR in animals (Chang et al., 1992). In adult dogs, ACD-CPR improved minute ventilation when compared to high-impulse manual CPR (Tucker et al., 1993a). The authors expressed their hope that with ACD-CPR physiological levels of minute ventilation could possibly be achieved, thereby obviating the need for mouth-to-mouth ventilation in a bystander arrest situation. In a recent animal study, Lindner et al. (1993) demonstrated a significant ($p < 0.05$) increase of myocardial and cerebral blood flow and coronary perfusion pressure with ACD CPR. End-tidal CO_2 increased as well, and was highly correlated to myocardial blood flow. Yet, after high-dose adrenaline (epinephrine), these differences disappeared, and ACD CPR was no longer superior to standard CPR. In patients, Cohen et al. (1993) reported an improved rate of initial resuscitation, survival at 24 h and neurological outcome with the ACD device when 62 patients with witnessed in-hospital arrest were resuscitated either with standard CPR or ACD CPR. As long-term studies with the ACD device are lacking completely, the results of current multicentre trials are needed to define the role of this device more accurately.

Open-chest CPR

Open-chest CPR (OCCPR) was routinely used until the early 1960s when efficacy of closed-chest compression was reported (Kouwenhoven et al., 1960; Jude et al., 1964). Until then, it had been used mainly in the operating room during surgery or anaesthesia-related cardiac arrest; recovery rates were reported as high as 28% (Stevenson et al., 1953). Although patients with out-of-hospital CPR are a different population, improved haemodynamic data during OCCPR point to a possible benefit with this technique. OCCPR produces higher diastolic pressure values while venous pressures are lower than with conventional closed-chest CPR. This mechanism results in higher perfusion pressures both in cerebral and coronary arteries.

In animal studies, cardiac output and coronary perfusion were found higher than pre-arrest values (Weiser et al., 1962; Barnett et al., 1986). Cerebral perfusion was between 63 and 94% of normal for up to 1 hour (Weiser et al., 1962). In dogs, OCCPR clearly produced a better neurological status during and after CPR than did conventional CPR or simultaneous ventilation-compression CPR. Pupillary reactivity and EEG-activity were maintained only with OCCPR, heart and brain returned rapidly to near-normal function (Bircher and Safar, 1985). In this study, less drug therapy was needed after 30 minutes of OCCPR than after immediate defibrillation after inducing VF. Recently, in a canine model, DeBehnke et al. (1991) reported OCCPR to produce higher resuscitation rates, but survival rates at 4 hours were similar when compared to conventional CPR. When untreated cardiac arrest persisted for more than 20 minutes, OCCPR did not produce long-term survival in dogs (Kern et al., 1991). These findings had been demonstrated earlier in man when emergency room OCCPR after 20 minutes of out-of-hospital CPR did not improve survival (Geehr and Auerbach, 1985).

Standard ACLS procedures will be effective in some groups of patients (as has been shown in the past), but in some patients OCCPR will be needed. The problem is in determining which patients will ultimately prove unresponsive to conventional CPR and should therefore receive OCCPR within 15 to 20 minutes. Some patients could receive OCCPR inappropriately because of their response to conventional CPR, and others will not benefit of OCCPR because it will be instituted too late. Yet, the scarcity of human data and controlled studies preclude the first line use of OCCPR.

Adrenaline

Debate continues as to whether adrenaline (epinephrine) should be given in doses higher than currently recommended by the American Heart Association (AHA, 1992). Animal data suggest improved cerebral and coronary blood flow as well as higher initial resuscitation rates when high-dose adrenaline is administered (Brown et al., 1986, 1987; Brunette and Jameson, 1990). Human data also indicate a dose-dependent vasopressor response with higher coronary perfusion pressures when higher adrenaline doses are given (Gonzalez et al., 1989). However, in a study on 1280 patients in cardiac arrest randomly assigned to receive either adrenaline 0.02 mg/kg or 0.2 mg/kg, respectively, no differences in the rate of return of spontaneous circulation, survival and neurological outcome was found (Brown et al., 1992). Yet, in the subgroup of patients who received adrenaline within 10 minutes of the arrest, a trend towards higher rates of hospital discharge was noted in the high-dose group. Likewise, when electromechanical dissociation was the first ECG rhythm recorded, return of spontaneous circulation was also more likely in the high-dose adrenaline group.

In another recent study including 650 patients, no benefit of high-dose adrenaline therapy could be demonstrated (Stiell et al., 1992), although a mean administration time of 21 minutes for out-of-hospital patients was a shortcoming of this study. In the subgroup of patients who received high-dose adrenaline more than 10 minutes after the arrest, the resuscitation rate was even diminished compared to the standard-dose group. Other studies reported a higher initial resuscitation rate with high-dose adrenaline while hospital discharge rates were not altered (Barton and Callaham, 1991; Lindner et al., 1991). Results of the multi-centre BRCT-III study, comparing three different adrenaline dosing regimes in 2500 patients, should be available shortly. Obviously, patient subgroups with a potential benefit of high-dose adrenaline therapy will have to be identified by large studies before this therapy can be recommended. Paediatric patients may represent such a group (Goetting and Paradis, 1991).

Buffer Therapy

Acid–base balance in cardiac arrest becomes severely altered with the cessation of blood flow and respiration. Intracellular hypercarbia and lactic acidosis are responsible for depressed myocardial and cerebral function, a diminished response to catecholamines and a decreased fibrillation threshold. However, correction of acidosis with bicarbonate results in increased CO_2 production. CO_2 enters into the cells immediately and contributes to cellular acidosis; infusion of bicarbonate results in reduced myocardial oxygen use and decreased cardiac output (Graf et al., 1984; Bersin et al., 1989). Further side-effects are hypernatraemia, hyperosmolarity with hypotension and reduced myocardial perfusion pressure, increase in intracranial pressure, and induction of alkalosis with subsequent shift of the oxygen-binding curve to the left and increased haemoglobin-oxygen affinity. In 1974, AHA standards routinely recommended bicarbonate infusion (AHA, 1974) because of pathological laboratory findings, but neither arterial nor venous pH values represent intracellular acidosis correctly during CPR (Kette et al., 1990). Buffering agents have not been shown to affect overall outcome (AufderHeide et al., 1992b). When Bishop and Weisfeldt (1976) demonstrated correction of arterial acidosis by artificial respiration for more than 30 minutes under CPR conditions, AHA guidelines began to change. 1986 guidelines classify bicarbonate as helpful in patients with known pre-existing hyperkalaemia and/or drug overdose. The mainstay of therapy during CPR is still ventilation, adrenaline administration and early defibrillation. Newer agents such as carbicarb (sodium bicarbonate and sodium carbonate) reduce the amount of released CO_2, but there is still lack of evidence of their superiority to bicarbonate (Blecic et al., 1991). In acidotic patients who still exhibit contractile functions, buffer therapy seems warranted because bicarbonate can reach the myocardium and reverse intracellular acidosis (Pagani et al., 1990).

Cerebral Resuscitation

As it is the ultimate goal of all resuscitation efforts to preserve intact neurological function, special attention has been paid to brain resuscitation after sucessful CPR in the last few years. Various early and late post-resuscitative disorders have been identified, and many animal and a few human studies have investigated the possible improvement of neurological function after therapy with prostaglandin inhibitors (Sasaki et al., 1988), NMDA antagonists (Meldrum, 1990), GABA agonists (Saji and Reis, 1987), barbiturates, naloxone (Dalkara et al., 1989), or free-radical scavengers, to name only a few. As intracellular calcium overload is the final pathway of cellular damage (Siesjö and Bengtsson, 1989), therapy with calcium antagonists appeared very promising. In primates, nimodipine improved neurological outcome (Steen et al., 1985), and in pigs even higher initial CPR success rates have been reported (Schindler et al., 1992). However, nimodipine did not prevent brain damage in a global ischaemia model in the rat (Calle et al., 1993). Nimodipine has been tested in patients with out-of-hospital VF but, apart from an increased rate of survivors in the subgroup with long ACLS delays, no positive effects could be confirmed (Roine et al., 1990). Despite continuing debate, nimodipine therapy is not warranted at the moment for brain protection after cardiopulmonary arrest.

PREHOSPITAL THROMBOLYSIS

Thrombolytic treatment of acute myocardial infarction is clearly associated with a limitation of infarction size, improved ventricular function, and a reduction in mortality (Simoons et al., 1986; Wilcox et al., 1988; Gulba et al., 1990). Both the GISSI and the ISIS studies have demonstrated the most striking reduction in mortality in patient subgroups with thrombolytic therapy within 1 h of the onset of pain symptoms (GISSI, 1987; ISIS, 1988). Thus, the earlier systemic thrombolysis is carried out, the greater the benefit to patients. For pre-hospital thrombolysis, it has been demonstrated that up to 45% of patients with relevant symptoms can be treated with benefit and complication rates similar to in-hospital treatment (GISSI, 1987; Galien et al., 1989; Arntz et al., 1990, 1992; GREAT, 1992).

Accuracy of pre-hospital thrombolytic candidate selection by paramedics together with telemetric ECG evaluation by emergency physicians was shown by AufderHeide et al. (1992a). Unfortunately this did not demonstrate the superiority of pre-hospital lysis over in-hospital thrombolytic therapy as far as objective end-points (infarct size, LV-function, mortality) were concerned. This was recently supported by the results of a large multi-centre study which enrolled 5469 patients in 15 European countries and Canada (EMIP, 1993). Though patients in the pre-hospital group received therapy 55 minutes earlier than those in the hospital group, overall mortality at 30 days was not significantly reduced. Only mortality from cardiac causes was 16% lower in the pre-hospital group. Just one open, randomized study has found a significant reduction in 14-day and 1-year mortality from pre-hospital thrombolysis (McAleer et al., 1992). Mean delay time to treatment was 138 min. in the pre-hospital group vs. 172 min. for the in-hospital group. Fourteen-day mortality was 2.3% vs. 11.7% ($p < 0.05$). This has not been confirmed by other authors (Castaigne et al., 1989; McNeill et al., 1989; Roth et al., 1990), probably because of the long interval between onset of pain to activation of the EMS system or patient presentation to hospital. Fifty-eight per cent of mean delay time to treatment is attributable to the patients and transport times account for only 14% of delay (Rustige et al., 1990). Thus, pre-hospital thrombolysis seems only justified when long transport times can be expected (Brugemann et al., 1992).

NEW DRUGS

Adenosine

Adenosine is an endogenous nucleoside. It depresses atrioventricular (AV) node and sinus node activity, and therefore inhibits supraventricular re-entry tachycardias running through the AV node or sinus node (DiMarco et al., 1983). Until recently, verapamil has been the drug of choice for patients with (paroxysmal) SVTs, but in patients with a Wolff–Parkinson–White syndrome this drug might exhibit deleterious side-effects by accelerating the refractory period of accessory pathways, thereby inducing ventricular fibrillation. This does not occur with adenosine. In addition, verapamil will further compromise contractility in patients with congestive heart failure. No negative side-effects were seen in patients who were actually in ventricular tachycardia (VT), but received adenosine inappropriately (McCabe et al., 1992), but with the increasing use of adenosine, more untoward side-effects (accelerating PSVT, bradyasystole, sinus arrest) have been reported (Reed et al., 1991; Orebaugh and Handy, 1992; Webster and Daar, 1993).

Because of its short half-life of only 5 seconds, adenosine will produce short-lived AV, or ventriculoatrial blockade, when given to patients not in (P)SVT and will help to clarify the diagnosis (DiMarco et al., 1985). As episodes of SVT may recur, definitive treatment with calcium channel blockers may be necessary later.

Magnesium

Magnesium stabilizes cell membranes, dilates coronary arteries, decreases platelet aggregation, and protects against catecholamine-induced myocardial necrosis (Horner, 1992; Woods et al., 1992). Magnesium deficiency results in cellular potassium depletion, and potassium repletion requires magnesium as a cofactor for sodium-potassium transport. Magnesium depletion is thought to be a major cause of supraventricular and ventricular arrhythmias (Gettes, 1992; Tso and Baish, 1992), at least in conjunction with other electrolyte disorders such as hypokalaemia (Gettes, 1992; Millane et al., 1992). Other effects of low Mg^{2+} levels include cardiac ischaemia, vasospasm, seizures, tetany, and coma. Hypomagnesaemia is most likely in patients who are on diuretics, in alcoholics, and in those with diabetic ketoacidosis (Tso and Barish, 1992). Sudden death is common in areas with a low water Mg^{2+} content, and myocardial Mg^{2+}

content is low in victims of sudden death (Eisenberg, 1992). The antiarryhthmic action of magnesium is separate from the overall magnesium balance (Millane, 1992).

In several studies, magnesium has been shown to increase survival in patients with acute myocardial infarction (Smith et al., 1986). In a meta-analysis of several randomized controlled trials including 930 patients, Horner (1992) found a 49% reduction in ventricular tachycardia and fibrillation in patients with acute myocardial infarction (AMI) after intravenous magnesium administration. The incidence of cardiac arrest was reduced by 58%, and reduction in mortality was 54%. In the LIMIT–2 trial including 2316 patients with suspected AMI, the incidence of left ventricular failure was reduced by 25% in the magnesium group, and 28-day mortality was 7.8% for the Mg^{2+} group vs. 10.3% for the placebo group (Woods et al., 1992). These findings were not supported by the results of the ISIS-4 study, when application of Mg^{2+} did not decrease mortality in the first 35-days (ISIS-4, 1994). However, patients in the LIMIT study received Mg^{2+} very early whereas in the ISIS study this drug was not given before 8–12 hours after the onset of symptoms. Craddock et al. (1991) reported a patient in VF/VT who was resuscitated for 70 min; after 8 g $MgSO_4$ had been administered intravenously, a stable pulse could be restored. Outcome is also improved in patients with non-occlusive coronary artery disease (Salem et al., 1991), and post-infarction arrhythmias are prevented by magnesium (Ceremúzynski et al., 1989; Teo et al., 1991). Thus, its use in patients with AMI seems increasingly justified, but more controlled randomized larger studies are needed to support its pre-hospital use. There is no question that magnesium is the treatment of choice in patients with torsades des pointes (Perticone et al., 1986; Tzivoni et al., 1988).

QUALITY ASSESSMENT, GUIDELINES, AND REPORTING

Quality control and the measurement of cost–benefit ratios in medicine are increasingly important. Patients must receive quality emergency medical care at justifiable expense. The familiar trinity of structure, process and outcome applies also to the EMS system. Process quality is probably of predominant importance as standards or guidelines can be developed, and deviation from these can be easily detected (e.g. ACLS, ATLS). Non-adherence to or deficiencies of standards could bias outcome analysis, and this again would influence structural defects and education of paramedics and emergency physicians. Quality improvement programmes have been shown to improve chart documentation and behaviour of paramedics (O'Connor and Megargel, 1994). Yet, outcome analysis is invariably linked to the patients' in-hospital course and will not adequately reflect EMS quality because post-resuscitation support will differ from hospital to hospital. For this reason, intermediate outcome analysis has been suggested (Thomas and Cayten, 1986). Hennes et al. (1993) divided EMS care quality into primary, secondary and tertiary efficacy. An index for the evaluation of primary efficacy (until admission to hospital) has been developed already (Hennes et al., 1992). In order to facilitate standardization of in-hospital treatment, it would be helpful if the EMS medical director was the supervising physician at the same time.

Guidelines such as ACLS or ATLS have been developed as a processing protocol for well-defined situations. They represent the consensus views of experts in this particular field, but this does not imply that they have to be applied in each and every situation. The term *standards and guidelines* has been changed by the AHA into *guidelines* to emphasize the flexibility for deviation from the protocol whenever it seems medically sound (AHA, 1992). Furthermore, 'standards' implicates a legal notion the term was never intended to have. Unfortunately, AHA and European Resuscitation Council (ERC) guidelines differ in a few essentials and a variety of details, creating confusion particularly among those responsible for teaching and training. This problem should soon be solved by a Joint Committee of both organizations.

Uniform reporting of EMS runs is mandatory for comparability. In Germany, a run sheet recently was adopted by the DIVI (German interdisciplinary association for intensive care and emergency medicine) which applies both to physicians and paramedics. Statistical evaluation based upon this sheet will provide important data for process evaluation. For the field of CPR, the European Resuscitation Council has presented a registration form (Delooz, 1992); an international working group has proposed 'guidelines for uniform reporting of data from out-of-hospital arrest: "Utstein style"' (Cummins et al., 1991).

REFERENCES

Alexander, R., Hodgson, P., Lomax, D., Bullen, C. (1993) A comparison of the laryngeal mask airway and Guedel airway, bag and facemask for manual ventilation following formal training. *Anaesthesia* **48**(3): 231–234.

American Heart Association (1974) Standards and Guidelines for cardiopulmonary resuscitation and emergency cardiac care. *Journal of the American Medical Association* **227**: 833–868.

American Heart Association (1992) Guidelines for cardiopulmonary resuscitation and emergency cardiac care. *Journal of the American Medical Association* **268**: 2171–2297.

Arntz, H.R., Storch, W.H., Völler, H. et al. (1990) Thrombolyse bei akutem Infarkt in der Prähospitalphase. *Intensivmed* **27**: 150–154.

Arntz, H.R., Stern, R., Linderer, T., Schröder, R. (1992) Efficiency of a physician-operated mobile intensive care unit for prehospital thrombolysis in acute myocardial infarction. *American Journal of Cardiology* **70**: 417–420.

Atherton, G.L., Johnson, J.C. (1993) Ability of paramedics to use the combitube in prehospital cardiac arrest. *Annals of Emergency Medicine* **22**: 1263–1268.

AufderHeide, T.P., Keelan, M.H., Hendley, G.E. et al. (1992a) Milwaukee prehospital chest pain project – phase I: feasibility and accuracy of prehospital thrombolytic candidate selection. *American Journal of Cardiology* **69**: 991–996.

AufderHeide, T.P., Martin, D.R., Olson, D.W. et al. (1992b) Prehospital bicarbonate use in cardiac arrest: A 3-year experience. *American Journal of Emergency Medicine* **10**: 4–7.

Barnett, W.M., Alifimoff, J.K., Paris, P.M. et al. (1986) Comparison of open-chest cardiac massage techniques in dogs. *Annals of Emergency Medicine* **15**: 408–411.

Bartlett, R.L., Martin, S.D., McMahon, J.M. Jr et al. (1992) A field comparison of the pharyngotracheal lumen airway and the endotracheal tube. *Journal of Trauma* **32**: 280–284.

Barton, C.W., Callaham, M.L. (1988) Successful prediction by capnometry of resuscitation from cardiac arrest. Abstr. *Annals of Emergency Medicine* **17**: 393–394.

Barton, C.W., Callaham, M.L. (1991) High-dose epinephrine improves the return of spontaneous circulation rates in human victims of cardiac arrest. *Annals of Emergency Medicine* **20**: 722–725.

Bersin, R.M., Chatterjee, K., Arieff, A.I. (1989) Metabolic and hemodynamic consequences of sodium bicarbonate administration in patients with heart disease. *American Journal of Medicine* **87**: 7–14.

Bircher, N., Safar, P. (1985) Cerebral preservation during cardiopulmonary resuscitation. *Critical Care Medicine* **13**: 185–190.

Bishop, R.L., Weisfeldt, M.L. (1976) Sodium bicarbonate administration during cardiac arrest. *Journal of the American Medical Association* **235**: 506–509.

Blecic, S., De Backer, D., Deleuze, M., Vachiery, J.L., Vincent, J.L. (1991) Correction of metabolic acidosis in experimental CPR: A comparative study of sodium bicarbonate, carbicarb, and dextrose. *Annals of Emergency Medicine* **20**: 235–238.

Brown, C.G., Werman, H.A., Davis, E.A. et al. (1986) Comparative effects of graded doses of epinephrine on regional brain blood flow during CPR in swine. *Annals of Emergency Medicine* **15**: 1138–1144.

Brown, C.G., Werman, H.A., Davis, E.A., Hobson, J., Hamlin, R.L. (1987) The effects of graded doses of epinephrine on regional myocardial blood flow during cardiopulmonary resuscitation in swine. *Circulation* **75**: 491–497.

Brown, C.G., Martin, D.R., Pepe, P.E. et al. (1992) A comparison of standard-dose and high-dose epinephrine in cardiac arrest outside the hospital. *New England Journal of Medicine* **327**: 1051–1055.

Brugemann, J., vanderMeer, J., deGraeff, P.A., Takens, L.H., Lie, K.I. (1992) Logistical problems in prehospital thrombolysis. *European Heart Journal* **13**: 787–788.

Brunette, D.D., Jameson, S.J. (1990) Comparison of standard versus high-dose epinephrine in the resuscitation of cardiac arrest in dogs. *Annals of Emergency Medicine* **19**: 8–11.

Calder, I., Ordman, A.J., Jackowski, A., Crockard, H.A. (1990) The brain laryngeal mask airway. An alternative to emergency tracheal intubation. *Anaesthesia* **45**: 137–139.

Callaham, M., Barton, C. (1990) Prediction of outcome of cardiopulmonary resuscitation from end-tidal carbon dioxide concentration. *Critical Care Medicine* **18**: 358–362.

Calle, P.A., Paridaens, K., De Ridder, L.I., Buylaert, W.A. (1993) Failure of nimodipine to prevent brain damage in a global brain ischemia model in the rat. *Resuscitation* **25**: 59–71.

Castaigne, A.D., HervÇ, C., Duval-Moulin, A.M. et al. (1989) Prehospital use of APSAC: Results of a placebo-controlled study. *American Journal of Cardiology* **64**: 30A–33A; discussion 41A–42A.

Ceremúzynski, L., Juriel, R., Kulakowski, P., Gebalska, J. (1989) Threatening arrhythmias in acute myocardial infarction are prevented by intravenous magnesium sulfate. *American Heart Journal* **118**: 1333–1334.

Chang, M.W., Coffeen, P., Lurie, K.G. et al. (1992) Tissue perfusion during standard vs. active compression-decompression CPR in the dog (abstract). *Circulation* **86**: 1233.

Cohen, T.J., Tucker, K.J., Redberg, R.F. et al. (1991) Active compression–decompression resuscitation: a new method of cardiopulmonary resuscitation. *Circulation* **84**: II–9. Abstract.

Cohen, T.J., Tucker, K.J., Lurie, K.G. et al. (1992) Active compression–decompression: a new method of cardiopulmonary resuscitation. *Journal of the American Medical Association* **267**: 2916–2923.

Cohen, T.J., Goldner, B.G., Maccaro, P.C. et al. (1993) A comparison of active compression–decompression cardiopulmonary resuscitation with standard cardiopulmonary resuscitation for cardiac arrests occurring in the hospital. *New England Journal of Medicine* **329**: 1918–1921.

Craddock, L., Miller, B., Clifton, G., Krumbach, B., Pluss, W. (1991) Resuscitation from prolonged cardiac arrest with high-dose intravenous magnesium sulfate. *Journal of Emergency Medicine* **9**: 469–476.

Cummins, R.O., Chamberlain, D.A., Abramson, N.A. et al. (1991) Recommended guidelines for uniform reporting of data from out-of-hospital cardiac arrest: the 'Utstein style'. *Circulation* **84**: 960–975.

Dalkara, T., Namer, I.J., Onur, R. Zileli, T. (1989) Intravenously and iontophoretically administered naloxone reverses ischemic changes in rat hippocampus. *Stroke* **20**: 1059–1064.

Davies, P.R., Tighe, S.Q., Greenslade, G.L., Evans, G.H. (1990) Larnygeal mask airway and tracheal tube insertion by unskilled personnel. *Lancet* **336**: 977–979.

DeBehnke, D.J., Angelos, M.G., Leasure, J.E. (1991) Comparison of standard external CPR, open-chest CPR, and cardiopulmonary bypass in a canine myocardial infarct model. *Annals of Emergency Medicine* **20**: 754–760.

Delooz, H.H., Mullie, A., Dick, W.F. (1992) Forms for registration of CPR efforts and outcome, respectively for out-of-hospital and in-hospital cardiac arrest. *Resuscitation* **24**: 155–166.

DiMarco, J.P., Sellers, T.D., Berne, R.M., West, G.A., Belardinelli, L. (1983) Adenosine: electrophysiologic effects and therapeutic use for terminating paroxsysmal supraventricular tachycardia. *Circulation* **68**: 1254–1263.

DiMarco, J.P., Sellers, T.D., Lerman, B.B. et al. (1985) Diagnostic and therapeutic use of adenosine in patients with supraventricular tachyarrhythmias. *Journal of the American College of Cardiology* **6**: 417–425.

Eichinger, S., Schreiber, W., Heinz, T. et al. (1992) Airway management in a case of neck impalement: use of the esophageal tracheal combitube airway. *British Journal of Anaesthesiology* **68**: 534–535.

Eisenberg, M.J. (1992) Magnesium deficiency and sudden death (editorial). *American Heart Journal* **124**: 544–549.

Ellinger, K., Striebel, J.P., Danner, W. (1988) Pulsoximetrie – Sinnvolles und praktikables nichtinvasives Monitoring in der präklinischen Phase. *Anästhesist* **37**(suppl.): 252.

European Myocardial Infarction Project Group (1993) Prehospital thrombolytic therapy in patients with suspected acute myocardial infarction. *New England Journal of Medicine* **329**: 383–389.

Galien, Avd., Takens, L.H., Lie, K.I. (1989) Pre-hospital thrombolytic treatment in acute myocardial infarction: percentage of evaluable patients and pitfalls. Results of a dutch multicenter pre-hospital study. Abstr. *European Heart Journal* **10**(suppl.): 122.

Geehr, E.C., Auerbach, P.S. (1985) Open-chest cardiac massage for victims of medical cardiac arrest (abstract). *Annals of Emergency Medicine* **14**: 499.

Gettes, L.S. (1992) Electrolyte abnormalities underlying lethal and ventricular arryhthmias. *Circulation* **85**(suppl. 1): I70–6.

Goetting, M.G., Paradis, N.A. (1991) High-dose epinephrine improves outcome from pediatric cardiac arrest. *Annals of Emergency Medicine* **20**: 22–8.

Gonzalez, E.R., Ornato, J.P., Garrett, A.R. et al. (1989) Dose-dependent vasopressor response to epinephrine during CPR in human beings. *Annals of Emergency Medicine* **18**: 920–926.

Graf, H., Leach, W., Arieff, A.I. (1984) Evidence for a detrimental effect of bicarbonate therapy in hypoxic lactic acidosis. *Science* **227**: 754–756.

GREAT Group (1992). Feasibility, safety, and efficacy of domiciliary thrombolysis by general practitioners: Grampian region early anistreplase trial. *British Medical Journal* **305**: 548–553.

Greene, M.K., Roden, R., Hinchley, G. (1992) The laryngeal mask airway. Two cases of prehospital trauma care. *Anaesthesia* **47**: 688–689.

Gruppo italiano per lo studio della streptochinase nell'infarto miocardico (GISSI) (1987) Long-term effects of intravenous thrombolysis in acute myocardial infarction: Final report of the GISSI study. *Lancet* **ii**: 871–874.

Gulba, D.C., Westhoff-Bleck, M., Reil, G.H. (1990) Thrombolysetherapie des akuten Herzinfarktes – Ergebnisse und neue Entwicklungen. *Dtsch Med Wschr* **115**: 187–195.

Hankins, D.G., Carruthers, N., Frascone, R.J., Long, L.A., Campion, B.C. (1993) Complication rates for the esophageal obturator airway and endotracheal tube in the prehospital setting. *Prehospital Disaster Medicine* **8**: 117–121.

Hennes, H.J., Reinhardt, T., Dick, W. (1992) Beurteilung des Notfallpatienten mit dem Mainz Emergency Evaluation Score. *Notfallmedizin* **18**: 130–136.

Hennes, H.J., Reinhardt, T., Otto, S., Dick, W. (1993) Die Effektivität der präklinischen Versorgung – Bedeutung, Begriffsbestimmung, Voraussetzungen. *Notfallmedizin* **19**: 76–78.

Horner, S.M. (1992) Efficacy of intravenous magnesium in acute myocardial infarction in reducing arrhythmias and mortality. *Circulation* **86**: 774–779.

ISIS-2-collaborative group (1988) Randomized trial of intravenous streptokinase, oral aspirin, both, or neither among 17,187 cases of suspected myocardial infarction: ISIS-2. *Lancet* **ii**: 349–360.

ISIS-4 (1994) Captopril, Isosorbidmononitrat und Magnesium beim akuten Myokardinfarkt. Der Arzneimittelbrief **28**: 5–6.

Jantzen, J.P., Hennes, H.J. (1991) Präklinische Kapnometrie – ein richtungsweisender Fortschritt. *Notfallmedizin* **17**: 450–456.

Jude, J.R., Kouwenhoven, W.B., Knickerbocker, G.G. (1964) External cardiac resuscitation. *Monographs in Surgical Science* **1**: 59–117.

Kern, K.B., Sanders, A.B., Janas, W. et al. (1991) Limitations of open-chest cardiac massage after prolonged, untreated cardiac arrest in dogs. *Annals of Emergency Medicine* **20**: 761–767.

Kette, F., Weil, M.H., von Planta, M., Gazmuri, R.J., Rackow, E.C. (1990) Buffer agents do not reverse intramyocardial acidosis during cardiac resuscitation. *Circulation* **81**: 1660–1666.

Klauser, R., Roggla, G., Pidlich, J. et al. (1992) Massive upper airway bleeding after thrombolytic therapy: sucessful airway management with the Combitube. *Annals of Emergency Medicine* **21**: 431–433.

Koehli, N. (1991) Aspiration and the laryngeal mask airway. *Anesthesia* **46**: 419.

Kokkinis, K. (1994) The use of the laryngeal mask airway in CPR. *Resuscitation* **27**: 9–12.

Kouwenhoven, W.B., Jude, J.R., Knickerbocker, G.G. (1960) Closed-chest cardiac massage. *Journal of the American Medical Association* **173**: 1064–1067.

Lindner, K.H., Ahnefeld, F.W., Prengel, A.W. (1991) Comparison of standard and high-dose adrenaline in the resuscitation of asystole and electromechanical dissociation. *Acta Anaesthesiologica Scandinavica* **35**: 253–256.

Lindner, K.H., Pfenninger, E.G., Lurie, K.G. et al. (1993) Effects of active compression–decompression resuscitation on myocardial and cerebral blood flow in pigs. *Circulation* **88**: 1254–1263.

Lurie, K.G., Lindo, C., Chin, J. (1990) CPR: the P stands for plumber's helper. *Journal of the American Medical Association* **264**: 1661.

McAleer, B., Ruane, B., Burke, E. et al. (1992) Prehospital thrombolysis in a rural community: short- and long-term survival. *Cardiovascular Drugs Therapy* **6**: 369–372.

McCabe, J.L., Adhar, G.C., Menegazzi, J.J., Paris, P.M. (1992) Intravenous adenosine in the prehospital treatment of paroxysmal supraventricular tachycardia. *Annals of Emergency Medicine* **21**: 358–361.

McGuire, T.J., Pointer, J.E. (1988) Evaluation of pulse oximeter in the prehospital setting. *Annals of Emergency Medicine* **17**: 1058–1093.

McNeill, A.J., Cunningham, S.R., Flannery, D.J. et al. (1989) A doubleblind placebo controlled study of early and late administration of recombinant tissue plasminogen activator in acute myocardial infarction. *British Heart Journal* **61**: 316–21.

Maltby, J.R., Loken, R.G., Watson, N.C. (1990) The laryngeal mask airway: clinical appraisal in 250 patients. *Canadian Journal of Anaesthesiology* **37**: 509–513.

Martin, G.B., Gentile, N.B., Paradis, N.A. (1990) Effect of epinephrine on end-tidal carbon dioxide monitoring during CPR. *Annals of Emergency Medicine* **19**: 396–398.

Meldrum, B. (1990) Protection against ischemic neuronal damage by drugs acting on excitatory neurotransmission. *Cerebrovascular and Brain Metabolism Reviews* **2**: 27–57.

Mertzlufft, F. (1990) Was die Puls-Oxymetrie für die Notfallmedizin bringt. *Notfallmedizin* **16**: 637–643.

Millane, T.A., Ward, D.E., Camm, A.J. (1992) Is hypomagnesemia arrhythmogenic? *Clinical Cardiology* **15**: 103–108.

O'Connor, R.E., Megargel, R.E. (1994) The effect of a quality improvement feedback loop on paramedic skills, charting, and behavior. *Prehospital Disaster Medicine* **9**: 35–39.

Orebaugh, S.L., Handy, M. (1992) Intravenous adenosine therapy accelerating rate of paroxsysmal supraventricular tachycardia. *American Journal of Emergency Medicine* **10**: 326–330.

Ornato, J.P., Shipley, J.B., Racht, E.M. et al. (1992) Multicenter study of a portable, hand-size, colorimetric end-tidal carbon dioxide detection device. *Annals of Emergency Medicine* **21**: 518–523.

Pagani, F.D., Baker, L.S., Cheng, H. et al. (1990) The correction of intramyocardial respiratory acidosis with sodium bicarbonate ($NaHCO_3$). *Circulation* **82**: 484 (abstract).

Paradis, N.A., Martin, G.B., Rivers, E.P. (1990) End-tidal CO_2 and high dose epinephrine during cardiac arrest in humans. Abstr. Oral presentations, cardiopulmonary resuscitation. *Critical Care Medicine* **18**: 276.

Pennant, J.H., Gajraj, N.M., Pace, N.A. (1992) Laryngeal mask airway in cervical spine injuries (letter). *Anesthesia and Analgesia* **75**: 1074–1075.

Perticone, F., Adinolfi, L., Bonaduce, D. (1986) Efficacy of magnesium sulfate in the treatment of torsades des pointes. *American Heart Journal* **112**: 847–849.

Reed, R., Falk, J.L., O'Brien, S. (1991) Untoward reaction to adenosine therapy for supraventricular tachycardia. *American Journal of Emergency Medicine* **9**: 566–570.

Reinhard, M., Luxem, J. (1992) Pulsoxymeter. *Notfallmedizin* **18**: 170–176.

Roine, R.O., Kaste, M., Kinnunen, A. et al. (1990) Nimodipine after resuscitation from out-of-hospital ventricular fibrillation. *Journal of the American Medical Association* **264**: 3171–3177.

Roth, A., Barbash, G.I., Hod, H. et al. (1990) Should thrombolytic therapy be administered in the mobile intensive care unit in patients with evolving myocardial infarction? A pilot study. *Journal of the American College of Cardiology* **15**: 932–936.

Rustige, J., Burczyk, U., Werner, A., Senges, J. (1990) Akuter Herzinfarkt: Verkürzung der Prähospitalphase durch Massenaufklärung möglich. *Deutsches Ärzteblatt* **87**: 906.

Salem, M., Munoz, R., Chernow, B. (1991) Hypomagnesemia in critical illness – a common and clinically important problem. *Critical Care Clinics* **7**: 225–252.

Sanders, A.B., Kern, K.B., Otto, C.W. et al. (1989) End-tidal carbon dioxide monitoring during cardiopulmonary resuscitation. A prognostic indicator for survival. *Journal of the American Medical Association* **262**: 1347–1351.

Saji, M., Reis, D.J. (1987) Delayed transneuronal death of substantia nigra neurons prevented by alpha-aminobutyric acid agonist. *Science* **235**: 66–69.

Sasaki, T., Nakagomi, T., Kirino, T. et al. (1988) Indomethacin ameliorates ischemic neuronal damage in the gerbil hippocampal CA1 sector. *Stroke* **19**: 1399–1403.

Schindler, I., Mauritz, W., Weindlmayr-Goettel, M. (1992) Effects of nimodipine administration during cardiopulmonary resuscitation in pigs. *European Journal of Anaesthesiology* **9**: 411–418.

Siesjö, B.K., Bengtsson, F. (1989) Calcium fluxes, calcium antagonists, and calcium-related pathology in brain ischemia, hypoglycemia, and spreading suppression: a unifying hypothesis. *Journal of Cerebral Blood Flow and Metabolism* **9**: 127–140.

Simoons, M.L., Serrnys, P.W., van den Brand, M. et al. (1986) Early thrombolysis in acute myocardial infarction: Limitation of infarct size and improved survival. *Journal of the American College of Cardiology* **7**: 717–728.

Smith, I., White, P.F. (1992) Use of the laryngeal mask airway as an alternative to a face mask during outpatient arthroscopy. *Anesthesiology* **77**: 850–855.

Smith, L.F., Heagerty, A.M., Bing, R.F. et al. (1986) Intravenous infusion of magnesium sulfate after acute myocardial infarction: Effects on arrhythmias and mortality. *International Journal of Cardiology* **12**: 175–183.

Staudinger, T., Brugger, S., Watschinger, B. et al. (1993) Emergency intubation with the combitube: comparison with the endotracheal airway. *Annals of Emergency Medicine* **22**: 1573–1575.

Steen, P.A., Gisvold, S.E., Milde, J.H. et al. (1985) Nimodipine improves outcome when given after complete cerebral ischemia in primates. *Anaesthesiology* **62**: 406–414.

Stevenson, H.E., Reid, L.C., Hinton, J.W. (1953) Some common denominators in 1200 cases of cardiac arrest. *Annals of Surgery* **137**: 731–744.

Stiell, I.G., Hebert, P.G., Weitzman, B.N. et al. (1992) High-dose epinephrine in adult cardiac arrest. *New England Journal of Medicine* **327**: 1045–1050.

Strunin, L., Williams, T. (1989) The FEF end-tidal carbon dioxide detector. *Anesthesiology* **71**: 621–622.

Teo, K.K., Yusuf, S., Collins, R., Held, P.H., Peto, R. (1991) Effects of intravenous magnesium in suspected acute myocardial infarction: an overview of randomised trials. *British Medical Journal* **303**: 1499–1503.

Tinker, J.H., Dull, D.L., Caplan, R.A., Ward, R.J., Cheney, F.W. (1989) Role of monitoring devices in prevention of anesthetic mishaps: a closed claims analysis. *Anesthesiology* **71**: 541–546.

Thomas, J.W., Cayten, C.G. (1986) EMS system planning and control. In Schwartz, G.R. (ed.) *Emergency Medicine*, pp 566–576. Philadelphia, WB Saunders.

Tolley, P.M., Watts, A.D., Hickman, J.A. (1992) Comparison of the use of the laryngeal mask and face mask by inexperienced personnel. *British Journal of Anaesthesiology* **69**: 320–321.

Trillo, G., Planta, Mv., Kette, F. (1994) $ETCO_2$ monitoring during low flow states: clinical aims and limits. *Resuscitation* **27**: 1–8.

Tso, E.L., Barish, R.A. (1992) Magnesium: clinical considerations. *Journal of Emergency Medicine* **10**: 735–745.

Tucker, K.J., Khan, J.H., Savitt, M.A. (1993) Active compression–decompression resuscitation: effects on pulmonary ventilation. *Resuscitation* **26**: 125–131.

Tucker, K.J., Redberg, R.F., Schiller, N.B., Cohen, T.J. (1993b) Active compression–decompression resuscitation: analysis of transmitral flow and left ventricular volume by transesophageal echocardiography in humans. *Journal of the American College of Cardiology* **22**: 1485–1493.

Tzivoni, D., Banai, S., Schuger, C. et al. (1988) Treatment of torsades des pointes with magnesium sulfate. *Circulation* **77**: 392–397.

Vogel, K., Silvanus, M.T., Stopfkuchen, H., Mertzlufft, F., Zander, R. (1988) Zuverlässigkeit und Wertigkeit von kutaner Sauerstoffpartialdruckmessung und Pulsoxymetrie an Früh und Termingeborenen. *Kliuische Pádiatrie* **200**: 150–151.

Webster, D.P., Daar, A.A. (1993) Prolonged bradyasystole and seizures following intravenous adenosine for supraventricular tachycardia. *American Journal of Emergency Medicine* **11**: 192–194.
Weiser, F.M., Adler, A.N., Kuhn, L.A. (1962) Hemodynamic effects of closed and open-chest cardiac resuscitation in normal dogs and those with myocardial infarction. *American Journal of Cardiology* **10**: 55.
Wilcox, R.G., von der Lippe, G., Olsson et al. (1988) Trial of tissue plasminogen activator for mortality reduction in acute myocardial infarction. Anglo-Scandinavian Study of Early Thrombolysis (ASSET). *Lancet* **ii**: 525–530.
Woods, K.L., Fletcher, S., Roffe, C., Haider, Y. (1992) Intravenous magnesium sulphate in suspected acute myocardial infarction: results of the second Leicester intravenous magnesium intervention trial (LIMIT-2). *Lancet* **339**: 1553–1558.

2

Pulmonary Vasomotor Dysfunction in Acute Lung Injury

Marc Leeman, Robert Naeije

INTRODUCTION

Acute lung injury, including its most severe form, the adult respiratory distress syndrome (ARDS), complicates several diseases such as sepsis, circulatory shock and trauma. Whatever the aetiology, increased pulmonary microvascular permeability leads to non-cardiogenic ('permeability') oedema. The pulmonary circulation plays a central role in the pathogenesis of lung injury. First, especially when the precipitating event does not involve the lung directly, it is submitted to the effects of the circulating inflammatory mediators that will trigger microcirculatory damage with resulting pulmonary oedema and hypertension. Second, abnormal pulmonary vasomotor tone contributes to the mismatching of perfusion to ventilation, responsible for arterial hypoxaemia.

In 1977, Zapol and Snider emphasized the constant occurrence of pulmonary hypertension in 30 patients with ARDS, even when hypoxaemia was corrected by mechanical ventilation or extracorporeal membrane oxygenation (Zapol and Snider, 1977). Pulmonary hypertension has been confirmed in recent reports on larger groups of ARDS patients (Table 2.1). The magnitude of pulmonary hypertension does not seem to predict mortality. In a group of 162 ARDS patients, initial mean pulmonary artery pressure (*P*pa) was 26 ± 8 (SE) and 27 ± 11 mmHg, and highest *P*pa was 37 ± 9 and 39 ± 12 mmHg, respectively in survivors and non-survivors (Suchyta et al., 1992). However, non-survivors developed a progressive worsening of their pulmonary hypertension (Sloane et al., 1992).

Pulmonary vessels are able to dilate during lung injury (Zapol et al., 1985; Mélot et al., 1987, 1989; Leeman, 1991). They can also constrict further: an ARDS patient may markedly increase his *P*pa when inadvertently disconnected from the ventilator (Zapol et al., 1985), indicating that a pressor response (at least to hypoxia)

Table 2.1 Haemodynamic measurements in ARDS patients

Reference	Zapol and Snider (1977)	Bernard et al. (1987)	Bone et al. (1989)	Sloane et al. (1992)	Suchyta et al. (1992)
n	30	99	74	153	162
*P*pa, mmHg	22–27 (*) 27–>35 (†)	25	27–29	27–28	26–27 (‡) 37–39 (§)
*P*pao, mmHg	10–12	12	NR	13–14	NR
Q, 1/min	variable	6.4	NR	7–8	NR
*P*EEP, cmH_2O	5–40	8	10	8	NR

*P*pa, mean pulmonary artery pressure. *P*pao, pulmonary artery occlusion pressure. Q, cardiac output. *P*EEP, positive end-expiratory pressure. NR, not reported. (*) No hypoxaemia. (†) hypoxaemia. (‡) initial *P*pa. (§) highest *P*pa.

remains possible. This chapter reviews the factors affecting the state of the pulmonary circulation in lung injury, and the relationship between pulmonary vascular tone and gas exchange.

NATURE OF PULMONARY HYPERTENSION IN LUNG INJURY

Zapol et al. (1985) observed that variations in cardiac output (Q), induced by isoprenaline (isoproterenol) infusion or by changes in bypass flow during extracorporeal oxygenation, had no effect on *P*pa. In other words, the *P*pa–Q relationship was nearly horizontal and the extrapolated pressure intercept was largely higher than left atrial pressure (*P*la). A suggested explanation is the occurrence of a pulmonary vascular closing pressure superior to *P*la.

Pulmonary vessels are collapsible and have tone so that they present with a closing pressure. Vascular closure occurs if the pressure generated by tone exceeds inflow pressure (*P*pa) or if surrounding pressure exceeds intravascular pressure. If the closing pressure is higher than *P*la, it becomes the effective outflow pressure and the linear extrapolation of the *P*pa–Q relationship will cross the pressure axis at the level of the mean closing pressure of the pulmonary vascular bed. Another consequence of a closing pressure superior to *P*la is that, under conditions of constant Q, increases in *P*la will affect *P*pa only when *P*la exceeds closing pressure (Permutt and Riley, 1963; Lopez-Muniz et al., 1968; Graham et al., 1982; Mitzner and Chang, 1989).

The presence of a closing pressure has been investigated in anaesthetized dogs with oleic acid lung injury (Boiteau et al., 1986; Leeman et al., 1990a). This injury bears close histological and pathophysiological similarities to the early stages of clinical ARDS (Schoene et al., 1984; Leeman et al., 1987a; Schuster, 1994). Venous return, and hence Q, was manipulated by inflating an inferior vena caval balloon catheter or by opening a femoral arterio-venous bypass, and *P*la was adjusted using a balloon catheter inserted into the left atrium.

The *P*pa–Q plots were essentially linear, suggesting full recruitment of pulmonary vessels over the range of Q studied (Leeman et al., 1989). Before oleic acid, the extrapolated pressure intercept of the *P*pa–Q plots approximated *P*la, and increases in *P*la at constant Q induced a proportional increase in *P*pa, indicating that *P*la was indeed the effective outflow pressure of the pulmonary circulation (Figure 2.1). After oleic acid lung injury, however, the *P*pa–Q relationship was shifted in parallel toward higher pressures (indicating pulmonary hypertension), so that the extrapolated pressure intercept was higher than *P*la (Figure 2.1a). Additionally, *P*la could be increased by several mmHg before affecting *P*pa (Figure 2.1b). These data suggest that lung injury increases the pulmonary vascular closing pressure, which becomes higher than *P*la and accounts for the

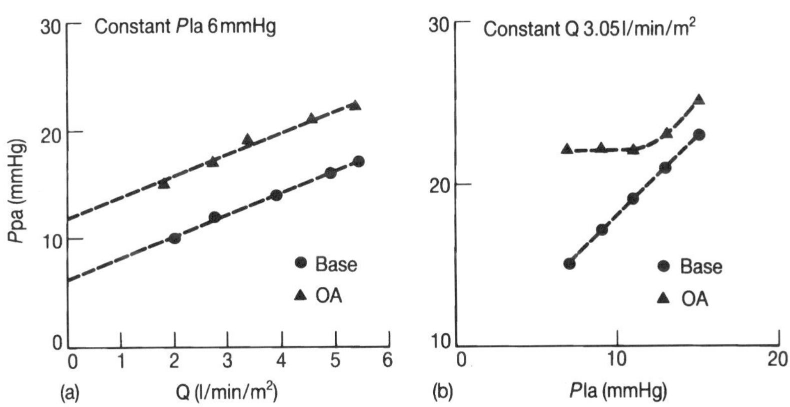

Figure 2.1. Illustrative experiments of mean pulmonary artery pressure (*P*pa) – cardiac index (Q) plots at constant left atrial pressure (*P*la) and of *P*pa–*P*la plots at constant Q, in dogs, before and after oleic acid lung injury (OA). Lung injury increased the extrapolated pressure intercept of the *P*pa–Q relationship (left) and caused a functional dissociation between *P*pa and *P*la (right), both suggestive of an increased closing pressure accounting for pulmonary hypertension in this model of ARDS. (Adapted from Leeman et al., 1990a.)

pulmonary hypertension (Leeman et al., 1990a). The functional dissociation between changes in *P*pa and in alveolar pressure observed after oleic acid lung injury suggests that the site of vascular closure is extra-alveolar (Leeman et al., 1990b). Minimal effect of positive end-expiratory pressure (up to 20 cmH_2O) on *P*pa had been noted in patients with ARDS (Zapol and Snider, 1977).

MECHANISMS OF PULMONARY HYPERTENSION IN LUNG INJURY

Pulmonary hypertension in acute lung injury results from functional (hypoxia and mediator-induced vasoconstriction) and mechanical (vascular compression by oedema fluid or fibrosis, vascular wall remodeling, thromboembolism, reduced lung volume) factors (Zapol et al., 1985; Leeman, 1991).

Active vasoconstriction is a major determinant of pulmonary hypertension in lung injury. Several vasodilators have been shown to reduce *P*pa in clinical as well as in experimental ARDS (Zapol et al., 1985; Leeman, 1991). For example, prostaglandin E_1 reduced by about 50% the extrapolated pressure intercept of *P*pa–Q plots constructed in dogs with oleic acid lung injury (Leeman et al., 1988a)

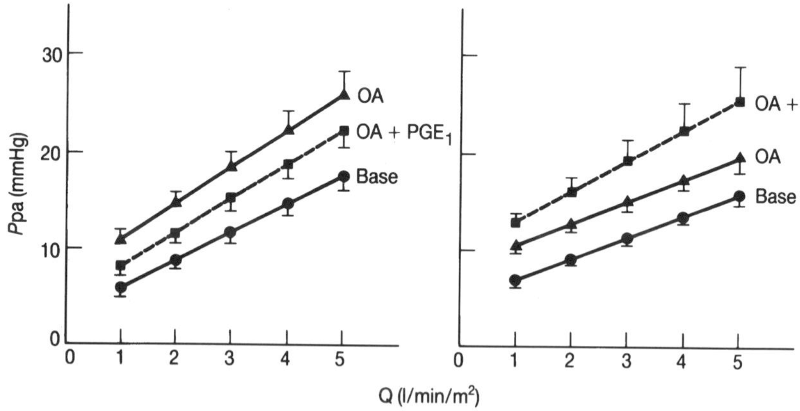

Figure 2.2. Composite mean pulmonary artery pressure (*P*pa) – cardiac index (Q) plots in dogs before and after oleic acid lung injury (OA), and then after prostaglandin E_1 (PG-E_1, $n = 8$) or after acetylsalicylic acid (ASA, $n = 8$). Injured pulmonary circulation remains able to dilate (left) and to constrict further (right). (Adapted from Leeman et al., 1988a, 1988b.)

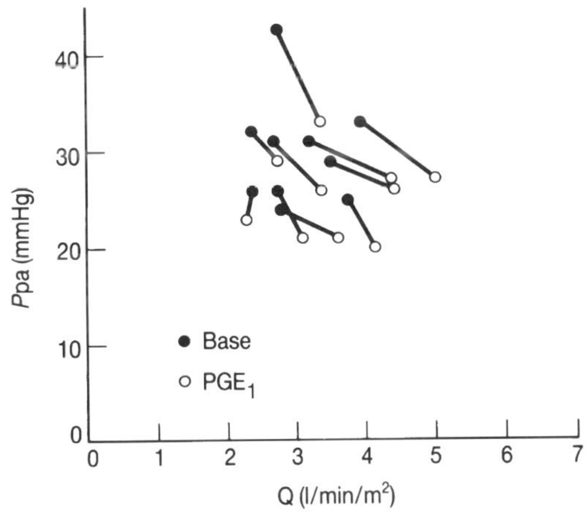

Figure 2.3. Mean pulmonary artery pressure (*P*pa) and cardiac index (Q) in 10 patients with ARDS, before and after infusion of prostaglandin E_1, which induced pulmonary vasodilation. (Adapted from Mélot et al., 1989.)

(Figure 2.2). In the same experimental model, metabolic alkalosis (arterial pH 7.60, arterial PCO_2 40 Torr), obtained by administration of Carbicarb (Na_2CO_3 + $NaHCO_3$), almost completely reversed the oleic acid-induced pulmonary hypertension (Brimioulle et al., 1991). In patients with ARDS, prostaglandin E_1 0.02 to 0.04 μg/kg/min intravenously reduced *P*pa and increased Q, indicating unequivocal pulmonary vasodilation (Mélot et al., 1989; Figure 2.3).

Several vasoconstrictor mediators have been implicated in the development of pulmonary hypertension in lung injury (Repine, 1992). Eicosanoids such as thromboxane A_2 and leukotrienes are pulmonary vasoconstrictors and contribute to pulmonary hypertension in various models of lung injury. In clinical studies, however, the thromboxane A_2 synthase inhibitor dazoxiben had no effect on *P*pa in patients with established ARDS, despite 75% inhibition of platelet thromboxane production (Leeman et al., 1985; Reines et al., 1985). Platelet-activating factor is another lipid mediator that causes pulmonary vasoconstriction (Chung, 1992; Henson et al., 1992). Platelet-activating factor receptor antagonists prevented pulmonary hypertension in experimental lung injury (Sessler et al., 1988). More recently, endothelin-1 has been identified as a potential mediator of pulmonary hypertension in patients with ARDS (Druml et al., 1993; Langleben et al., 1993).

VASODILATOR RELEASE IN LUNG INJURY

Numerous vasoactive substances are released during lung injury, not only vasoconstrictors (see above), but also vasodilators, which attenuate pulmonary hypertension. Administration of cyclooxygenase inhibitors, such as aspirin, indomethacin and meclofenamate, further increased *P*pa after oleic acid lung injury, suggesting that a vasodilating prostaglandin, presumably prostacyclin, is released in this model (Leeman et al., 1988b; Schulman et al., 1988) (Figure 2.2). Inhibition of nitric oxide (NO) synthesis (by *N*(G)-nitro-L-arginine) or effect (by methylene blue) also increased pulmonary vascular tone after oleic acid in dogs, suggesting that NO formation limits pulmonary hypertension (Leeman et al., 1993).

However, prostacyclin and NO could contribute to altered gas exchange in lung injury, by opening constricted vessels in hypoxic lung regions, in other words, by inhibiting hypoxic pulmonary vasoconstriction (Sprague et al., 1984; Leeman et al., 1987b, 1994). The ARDS lung is characterized by regions with near-normal ventilation and perfusion neighbouring loci of severe damage and alveolar collapse (Gattinoni et al., 1993). These poorly aerated regions remain perfused, leading to ventilation/perfusion mismatch and intrapulmonary shunt. Hypoxic pulmonary vasoconstriction is an intrapulmonary process that diverts blood flow away from hypoxic lung regions, resulting in a better matching of perfusion to ventilation and less hypoxaemia. Pulmonary vessels of ARDS patients obviously retain their capability to constrict in response to hypoxia (Zapol et al., 1985) but efficacy of hypoxic vasoconstriction may nevertheless be blunted in injured lungs.

Impairment of hypoxic pulmonary vasoconstriction has been described in models of pulmonary disease (Hales et al., 1981; Hutchinson et al., 1985; Gillespie and Bowdy, 1986; Graham et al., 1990; Johnson et al., 1993). The hypoxic vasomotor response has been examined by constructing *P*pa-inspiratory fraction of O_2 relationships (with Q kept constant) in anaesthetized dogs, before and during oleic acid lung injury (Leeman et al., 1992a). A transient inhibition of hypoxic pulmonary vasoconstriction was observed after oleic acid, which could be prevented by cyclooxygenase inhibitors (Figure 2.4). Dogs pre-treated with aspirin or indomethacin (and thus with preserved hypoxic pulmonary vasoconstriction), had less deterioration of gas exchange than controls after oleic acid (Leeman et al., 1992a). Pretreatment with indomethacin also prevented loss of hypoxic vasoconstriction in dogs with endotoxin lung injury (Hales et al., 1981).

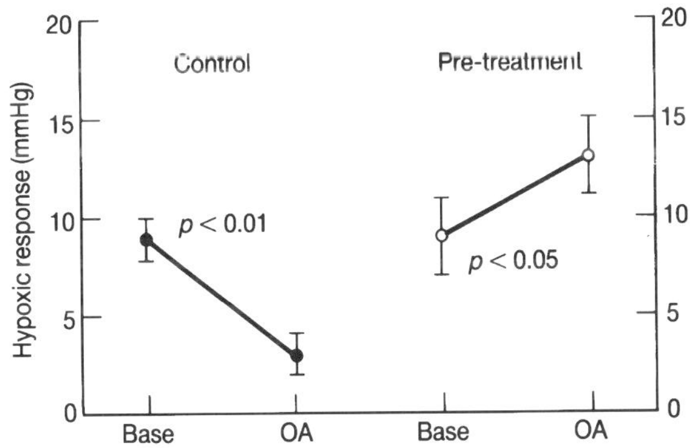

Figure 2.4 Mean pulmonary artery pressure (*P*pa) hypoxic response (*P*pa at inspiratory fraction of O_2 0.1 minus *P*pa at inspiratory fraction of O_2 0.4, at constant flow), before and after oleic acid lung injury (OA). After OA, hypoxic pulmonary vasoconstriction was blunted in untreated dogs (left, $n = 7$) but preserved (and even increased) in dogs pre-treated with aspirin ($n = 6$) or indomethacin ($n = 7$) (right). (Adapted from Leeman et al., 1992a.)

Treatment with cyclooxygenase inhibitors worsened pulmonary hypertension but improved gas exchange in oleic acid lung injury (Leeman et al., 1988b; Schulman et al., 1988). These drugs also improved arterial oxygenation in other models of pulmonary disease (Garrett and Thomas, 1983; Light, 1986; Hanly et al., 1987a; Bishop et al., 1988) and in patients with bacterial pneumonia (Hanly et al., 1987b), chronic lung disease (Adnot et al., 1987) and ARDS (Steinberg et al., 1990; Leeman et al., 1992b). In summary, many experimental and clinical data support the view that a vasodilating prostaglandin is released during lung injury, attenuates pulmonary hypertension, but contributes to altered gas exchange by inhibiting hypoxic pulmonary vasoconstriction.

The influence of endogenous NO on the hypoxic regulation of regional pulmonary perfusion in lung injury is less clear. In intact anaesthetized dogs with undiseased lungs, *N*(G)-nitro-L-arginine and methylene blue did not affect hyperoxic and normoxic pulmonary vascular tone, but increased it during hypoxia, thereby enhancing the pulmonary vasopressor response to hypoxia, suggesting that endogenous NO inhibits vasoconstriction (Leeman et al., 1994). As already mentioned, inhibition of NO synthesis or effect further increased pulmonary vascular tone after oleic acid lung injury, suggesting that NO release blunted pulmonary hypertension. However, methylene blue, but not *N*(G)-nitro-L-arginine, improved gas exchange after oleic acid (Leeman et al., 1993). Other L-arginine analogues did not restore loss of pulmonary vascular reactivity induced by tumour necrosis factor-α (Johnson et al., 1993) or by chronic pneumonia (Yaghi et al., 1993).

Pulmonary gas exchange can improve if blood flow is diverted from hypoxic to better oxygenated lung units. This can be achieved by further constricting vessels perfusing hypoxic areas (using cyclo-oxygenase inhibitors) and/or by dilating vessels in adequately ventilated units, using inhaled vasodilators. Preliminary studies with inhaled NO (Rossaint et al., 1993) or prostacyclin (Walmrath et al., 1993) in ARDS patients reported reduction in pulmonary hypertension, improvement in gas exchange and absence of systemic hypotension. These encouraging results should justify a controlled trial to evaluate the benefit of inhaled agents in the management of ARDS.

Intravenously administered vasodilators usually worsen arterial oxygenation (Zapol et al., 1985; Mélot et al., 1987, 1989; Leeman, 1991), possibly by relaxing contracted vessels in hypoxic lung units. On the other hand, pulmonary vasoconstriction is not always associated with better gas exchange (Leeman et al., 1988b, 1992c), indicating that some agents do not specifically constrict vessels perfusing hypoxic areas.

PULMONARY ENDOTHELIUM-DEPENDENT RELAXATION IN LUNG INJURY

We have seen that the pulmonary circulation is affected by widespread release of constricting and dilating mediators during lung injury, the net effect being pulmonary vasoconstriction and hypertension. Does the pulmonary vascular wall react normally to these mediators? In other words, could impaired endothelium-dependent relaxation contribute to pulmonary hypertension, as has been described in systemic arterial hypertension (Panza et al., 1990)?

Experimental (Schoene et al., 1984; Schuster, 1994) as well as clinical (Zapol et al., 1985) ARDS is associated with pulmonary endothelial cell damage. The endothelium modulates vascular tone by releasing compounds that mediate contraction or relaxation of the underlying vascular smooth muscle. Among important factors, NO, formed from L-arginine within the endothelial cell in response to several stimuli (shear stress, acetylcholine), mediates endothelium-dependent relaxation and is continuously released for precise adjustments of vascular tone (Moncada and Higgs, 1993).

The pulmonary vascular effects of the endothelium-dependent

Table 2.2 Pulmonary endothelium-dependent relaxation in lung injury

Reference	Model	Injury	Relaxation response to acetylcholine
Feddersen et al. (1986)	Isolated rat lung	ANTU Hyperoxia	Preserved Preserved
Coflesky and Evans (1988)	Rat PA	Hyperoxia	Decreased
Ito et al. (1988)	Rat PA	Monocrotaline	Decreased
Tracey et al. (1989)	Guinea-pig PA	O_2 radicals	Decreased (*)
Archer et al. (1990)	Isolated rat lung	Monocrotaline	Preserved
Chen and Gillis (1991)	Isolated rabbit lung	O_2 radicals	Decreased
Crawley et al. (1992)	Rat PA	Bleomycin	Preserved
Liu et al. (1992)	Isolated rat lung	TNF-α	Decreased

ANTU, α-naphthyl thiourea; PA, pulmonary artery; TNF, tumour necrosis factor.
(*) Relaxation response to acetylcholine was preserved in pulmonary venules.

dilator acetylcholine has been examined in several models of lung injury. Some studies displayed a blunted relaxant response to acetylcholine after lung injury, suggesting endothelial dysfunction, while in other studies, the response was preserved (Table 2.2). When examined, the endothelium-independent relaxation to sodium nitroprusside was retained (Coflesky and Evans, 1988; Chen and Gillis, 1991; Liu et al., 1992), indicating specific endothelial damage.

Release of NO has been suggested in the oleic acid model (Leeman et al., 1993), implicating maintained (or even enhanced) NO production. If endothelial dysfunction occurs in lung injury, the defect should then involve reduced expression of muscarinic (or other) receptors, or impaired signal transduction from receptor to NO synthase. On the other hand, since only few intact endothelial cells are needed to obtain acetylcholine-induced vessel relaxation (Furchgott and Zawadzky, 1980), endothelium-dependent dilation could be preserved, despite severe lung injury, if a sufficient number of endothelial cells escaped from damage.

SUMMARY

In acute lung injury:

1 Pulmonary hypertension is an almost constant occurrence and results from functional and mechanical factors.
2 The pulmonary circulation is influenced by widespread release of constricting and dilating mediators, the net effect being pulmonary vasoconstriction.
3 Pulmonary vessels retain their ability to dilate and to further constrict.
4 The release of endogenous vasodilators such as prostacyclin and nitric oxide attenuates pulmonary hypertension, but could contribute to the alteration of gas exchange by inhibiting hypoxic vasoconstriction. Accordingly, hypoxic pulmonary vasoconstriction is not maximally expressed in most models of lung injury.
5 Whether pulmonary endothelium-dependent relaxation is impaired remains uncertain.
6 Pulmonary gas exchange can be improved by vasodilating well ventilated lung units (using inhaled vasodilators) and/or by vasoconstricting the most hypoxic lung regions (using cyclooxygenase inhibitors). Controlled clinical trials are needed to evaluate the benefit of these strategies.

REFERENCES

Adnot, S., Defouilloy, C., Brun-Buisson, C. et al. (1987) Effects of indomethacin on pulmonary hemodynamics and gas exchange in patients with pulmonary artery hypertension. *American Review of Respiratory Diseases* **136**: 1343–1349.

Archer, S.L., Rist, K., Nelson, D.P. et al. (1990) Comparison of the hemodynamic effects of nitric oxide and endothelium-dependent vasodilators in intact lungs. *Journal of Applied Physiology* **68**: 735–747.

Bernard, G.R., Luce, J.M., Sprung, C.L. et al. (1987) High-dose corticosteroids in patients with the adult respiratory distress syndrome. *New England Journal of Medicine* **317**: 1565–1570.

Bishop, M.J., Artman, L.D., Cheney, F.W. (1988) Ibuprofen potentiates divertion of flow from hypoxic to normoxic lung. *Journal of Critical Care* **3**: 112–115.

Boiteau, P., Ducas, J., Schick, U., Girling, L., Prewitt, R.M. (1986) Pulmonary vascular pressure: flow relationship in canine oleic acid pulmonary edema. *American Journal of Physiology* **251**: H1163–H1170.

Bone, R.C., Maunder, R., Slotman, G. et al. (1989) An early test of survival in patients with the adult respiratory distress syndrome. *Chest* **96**: 849–851.

Brimioulle, S., Vachiéry, J.L., Lejeune, P. et al. (1991) Acid-base status affects gas exchange in canine oleic acid pulmonary edema. *American Journal of Physiology* **260**: H1080–H1086.

Chen, X., Gillis, C.N. (1991) Effects of free radicals on pulmonary vascular response to acetylcholine. *Journal of Applied Physiology* **71**: 821–825.

Chung, K.F. (1992) Platelet-activating factor in inflammation and pulmonary disorders. *Clinical Science* **83**: 127–138.

Coflesky, J.T., Evans J.N. (1988) Pharmacologic properties of isolated proximal pulmonary arteries after seven-day exposure to in vivo hyperoxia. *American Review of Respiratory Diseases* **138**: 945–951.

Crawley, D.E., McCormack, D.G., Evans, T.W. (1992) Bleomycin-induced acute lung injury in the rat does not influence pulmonary vascular responsiveness in vitro. *Critical Care Medicine* **20**: 641–644.

Druml, W., Steltzer, H., Waldhäusl, W. et al. (1993) Endothelin-1 in adult respiratory distress syndrome. *American Review of Respiratory Diseases* **148**: 1169–1173.

Feddersen, C.O., McMurtry, I.F., Henson, P., Voelkel, N.F. (1986) Acetylcholine-induced pulmonary vasodilation in lung vascular injury. *American Review of Respiratory Diseases* **133**: 197–204.

Furchgott, R.F., Zawadzky, J.V. (1980) The obligatory role of endothelial cells in relaxation of arterial smooth muscle by acetylcholine. *Nature* **288**: 373–376.

Garrett, R.C., Thomas III, H.M. (1983) Meclofenamate uniformly decreases shunt fraction in dogs with lobar atelectasis. *Journal of Applied Physiology* **54**: 284–289.

Gattinoni, L., D'Andrea, L., Pelosi, P. et al. (1993) Regional effects and mechanisms of positive end-expiratory pressure in early adult respiratory distress syndrome. *Journal of the American Medical Association* **269**: 2122–2127.

Gillespie, M.N., Bowdy, B.D. (1986) Impact of platelet activating factor on vascular responsiveness in isolated rat lung. *Journal of Pharmacology and Experimental Therapeutics* **236**: 396–402.

Graham, R., Skoog, C., Oppenheimer, L., Rabson, J., Goldberg, H.S. (1982) Critical closure in the canine pulmonary vasculature. *Circulation Research* **50**: 566–572.

Graham, L.M., Vasil, A., Vasil, M.L., Voelkel, N.F., Stenmark, K.R. (1990) Decreased pulmonary vasoreactivity in an animal model of chronic *Pseudomonas* pneumonia. *American Review of Respiratory Diseases* **142**: 221–229.

Hales, C.A., Sonne, L., Peterson, M., Kong, D., Miller, M., Watkins, W.D. (1981) Role of thromboxane and prostacyclin in pulmonary vasomotor changes after endotoxin in dogs. *Journal of Clinical Investigation* **68**: 497–505.

Hanly, P., Sienko, A., Light, R.B. (1987a) Effect of cyclooxygenase blockade on gas exchange and hemodynamics in *Pseudomonas* pneumonia. *Journal of Applied Physiology* **63**: 1829–1836.

Hanly, P., Dobson, K., Roberts, D., Light, R.B. (1987b) Effect of indomethacin on arterial oxygenation in critically ill patients with severe bacterial pneumonia. *Lancet* **i**: 351–354.

Henson, P.M., Barnes, P.J., Banks-Schlegel, S.P. (1992) Platelet-activating factor: role in pulmonary injury and dysfunction and blood abnormalities. *American Review of Respiratory Diseases* **145**: 726–731.

Hutchinson, A.A., Ogletree, M.L., Snapper, J.R., Brigham, K.L. (1985) Effect of endotoxemia on hypoxic pulmonary vasoconstriction in unanesthetized sheep. *Journal of Applied Physiology* **58**: 1463–1468.

Ito, K., Nakashima, T., Murakami, K., Murakami, T. (1988) Altered function of pulmonary endothelium following monocrotaline-induced vascular injury in rats. *British Journal of Pharmacology* **94**: 1175–1183.

Johnson, D., Hurst, T., Wilson, T. et al. (1993) *N*(G)-monomethyl-*L*-arginine does not restore loss of hypoxic pulmonary vasoconstriction induced by TNF-α. *Journal of Applied Physiology* **75**: 618–625.

Langleben, D., Demarchie, M., Laporta, D. et al. (1993) Endothelin-1 in acute lung injury and the adult respiratory distress syndrome. *American Review of Respiratory Diseases* **148**: 1646–1650.

Leeman, M. (1991) The pulmonary circulation in acute lung injury: a review of some recent advances. *Intensive Care Medicine* **17**: 254–260.

Leeman, M., Boeynaems, J.M., Degaute, J.P., Vincent, J.L., Kahn, R.J. (1985) Administration of dazoxiben, a selective thromboxane synthetase inhibitor, in the adult respiratory distress syndrome. *Chest* **87**: 726–730.

Leeman, M., Lejeune, P., Naeije, R. (1987a) Inhibition of angiotensin-converting enzyme by perindopril diacid in canine oleic acid pulmonary edema. *Critical Care Medicine* **15**: 567–573.

Leeman, M., Naeije, R., Lejeune, P., Mélot, C. (1987b) Influence of cyclo-oxygenase inhibition and of leukotriene receptor blockade on pulmonary vascular pressure–cardiac index relationship in hyperoxic and in hypoxic dogs. *Clinical Science* **72**: 717–724.

Leeman, M., Lejeune, P., Mélot, C., Naeije, R. (1988a) Pulmonary vascular pressure-flow plots in canine oleic acid pulmonary edema. Effects of prostaglandin E_1 and nitroprusside. *American Review of Respiratory Diseases* **138**: 362–367.

Leeman, M., Lejeune, P., Hallemans, R., Mélot, C., Naeije, R. (1988b) Effects of increased pulmonary vascular tone on gas exchange in canine oleic acid pulmonary edema. *Journal of Applied Physiology* **65**: 662–668.

Leeman, M., Closset, J., Vachiéry, J.L. et al. (1989) Sinoaortic deafferentation reduces intrapulmonary shunt in dogs with oleic acid lung injury. *Journal of Applied Physiology* **67**: 833–838.

Leeman, M., Lejeune, P., Closset, J. et al. (1990a) Nature of pulmonary hypertension in canine oleic acid pulmonary edema. *Journal of Applied Physiology* **69**: 293–298.

Leeman, M., Lejeune, P., Closset, J. et al. (1990b) Effects of PEEP on pulmonary hemodynamics in intact dogs with oleic acid pulmonary edema. *Journal of Applied Physiology* **69**: 2190–2196.

Leeman, M., Delcroix, M., Vachiéry, J.L., Mélot, C., Naeije, R. (1992a) Blunted hypoxic pulmonary vasoconstriction in oleic acid lung injury: effect of cyclooxygenase inhibitors. *Journal of Applied Physiology* **72**: 251–258.

Leeman, M., Mélot, C., Naeije, R. (1992b) L'inhibition de la cyclooxygénase améliore les échanges gazeaux dans le SDRA. *Réanimation et Urgences* **1**: 95 (abstract).

Leeman, M., Delcroix, M., Vachiéry, J.L., Mélot, C., Naeije, R. (1992c) Almitrine and doxapram in experimental lung injury. *American Review of Respiratory Diseases* **145**: 1042–1045.

Leeman, M., Zegers de Beyl, V., Gilbert, E., Mélot, C., Naeije, R. (1993) Is nitric oxide released in oleic acid lung injury? *Journal of Applied Physiology* **74**: 650–654.

Leeman, M., Zegers de Beyl, V., Delcroix, M., Naeije, R. (1994) Effects of endogenous nitric oxide on pulmonary vascular tone in intact dogs. *American Journal of Physiology* **266**: H2343–H2347.

Light, R.B. (1986) Indomethacin and acetylsalicylic acid reduce intrapulmonary shunt in experimental pneumococcal pneumonia. *American Review of Respiratory Diseases* **134**: 520–525.

Liu, S.F., Dewar, A., Crawley, D.E., Barnes, R.J., Evans, T.W. (1992) Effect of tumor necrosis factor on hypoxic pulmonary vasoconstriction. *Journal of Applied Physiology* **72**: 1044–1049.

Lopez-Muniz, R., Stephens, N.L., Bromberger-Barnea, B., Permutt, S., Riley, R.L. (1968) Critical closure of pulmonary vessels analyzed in terms of Starling resistor model. *Journal of Applied Physiology* **24**: 625–635.

Mélot, C., Naeije, R., Mols, P. et al. (1987) Pulmonary vascular tone improves gas exchange in the adult respiratory distress syndrome. *American Review of Respiratory Diseases* **136**: 1232–1236.

Mélot, C., Lejeune, P., Leeman, M., Moraine, J.J., Naeije, R. (1989). Prostaglandin E_1 in the adult respiratory distress syndrome. Benefit for pulmonary hypertension and cost for pulmonary gas exchange. *American Review of Respiratory Diseases* **139**: 106–110.

Mitzner, W., Chang, H.K. (1989) Hemodynamics of the pulmonary circulation. In Chang, H.K. & Paiva, M. (eds) *Respiratory Physiology, An Analytical Approach*, pp 561–631. New York: Marcel Dekker.

Moncada, S., Higgs, A. (1993) The L-arginine-nitric oxide pathway. *New England Journal of Medicine* **329**: 2002–2012.

Panza, J.A., Quyyumi, A.A., Brush, J.E. Jr., Epstein, S.E. (1990) Abnormal endothelium-dependent vascular relaxation in patients with essential hypertension. *New England Journal of Medicine* **323**: 22–27.

Permutt, S., Riley, R.L. (1963) Hemodynamics of collapsible vessels with tone: the vascular waterfall. *Journal of Applied Physiology* **18**: 924–932.

Reines, H.D., Halushka, P.V., Olanoff, L.S., Hunt, P.S. (1985) Dazoxiben in human sepsis and adult respiratory distress syndrome. *Clinical Pharmacology and Therapeutics* **37**: 391–395.

Repine, J.E. (1992) Scientific perspectives on adult respiratory distress syndrome. *Lancet* **339**: 466–469.

Rossaint, R., Falke, K., Lopez, F. et al. (1993) Inhaled nitric oxide for the adult respiratory distress syndrome. *New England Journal of Medicine* **328**: 399–405.

Schoene, R.B., Robertson, H.T., Thorning, D.R. et al. (1984) Pathophysiological patterns of resolution from acute oleic acid lung injury in the dog. *Journal of Applied Physiology* **56**: 472–481.

Schulman, L.L., Lennon, P.F., Ratner, S.J., Enson, Y. (1988) Meclofenamate enhances blood oxygenation in acute oleic acid lung injury. *Journal of Applied Physiology* **64**: 710–718.

Schuster, D.P. (1994) ARDS: clinical lessons from the oleic acid model of acute lung injury. *American Journal of Respiratory and Critical Care Medicine* **149**: 245–260.

Sessler, C.N., Glauser, F.L., Davis, D., Fowler, A.A. (1988) Effects of platelet-activating factor antagonist SRI 63–441 on endotoxemia in sheep. *Journal of Applied Physiology* **65**: 2624–2631.

Sloane, P.J., Gee, M.H., Gottlieb, J.E. et al. (1992) A multicenter registry of patients with acute respiratory distress syndrome. *American Review of Respiratory Diseases* **146**: 419–426.

Sprague, R.S., Stephenson, A.H., Lonigro, A.J. (1984) Prostaglandin I_2 supports blood flow to hypoxic alveoli in anesthetized dogs. *Journal of Applied Physiology* **56**: 1246–1251.

Steinberg, S.M., Rodriguez, J.L., Bitzer, L.G. et al. (1990) Indomethacin treatment of human adult respiratory distress syndrome. *Circulatory Shock* **30**: 375–384.

Suchyta, M.R., Clemmer, T.P., Elliott, C.G., Orme, J.F., Weaver, L.K. (1992) The adult respiratory distress syndrome. A report of survival and modifying factors. *Chest* **101**: 1074–1079.

Tracey, W.R., Hamilton, J.T., Craig, I.D., Paterson, N.A.M. (1989) Effect of endothelial injury on the responses of isolated guinea pig pulmonary venules to reduced oxygen tension. *American Review of Respiratory Diseases* **140**: 68–74.

Walmrath, D., Schneider, T., Pilch, J., Grimminger, F., Seeger, W. (1993) Aerosolized prostacyclin in adult respiratory distress syndrome. *Lancet* **342**: 961–962.

Yaghi, A., Paterson, N.A.M., McCormack, D.G. (1993) Nitric oxide does not mediate the attenuated pulmonary vascular reactivity of chronic pneumonia. *American Journal of Physiology* **265**: H943–H948.

Zapol, W.M., Snider, M.T. (1977) Pulmonary hypertension in severe acute respiratory failure. *New England Journal of Medicine* **296**: 476–480.

Zapol, W.M., Snider, M.T., Rie, M.A., Quinn, D.A., Fikker, M. (1985) Pulmonary circulation during adult respiratory distress syndrome. In Zapol, W.M. & Falke, K.J. (eds) *Acute Respiratory Failure*, pp 241–273. New York: Marcel Dekker.

3

Serious Illness in Pregnancy and Childbirth

Barry N.J. Walters

INTRODUCTION

Pregnant women are subject to the same medical calamities as may befall any member of the population, but in addition there are several problems unique to the gravid state. This chapter reviews a number of these gestational disorders which are likely to be seen in an intensive care unit.

BIOLOGICAL CHANGES IN PREGNANCY

Pregnancy is accompanied by changes in anatomy, physiology and pharmacokinetics which all have a profound influence upon the management of disease. These are too extensive to be reviewed here but the reader is referred to the definitive text of Hytten and Chamberlain (1991) which deals with the clinical physiology of pregnancy.

It must be appreciated that non-pregnant reference values are often quite inappropriate for pregnancy. Interpretation of laboratory and other investigations requires a knowledge of these changes and I have summarized many of relevance to the intensivist in Table 3.1. Cardiac output and blood volume increase by 40% and pulmonary capillary wedge pressure (*P*CWP) by about 15% (Clark et al., 1989). Combined with a 15% fall in colloid oncotic pressure, the safety margin against pulmonary oedema is decreased in pregnancy and this is a theme in several discussions to follow.

MEDICAL CARE OF PREGNANT WOMEN

Clinical care of the gravid or recently delivered woman requires a team approach involving the intensivist, the obstetrician and a

Table 3.1 Normal reference values for pregnancy

	Non-pregnant	Late pregnancy
Haemodynamics		
Cardiac output (l/min)	4–7	5.2–9.8
CVP (mmHg)	1–10	1–10
PCWP (mmHg)	3–10	3–10
PA pressure (mmHg)	9–16	9–16
SVR kPa.sec/litre	77–150	58–112
Respiratory		
Arterial pH	7.35–7.40	7.40–7.95
Aterial pO_2 (mmHg)	90–95	108–10
Arterial pCO_2 (mmHg)	28–40	27–32
Tidal volume (ml)	470–610	660–760
Functional residual capacity (ml)	2800	2300
Biochemistry		
Albumin (g/l)	33–36	24–28
AST (μ/l)	10–40	10–40
Calcium (total) (mEq/l)	2.2–12.7	2.15–2.45
Creatinine (μmol/l)	55–95	45–82
Osmolality (mOsm/kg)	289	280
Sodium (mEq/l)	139	137
Urea (mmol/l)	3.4–5.2	3.1–3.9
Haematology		
Hb (g/l)	125–155	110–130
WCC ($\times 10^9$/l)	4.5–11	3.5–16.5
Platelets ($\times 10^9$/l)	130–400	130–350

physician with experience in medical problems of pregnancy. The paediatrician is often also involved.

Psychological factors are paramount. At all times the pregnant woman and her husband must be reassured that procedures being undertaken and treatments given are not harmful to her baby. Where there is some small risk, as in radiological tests, it must be explained and measures taken to minimize the risk.

Changes in anatomy are so obvious in pregnancy, and yet their influence is often forgotten. For example, the mass of the gravid uterus in the last months causes aortocaval compression, and the supine hypotension syndrome is a genuine concern with up to 25% decrease in cardiac output (Kerr, 1965). Therefore, in nursing pregnant women, a pillow or other wedge should be used to ameliorate these effects. The woman is tilted towards her left, thereby displacing the uterus from the underlying vena cava.

Endotracheal intubation should always be performed by experienced personnel as it may be unexpectedly difficult in pregnant women. The risk of aspiration of gastric contents is much increased by increased intra-abdominal pressure and incompetence of the gastro-oesophageal sphincter, and prophylactic measures must be taken.

Metabolism in pregnancy is altered such that 'accelerated starvation' is observed with ketone bodies appearing even after brief periods of calorie deprivation (Metzger et al., 1982). Nutritional support should not be delayed.

Cardiopulmonary Resuscitation

All of these changes are of relevance in CPR. Particular recommendations have been formulated into a policy document (Barth, 1992). This document mentions the depressing but realistic possibility that perimortem caesarean delivery might be necessary. This should be kept in mind as it is unlikely that there will be sufficient time for detailed consideration should the occasion arise to save the life of an infant by rapid action in desperate circumstances (Katz et al., 1986).

SEVERE PRE-ECLAMPSIA AND ECLAMPSIA

Pre-eclamptic toxaemia (PET) as seen in an intensive care unit is the end result of a process of pathological derangement that has its genesis in early pregnancy (Khong et al., 1986) followed by a long pre-clinical asymptomatic stage. At the time of presentation, however, the disorder has caused or is effecting aberrations in multiple systems (Table 3.2).

Pathogenesis

Present concepts of pre-eclampsia place central importance upon vascular endothelial damage (Roberts et al., 1991) caused by circulating factors activating platelets (Ballegeer et al., 1992) and neutrophils (Greer et al., 1989), and adverse changes in the balance between prostacyclin and thromboxane. Loss of the normal endothelial contribution to control of vascular tone leads to hypertension from severely increased peripheral resistance. This is the most frequent abnormality in PET whilst proteinuria, sometimes of nephrotic degree, attests to the loss of glomerular capillary barrier function.

Table 3.2 Complications of severe pre-eclampsia

Neurological	Eclampsia Cerebral haemorrhage Cortical blindness Cerebral oedema
Ocular	Retinal detachment
Renal	Renal failure Nephrotic syndrome
Cardiovascular	Pulmonary oedema
Hepatic	Hepatic haemorrhage Focal liver infarction Liver rupture
Haematological	Thrombocytopenia Haemolysis Coagulopathy
Fetus/placenta	Fetal growth retardation Abruptio placentae Placental infarction

Disturbance of endothelial function leads to oedema of vasogenic origin and a propensity to pulmonary oedema secondary to both hypertension and vascular permeability changes. Colloid oncotic pressure measurements are often profoundly low in severe PET and measurements of interstitial fluid oncotic pressure (Oian et al., 1986) infer that substances responsible for intravascular oncotic pressure have transferred to the extravascular space.

Damage to the vascular endothelium also predisposes locally to intravascular thrombi which may lead to disturbances in many organs including the liver, placental bed, and perhaps brain whilst vasospasm is a major contributor (Visser and Wallenburg, 1991).

It follows from the above that debates about therapy to correct these problems by volume replacement (see below) are ingenuous and fail to appreciate that even fluids of high oncotic pressure have a much accelerated disappearance time when injected into the circulation of pre-eclamptic women (Oian et al., 1986).

Placenta

In the uteroplacental vascular bed (almost certainly the initial site of vascular disturbance in PET) there is focal occlusion of arteries supplying the placenta (Khong et al., 1986). This occurs stepwise over a period of days or weeks and results in placental ischaemia and/or infarction (Fox, 1988), both serious for the fetus and resulting in fetal death when widespread, or intrauterine growth retardation when sufficiently leisurely in progression to result in a state of chronic placental failure. The incidence of placental abruption is much increased in PET (Fox, 1988) because of these problems.

Clinical Features

PET is a syndrome, a final common pathway entered from many routes. Its combination of pathology varies, some displaying dominant renal aberrations, others haematological and still others placental. The disease may be primary, or secondary to an underlying medical disorder such as renal, endocrine, autoimmune, or vascular disease. The likelihood of secondary pre-eclampsia is greater in multiparous women with the disorder. In severe PET thrombocytopenia may be profound and may worsen for some days after delivery. Other coagulation abnormalities are usually not severe unless there has been major haemorrhage or liver involvement. With placental abruption there may be disseminated intravascular coagulation. Fibrinogen levels are increased in most cases but this may reflect an acute-phase reactant.

Liver involvement

Liver involvement is suggested by a characteristic, usually nocturnal pain in the epigastrium or subcostal region of overwhelming severity accompanied by elevated liver enzymes, particularly and often only the transaminases (Walters and Walters, 1991). Bilirubin elevation may be present, and will be pronounced if there is haemolysis (*H*) (a microangiopathic feature of severe PET) which often accompanies the liver abnormalities (*E*levated *L*iver enzymes) and thrombocytopenia (*L*ow *P*latelets). One observer has contributed the acronym 'HELLP' as a mnemonic to describe this combination of features in some women with PET (Weinstein, 1982); but there is no reason to regard this group differently from others with severe disease. Anaemia indicates either haemolysis, or intrahepatic haemorrhage, either multiple or coalescing into a large haematoma (Sheehan and Lynch, 1973). This is a potentially lethal complication and not often well visualized by ultrasound. CT and MRI are most suited to demonstrate haematoma, and fortunately this is a rare complication in developed nations.

Eclampsia

Eclampsia is the major cerebral manifestation of this disorder often heralded by less dramatic neurological disturbances, such as migrainous auras, dysphasia, teichopsia or acral paraesthesiae. The fits may be focal or generalized, are usually brief, but may proceed one upon the other to status eclampticus, potentially fatal where control is not achieved promptly. Cerebral haemorrhage is a major cause of death in PET and eclampsia (Department of Health, 1989) and results from the dangerous combination of severe hypertension and endothelial damage. It is often, but not always, a complication of eclampsia and control of hypertension is the most critical factor in preventing cerebral haemorrhage.

Therapy

Delivery is the only definitive treatment of PET and will invariably usher in the beginning of resolution. However, the pathological cascades remain active and potentially life-threatening for 24 to 72 hours post-partum (Sibai, 1988). This intrinsic self-limiting nature of the disease after delivery distinguishes it from most disorders seen in a general intensive care unit. By implication, therefore, most therapeutic and investigational manoeuvres must be supportive and corrective, and iatrogenic complications are all the more regrettable.

The critical requirements in care of these women are control of hypertension, avoidance of excessive fluid administration, and prevention of eclampsia, whilst awaiting resolution.

Fluid therapy

Whilst there may be some diversity in the haemodynamic profile of women presenting with severe PET (Macphail, 1992) the most common finding is a greatly increased systemic vascular resistance. This is usually combined with hyperdynamic ventricular function, low to normal CVP and normal pulmonary vascular resistance (Visser and Wallenburg, 1991) with low to very low COP. Whilst these observations are of great interest, most women can be treated without invasive haemodynamic monitoring and the American College of Obstetrics & Gynecology shares the view that benefits in excess of the risks of that procedure (pulmonary artery catheterization) have yet to be demonstrated (see Cunningham and Lindheimer, 1992). Nevertheless, such monitoring does have a limited place in certain circumstances (see below). Furthermore, it is likely that haemodynamic monitoring by non-invasive means (Doppler flow analysis) will soon be available, and the whole concept will warrant reassessment (Easterling et al., 1989).

Plasma volume expansion has been supported by the following process of reasoning, but there are no controlled trials of this therapy.

In the antepartum period, there is some evidence that uteroplacental perfusion may be compromised by dramatic falls in blood pressure induced by vasodilator drug treatment, with detriment to the baby. Such observations are rare (Vink et al., 1980) but concerns about maintaining placental and renal perfusion during the process of blood pressure control are well-founded. These have led to the contention that plasma volume expansion ought to be considered in therapy (Duncan, 1989; Wasserstrum et al., 1989). This recognizes the fact that many (but not all) pre-eclamptic women have a reduced circulating blood volume at presentation (Gallery et al., 1979) which will be aggravated by vasodilator therapy. The nostrum recommended, therefore, is judicious plasma volume expansion accompanying use of a vasodilating drug such as hydralazine. Invasive haemodynamic monitoring is accepted in these cases to negotiate the narrow channel between over-replacement leading to pulmonary oedema, or vasodilatation causing renal and placental hypoperfusion. Pulmonary oedema is well recognized as a major cause of death in PET (Sibai et al., 1987).

Invasive Monitoring

There is considerable experience with invasive haemodynamic monitoring in North America (Wasserstrum and Cotton, 1986) and Europe (Visser and Wallenburg, 1991) where hydralazine, diazoxide or other vasodilator agents are infused contemporaneously with colloid replacement and monitoring to limit and maintain pulmonary capillary wedge pressure.

There are no controlled trials of this form of monitoring, but considerable experience has accrued elsewhere avoiding invasive monitoring but with management using clinical monitoring, frequent observation, and empiric fluid therapy of 80–120 ml/h of mostly crystalloid solutions. Of course the use of epidural anaesthesia carries a need for more vigorous fluid loading (not more than 1 l crystalloid) but this is transient, not an ongoing necessity and by itself does not warrant use of the Swan–Ganz catheter. Epidural anaesthesia is the technique of choice for delivery in PET avoiding the hazards of general anaesthesia and may even enhance intervillous blood flow (Jouppila et al., 1982), but is contraindicated by coagulopathy.

Therefore when should invasive monitoring be used? Our practice is to consider it only when pulmonary oedema or major haemorrhage complicates severe PET, in which circumstances we have found it useful in selected cases.

Oliguria

Invasive monitoring has been recommended for management of oliguria in PET (Clark and Cotton, 1988). This is usually unnecessary as oliguria almost always occurs postpartum and will almost invariably be temporary. Continuation of a maintenance fluid infusion at the above rate is necessary together with an understanding that in the majority of cases, oliguria will resolve within 24 h of delivery without aggressive therapy. The priority is to avoid pulmonary oedema and one should err on the side of volume restriction where there is doubt. Occasionally, after 12 h or more of oliguria, frusemide may increase hourly urine output but there is no evidence it alters the prognosis, namely full return of renal function. Mannitol has theoretical hazards and may worsen pulmonary oedema or cerebral oedema by traversing a damaged blood–brain barrier (Donaldson, 1991). Thirdly, the use of low-dose dopamine for pre-eclamptic oliguria has been reported but is not widely used.

Perhaps 1% of cases will proceed to acute tubular necrosis and may require a limited period of dialysis but all of these in our experience have recovered full renal function within three weeks. There is no evidence that invasive monitoring can influence this outcome.

Blood Pressure Control

The aim in treating hypertension is to prevent the cerebral complications of PET, chiefly eclampsia and cerebral haemorrhage, which account for 30–40% of deaths from the condition (Department of Health, 1989). Both multiple petechial haemorrhages and large intracerebral haematomata may occur (Donaldson, 1991) with or without eclampsia. Whether the disorder is explained as hypertensive encephalopathy, which it closely resembles, or another vasogenic disorder may be a semantic argument. Certainly the evidence is compelling that blood pressure control is essential when greatly elevated, even though the occasional case is seen whose blood pressure is deemed modestly elevated, particularly when first seen post-ictally.

After eclampsia has occurred even once, however, the threshold for further seizures is lowered. Fits may recur unpredictably with no relationship to minute by minute changes in blood pressure, which may have been very high before the first fit. By then there are established vascular changes and cerebral irritability. Furthermore, a young woman whose resting non-gravid blood pressure is 90/50 may be in serious jeopardy at levels of 150–160 systolic in this disorder, so treatment thresholds need to be individualized.

Many hypotensive agents have been used to treat pre-eclamptic hypertension. Acute reduction may be effected orally with nifedipine (Walters and Redman, 1984) or parenterally using hydralazine, diazoxide or labetalol. Nitroprusside can only be used in an Intensive Care Unit and one or other of these agents will virtually always be effective. Once control is achieved, maintenance relies upon slower acting oral agents such as methyldopa, labetalol or atenolol (Redman, 1991) to any of which oral hydralazine may be added up to 200 mg daily.

Postnatal Complications

Severe hypertension often persists in the puerperium for several days (Walters and Walters, 1987) although there is generally a transient fall for the first 24 h. Late postpartum eclampsia (after 24 h) remains a small but definite risk up to about 120 h and attempts to control blood pressure should persist until that time, after which the risks are increasingly remote. Most cases of pulmonary oedema occur within 48 h of delivery as extravascular fluid re-enters the circulation.

Prevention and Treatment of Eclampsia

Is it possible that meticulous control of hypertension alone is sufficient to prevent eclampsia without prophylactic anticonvulsants? A recent very large but retrospective study in South Africa (Odendaal and Hall, 1994) showed the risk of eclampsia with strict blood pressure control in 996 parturients was 0.5%. Half received magnesium sulfate in addition and half no eclampsia prophylaxis with two seizures in one group, three in the other. However, at present prophylaxis against eclampsia is given in most centres, at least to some patients, combined with blood pressure control.

Magnesium sulphate is used extensively in the United States (Pritchard et al., 1984) but much less elsewhere. It may be given by the intravenous or intramuscular route with a regimen involving a loading dose followed by maintenance. Its chief effect may well be peripheral neuromuscular blockade (Ramanathan et al., 1988) and it may not even traverse the blood–brain barrier (Donaldson, 1991). Its maternal toxicity includes respiratory depression, muscular paralysis and cardiac arrest; hence close monitoring of serum levels is mandatory. Despite these caveats, the agent is widely, even universally used in the United States and clinical experience suggests toxicity is an unusual occurrence.

The agent most used elsewhere is phenytoin, given intravenously, but chlormethiazole is also used. Phenytoin is given slowly in a loading dose of 10 mg/kg then 5 mg/kg 2 h later (Slater et al., 1987). No controlled trials are available to determine the efficacy of either of these approaches and it is entirely possible, as suggested above, that anticonvulsant therapy is unnecessary.

For eclampsia, however, energetic and immediate drug control of fitting and the associated derangements is necessary. Mortality increases directly with the number of seizures. For seizure control, intravenous diazepam (10 mg boluses up to 50 mg) or clonazepam are undoubtedly effective and are familiar to all. Magnesium sulfate is also effective, although many neurologists are perplexed by its choice (Donaldson, 1991) as it does not have the usual pharmacological characteristics of an effective anticonvulsant. All of these agents may depress the newborn child and paediatric assistance in the delivery room is important.

Respiratory implications

In addition to hypotension and anticonvulsant agents, adequate ventilation must be assured as hypercarbia lowers the threshold for further seizures. However, intubation and mechanical ventilation need not always follow. Most women will maintain adequate ventilation and a margin of safety even after two or three convulsions. However, the most severely affected may require large doses of anticonvulsant medication such that neuromuscular depression becomes a concern. In status eclampticus, intubation will usually be required with transient ventilation until stabilized. Hyperventilation may be required if cerebral oedema is present. It should be noted that lateral tilt of the patient is necessary to reduce aortocaval compression.

Neurological imaging

Either CT or MRI is helpful, but not essential unless there is persisting neurological deficit or obtundation to suggest haemorrhage, or concern about alternative diagnoses. Secondary anticonvulsant prophylaxis, namely that given to prevent recurrence of seizures, must be maintained for at least 24 h after eclampsia, a time of continuing neurological and haemodynamic instability.

Post-partum Phase

Whilst delivery begins the process of resolution, it must be remembered that 30–50% of eclamptic seizures and 40–60% of deaths occur after delivery. Intensive monitoring should be maintained for 24–48 h and blood pressure may worsen on day 3–5, with a small but definite risk of late post-partum eclampsia. Many cases of the 'HELLP' variant of pre-eclampsia deteriorate temporarily after delivery. The platelet count may fall for up to four days and haemolysis may appear after delivery. Despite that, if the diagnosis is pre-eclampsia rather than thrombotic thrombocytopoenic purpura, haemolytic uraemic syndrome, or other disorder, resolution is invariable. Postnatal plasma exchange has been used in the situation of prolonged post-partum morbidity with this syndrome (Schwartz, 1986).

AMNIOTIC FLUID EMBOLISM

The syndrome of amniotic fluid embolism (AFE) comprises a dramatic set of haemodynamic and coagulation derangements that progress over minutes or up to an hour to a life-threatening state. Many deaths occur within the first 30 minutes. The classical case is said to occur in an older multiparous woman in tumultuous labour with a large fetus. However, the above stereotype accounts for less than 50% of cases and many have been recorded in unexpected clinical circumstances. These include early pregnancy termination, amniocentesis, during uncomplicated pregnancy, after closed abdominal trauma and particularly, during caesarean section.

AFE is a significant minority cause of maternal mortality accounting for up to 16% of maternal deaths in Sweden (Hogberg and Joelsson, 1985), 4.5% (54 deaths) in 20 years in Australia (Ratten, 1988) and 7% in the United States (Kaunitz et al., 1985) between 1974 and 1978. As death occurs in 40–85% of recognized cases (Morgan, 1979) the incidence of clinical AFE may be as high as 1:10 000 deliveries.

Diagnosis

This is difficult because there is no definitive diagnostic test. The diagnosis is made on clinical grounds and the differential diagnoses include pulmonary thromboembolism, air embolism, septic shock, aspiration pneumonia, placental abruption and myocardial infarction. This list indicates the frightening clinical scenario of heart failure, cyanosis, seizures, shock and massive haemorrhage that marks the fully developed syndrome. AFE results from the entry of amniotic fluid into the maternal circulation via small, usually unidentified tears in the uterus, cervix or vagina.

Clinical Features

AFE most frequently presents during labour or caesarean section (65%) with another 20% occurring very soon after (Ratten, 1988). In 10–20%, death occurred before the onset of labour and amniotic fluid entered the circulation then. The embolism to death interval was inferred from reports of 48 cases in the same study. Only four women lived beyond 24 h whilst 75% (36) died within 2 h of the event.

Symptoms

The initial symptom is often sudden dyspnoea and vascular collapse, perhaps with profound cyanosis. One or more seizures follow in 10–20%, probably hypoxic. In women undergoing electronic fetal monitoring, the initial sign may be of fetal distress on the cardiotocograph. The onset of widespread bleeding is the initial aberration in 10–20% but overall is seen in at least 40%, most following the cardiorespiratory collapse. Disseminated intravascular coagulation is observed and, particularly immediately after delivery of the child, major and unrelenting vaginal haemorrhage may ensue with failure of uterine contractions. After caesarean section the bleeding may be intra-abdominal.

Blood pressure usually falls dramatically, unrelated to and usually before the bleeding, with evidence of respiratory failure. Pulmonary oedema may be diagnosed, or pulmonary thromboembolism.

Pathophysiology

Given the rarity of this condition, it is understandable that there are no reports of acute studies in humans, and the handful of haemodynamic studies that are available (Clark et al., 1988) were all of women at least 2–3 h after the event. There have been a few experimental studies of pregnant animals, but only two used autologous amniotic fluid and obtained haemodynamic measurements (Reis et al., 1965; Hankins et al., 1993). The former study using sheep found marked pressor responses in the pulmonary circulation and concluded that AFE results in acute pulmonary hypertension and cor pulmonale subsequent to pulmonary arterial spasm or mechanical occlusion of the lung circulation. Mean PA pressure rose 90%. For many years, therefore, from this and similar studies, therapy in the human was based upon attempts to relieve PA spasm.

Clinical and haemodynamic observations in humans (Hankins et al., 1993), however, were at variance with the expectations from early animal studies and have shown only mild or modest increase in PA pressures but considerable evidence of left ventricular dysfunction. This has led to the contention (Clark et al., 1988) that left heart failure is the dominant disturbance, at least in those who survive long enough to enter an ICU and undergo haemodynamic monitoring. In fact of the 14 adequately documented cases reported by 1993, PCWP exceeded the mean for normal pregnancy by at least three standard deviations in 85% (see Hankins et al., 1993). In half, wedge pressure exceeded 17 mmHg, and clinical pulmonary oedema is detailed in many reports.

A recent detailed haemodynamic study of pregnant goats given their own amniotic fluid with or without meconium is valuable (Hankins et al., 1993). Acute major increases (900–1000% by 10 min) in both systemic and pulmonary vascular resistance (PVR) were seen in the group given amniotic fluid containing meconium, and wedge pressure increased 1000% by 10 min falling to 300% by one hour. Without meconium, systemic vascular resistance (SVR) and cardiac output did not change, but pulmonary vascular resistance (PVR) increased 400% at 10 min returning to baseline by 30 min, with little change in wedge pressure.

The above dilemma can be reconciled by a scheme involving two haemodynamic phases to the illness (Clark et al., 1985). In the first phase, amniotic fluid enters the pulmonary circulation and causes transient pulmonary and systemic arterial spasm. This causes hypoxaemia, acidosis and perhaps coronary artery spasm followed by the second phase of pulmonary capillary damage and left ventricular failure. Most women enter an ICU during the second phase, by which time acute respiratory distress syndrome (ARDS) coexists with left ventricular failure, and pulmonary oedema is prominent.

Coagulopathy

A major element of this syndrome is coagulopathy and occasionally it is the presenting feature and may be overwhelming. This disturbance is attributed to the thromboplastic activity of amniotic fluid (Yaffe et al., 1977) which stimulates intravascular coagulation with avid consumption of clotting factors.

Pathogenesis

The most recent study (Hankins et al., 1993) and others have suggested that the presence of meconium, specifically particulate matter, is necessary for the most profound and damaging changes. There is, therefore, the possibility that mechanical obstruction of pulmonary vessels by fetal squames and lanugo hair is important. However, pulmonary vascular cytology of women without AFE has also shown squames (see below) and it may well be that some other component of amniotic fluid is the trigger for this syndrome. The suggestion that abnormal amniotic fluid is necessary (Clark, 1985) seems less attractive; a component, ‘tissue factor’, may account for most of the procoagulant activity and has been proposed as a possible trigger of the other changes as well (Lockwood et al., 1991). It has been proposed that there is widespread occlusion of the vessels by platelet fibrin thrombi leading to shock and respiratory failure. The normal fibrinolytic response of the lung vessels presumably clears such thrombi if the patient survives the massive initial upheaval.

Cytological Diagnosis

Diagnosis is largely on clinical grounds and relies on exclusion of imitators. There is some conviction that characteristic embolic material can be identified in a sample of fluid drawn from a wedged PA catheter (Masson and Ruggieri, 1985). Slides are stained by the

Papanicolaou method revealing fetal squames which may be surrounded by maternal neutrophils.

Despite these findings, others contend that squamous cells may be found in pulmonary blood in many situations and may originate from the maternal puncture site (Lee et al., 1986).

Treatment

Arrest of haemorrhage with correction of oxygenation and of cardiac failure are the immediate priorities. As large volumes of fluid may be required, and the pulmonary capillary permeability and ventricular dysfunction predispose to oedema, haemodynamic monitoring by PA catheter is very helpful. Uterine bleeding may be torrential, uterine atony is frequent and ongoing obstetric assistance is critical in these cases. Even so, surgery to correct haemorrhage should be withheld if possible as it is extremely hazardous until the coagulopathy is resolving. Intramyometrial prostaglandin may be helpful in this situation.

Platelets and fresh frozen plasma are often required, and the freshest available blood should be used. The role of heparin in this scenario has been debated for many years (Bonnar, 1973; Chung and Merkatz, 1973). In theory it seems rational to break the vicious cycle of DIC when the circulation is intact. However, the presence of a large bleeding placental site mandates considerable circumspection in the use of heparin. Until controlled trial evidence is available, therefore, the use of heparin must be regarded as experimental and reserved for cases where conventional therapy has failed.

ACUTE FATTY LIVER OF PREGNANCY (AFLP)

This is a rare disorder with an incidence of approximately 1:10 000 pregnancies (Purdie and Walters, 1988). Pathologically it is characterized by the presence of microvesicular steatosis in hepatocytes as is seen in Reye's syndrome in children and tetracycline toxicity (Allen and Brown, 1966). The latter was a major cause of AFLP in pregnancy up to about 1970.

The prognosis of AFLP used to be poor. Before 1980, 50–70% of reported cases were fatal. Since then, either because of earlier diagnosis, reporting of milder cases, or improvements in management, mortality is less than 25% (Pockros et al., 1984). Perinatal mortality rate, however, remains appreciable, greater than 25%.

Diagnosis

The chief presenting feature in almost all cases is persistent vomiting in the third trimester of pregnancy (Purdie and Walters, 1988). This is usually accompanied by a systemic illness with prominent tiredness and malaise for days or weeks followed by jaundice with drowsiness or confusion. An unusual but frequent symptom is polydipsia which may be extreme, with pseudo-diabetes insipidus. Upper abdominal pain is also present in many cases, but severe pain is suggestive of pre-eclamptic liver disease (Walters and Walters, 1991).

On presentation severe cases are jaundiced with deteriorating conscious state leading to hepatic encephalopathy (Burroughs et al., 1982). This is accompanied by renal failure, acidosis, coagulation failure and occasionally pancreatitis (Rolfes and Ishak, 1985). Gastrointestinal haemorrhage is common and hypoglycaemia may be profound.

Differential diagnosis

AFLP may appear very similar to pre-eclamptic liver disease as described above ('HELLP' variant). Further confusion arises as some hypertension and proteinuria are present in about 40% of cases (Burroughs et al., 1982). If these features are severe, however, PET is more likely.

Acute viral hepatitis may be similar and viral serology should always be ordered urgently. The transaminase elevation, however, is usually more severe in hepatitis than in AFLP.

Accurate diagnosis requires liver biopsy, but it must be stressed that coagulopathy usually precludes the percutaneous route. Moreover, unless an alternative diagnosis can be made quickly and with certainty, delivery must be recommended as delay is life-threatening for both mother and baby. To await biopsy confirmation cannot be justified in this clinical setting based on the clinical diagnosis.

Laboratory Features

There are striking abnormalities in biochemistry and haematology which may strongly suggest the diagnosis (Purdie and Walters, 1988). The liver enzymes present a combination of hepatocellular and obstructive disturbance. AST and ALT are usually modestly elevated only. Bilirubin is elevated and albumin decreased considerably. Hypoglycaemia may be pronounced. The blood film may show leukaemoid or leukoerythroblastic change (Burroughs et al., 1982) and thrombocytopoenia (Kaplan, 1985). Liver-dependent clotting tests are deranged and the bleeding diathesis may be severe. Uric acid elevation is often extreme (Hague et al., 1983).

Aetiology

The cause(s) and pathogenesis of this disorder are not understood. Tetracycline is no longer observed as a cause, either because it is avoided in pregnancy, or it has changed. AFLP occurred in one mother of infants with an acyl-fatty acid oxidation defect (Schoeman et al., 1991) but this must constitute a rare clinical finding as virtually all reported surviving babies have been normal. The lack of recurrence in subsequent pregnancies (Burroughs et al., 1982; Purdie and Walters, 1988) argues against an underlying maternal metabolic disease. Microvesicular fatty infiltration is seen in a number of organs at autopsy, including the kidneys (Rolfes and Ishak, 1986). With appropriate management, however, the liver returns to normal within months of delivery.

Management

As in PET, the essential prerequisite for recovery of the mother, and for fetal survival, is delivery. There are no cases reported of resolution of this disease before delivery. For these reasons, most cases will arrive at the ICU post-partum. Delivery, however, does not guarantee survival and many of the reported deaths have occurred in women who continued to deteriorate in the puerperium. Even so, the prognosis is good where diagnosis and delivery occur before liver failure and the major complications have occurred.

No studies are available to support a choice between vaginal or caesarean delivery and that decision must rest on clinical assessment of mother and baby at the time.

Management of the liver failure is along usual lines, providing optimal nutrition in the form of parenteral glucose (Davies et al., 1980) to reduce protein catabolism and subsequent nitrogenous waste and to prevent life-threatening hypoglycaemia. Treatment with oral lactulose and neomycin are intended to evacuate the bowel and reduce production of ammonia by bacteria, and protein is excluded from the diet.

Coagulopathy will need correction with vitamin K, platelets, fresh frozen plasma and blood transfusion will often prove necessary. The coagulopathy may preclude use of epidural anaesthesia and narcotics may worsen encephalopathy so pain relief for labour and delivery needs careful consideration by the anaesthetist. Oxygenation must be assured by mechanical ventilation if necessary. Infection and gastro-intestinal haemorrhage are to be anticipated and measures taken to prevent or control them. Finally, acute liver transplantation would be a consideration if all modalities failed.

PULMONARY OEDEMA DUE TO TOCOLYTIC THERAPY

Pre-term delivery is a major contributor to perinatal morbidity and mortality, and long-term handicap of the child. For these reasons the obstetrician will want to inhibit premature labour. A number of pharmacological agents are used including magnesium sulfate and alcohol, but those most favoured are the beta sympathomimetic agents.

Beta Stimulants

Salbutamol, ritodrine, terbutaline, and others have a direct relaxant effect on uterine muscle when given in large doses by intravenous infusion. The tocolytic effect is β_2 receptor mediated, but it has not been possible to separate this from β_1 activity. Increased cardiac output accompanies the use of these drugs. This may be a reflex response to the lowered diastolic blood pressure together with direct stimulation of cardiac β_1 receptors. The second category of adverse effects is metabolic, as detailed below.

Metabolic Effects

Beta agonist agents stimulate glucagon secretion (Lipshitz and Vinik, 1978) resulting in glycogenolysis and hyperglycaemia. Mobilization of free fatty acids and enhanced production of ketone bodies are also seen (Lunell et al., 1977), accounting for ketonuria, but significant acidosis is unusual.

A transmembrane shift of potassium into cells occurs, sometimes resulting in hypokalaemia as a result of beta stimulation (Young et al., 1983; Cano et al., 1985). This is not usually treated, but requires monitoring.

These agents also cause a decrease in free water clearance by increased sodium reabsorption (Kleinman et al., 1984) resulting from enhanced renin secretion. A fall in haematocrit due to haemodilution by this mechanism is often seen. It is possible that the water retention may be reduced if less sodium is available for reabsorption, as when using 5% dextrose (Philipsen et al., 1981).

Cardiorespiratory Risk Factors

Infection is a common precipitant of pre-term labour (30%) and chorioamnionitis, pyelonephritis, etc., may lead to release of cytokines and other vasoactive substances contributing to pulmonary oedema by capillary membrane injury (MacLennan et al., 1985).

Multiple gestation is present in 10–15% of cases of pre-term labour, and in twin pregnancy, blood volume is elevated by 50–60% compared with non-pregnant levels.

Even in singleton pregnancy, blood volume expands 40%, such that the intravenous volume load that may be given by infusing beta stimulants to inhibit labour may contribute to pulmonary oedema.

Where haemorrhage complicates pre-term labour, and it often will, the addition of blood transfusion further stresses the pregnant cardiovascular system. Furthermore, labour alone accounts for an increase in cardiac output of 30–50%.

Thus, it can be seen that even without β-adrenergic stimulation, women in pre-term labour may be at risk of heart failure. The chronotropic, inotropic, volume-expanding and possibly ischaemic effects on the heart of these agents, will contribute to the risk of death (Katz et al., 1981).

Pulmonary Oedema

Pulmonary oedema may occur in women given these agents and presents as dyspnoea, orthopnoea and often, cough. Chest pain is reported by a fifth of women and evidence of myocardial ischaemia may be found (Cohen et al., 1988). Sinus tachycardia is universal and not surprising given that it is standard obstetric practice to maintain the infusion at a rate to ensure maternal heart rate does not fall below 120 min. Ventricular and supraventricular extrasystoles are likely (Benedetti, 1986). The tachycardia is particularly dangerous in a woman with a cardiac lesion, such as mitral stenosis and maternal cardiac disease is a contraindication to the use of beta stimulants for tocolysis.

A literature review (Pisani and Rosenow, 1989) found 58 cases in the decade to 1989. Clearly these represent only a proportion of many cases that must have occurred. Attention has been drawn to a high risk (3%) of pulmonary oedema in cases where there is pre-term labour in the presence of infection (Hatjis and Swain, 1988). The risk remains for a few hours after beta stimulant therapy has been stopped.

The mean duration of treatment before diagnosis was 54 h and no cases occurred in less than 17 h. Thus pulmonary oedema rarely develops rapidly and usually there has been a long period of fluid and drug administration. Fluid overload was diagnosed in 70% of the cases analysed. Twins were present in 25% of cases.

Haemodynamic measurements were sparse in this set of patients. Echocardiography was normal where reported, and elevated wedge pressure was found in a minority only. Thus the accumulation of alveolar fluid is multifactorial in cause. On balance, however, the evidence suggests that the dominant disorder is myocardial fatigue resulting from prolonged tachycardia, fluid overload and further myocardial stimulation when the heart is already operating near its limits.

Therapy

When a woman develops chest pain, dyspnoea, cough or any suggestion of pulmonary oedema, the fluid and beta stimulant should be ceased immediately. High flow oxygen should be given and morphine is therapeutic in small doses. Of course, upright posture is important. Diuretic use will usually result in considerable clearance of fluid overload. Rarely these measures do not suffice and intubation with ventilatory support is necessary.

The possibility of infection in such cases must be considered carefully. A pulmonary capillary permeability effect may result from intrauterine, or other infection, and greatly increases susceptibility to volume overload.

PULMONARY INJURY COMPLICATING PYELONEPHRITIS IN PREGNANCY

Sepsis at any time is a potential cause of respiratory distress but in late pregnancy there appears to be a predilection for lung involvement with pyelonephritis (Cunningham et al., 1987) and also with chorioamnionitis. This is described as a non-hydrostatic permeability pulmonary oedema and may result largely from fluid overload (Towers et al., 1991). In addition, endotoxin and cytokines generated by serious infection are postulated as injurious to the lung and myocardium (Parrillo, 1993).

During acute uncomplicated pyelonephritis in a study of 37 pregnant women, a 30% decrease in systemic vascular resistance was found combined with a similar increase in cardiac output (Twickler et al., 1994). The stress of sepsis added to the physiological changes of pregnancy increases susceptibility to fluid overload.

Clinical Features

Respiratory distress and pulmonary infiltrates on radiology developed a mean of 30 h after admission in 15 patients (Cunningham et al., 1987) with varying degrees of hypoxia and hypercarbia. Even though loin pain and tenderness are usually obvious features, in some cases respiratory symptoms have overshadowed these and pneumonia was the first, erroneous, diagnosis.

There is often mild thrombocytopaenia, consumption coagulopathy and haemolysis. Renal dysfunction is frequent. *E. coli* or *Klebsiella* are often grown in blood cultures and urine. Severe pyrexia is almost always present.

This disorder is very rare in early pregnancy, most cases occurring after 20 weeks (Ridgway et al., 1991). This supports a contributory role of low colloid osmotic pressure.

Prediction of risk is imprecise. In one study (Towers et al., 1991) pulmonary injury was more likely to complicate pyelonephritis where pulse rate exceeded 110 beats per minute and temperature exceeded 39.4°C. Gestational age was above 20 weeks in all patients. Use of tocolytic agents was noted in many cases and occasionally there was evidence of fluid overload.

Treatment

Appropriate antibiotic therapy clearly is essential. Oxygenation may require intubation and ventilation using 100% oxygen and positive end-expiratory pressure. Judicious attention to fluid balance is mandatory to avoid over hydration even though this was not often seen in the study of Cunningham et al. (1987). Fluid restriction to 40–60 ml per hour is prudent, or certainly avoidance of aggressive hydration. Beta stimulant tocolysis is contra-indicated and should not be used in general in patients with pyelonephritis even where respiratory distress does not exist.

Usually there is cardiomegaly on X-ray but not accompanied by haemodynamic evidence of ventricular failure. In the above series, pulmonary capillary wedge pressure was 0–12 mmHg in the five women studied.

CONCLUSION

The pregnant woman and her baby are subject to certain pathologies quite different from those seen in non-gravid individuals. Some of these have been discussed.

In the management of serious illness in pregnancy, care of the fetus includes maintenance of placental blood flow and oxygenation, and should involve consultation with an obstetrician. Obstetric input is essential in all antenatal cases as decisions about the timing and mode of delivery may be critical. An understanding of the altered physiology in pregnancy and the puerperium is necessary in the care of these cases.

In almost all cases, however life-threatening, the pregnancy-induced diseases discussed above are reversible and the woman should return to full health. Often, intensive care implies achieving physiological stabilization, avoiding iatrogenic complications, and awaiting the expected resolution of the disease process.

REFERENCES

Allen, E.S., Brown, W.E. (1966) Hepatic toxicity of tetracycline in pregnancy. *American Journal of Obstetrics and Gynecology* **95**: 12–22.

Ballegeer, V.C., Spitz, B., De Baene, L.A. et al. (1992) Platelet activation and vascular damage in gestational hypertension. *American Journal of Obstetrics and Gynecology* **166**: 629–33.

Barth, W.H. (1992) Special resuscitation situations: pregnancy. *Journal of the American Medical Association* **268**: 2249–2250.

Benedetti, T.J. (1986) Life-threatening complications of betamimetic therapy for preterm labour inhibition. *Clinics in Perinatology* **13**: 843–852.

Bonnar, J. (1973) Blood coagulation and fibrinolysis in obstetrics. *Clinics in Haematology* **2**: 213–233.

Burroughs, A.K., Seong, N.H., Dojcinow, D.M. et al. (1982) Idiopathic acute fatty liver of pregnancy in 12 patients. *Quarterly Journal of Medicine* **51**: 481–496.

Cano, A., Tovar, I., Parrilla, J.J., Abad, L. (1985) Metabolic disturbances during intravenous use of ritodrine: increased insulin levels and hypokalaemia. *Obstetrics and Gynecology* **65**: 356–360.

Chung, A.F., Merkatz, I.R. (1973) Survival following amniotic fluid embolism with early heparinization. *Obstetrics and Gynecology* **42**: 809–814.

Clark, S.L. (1985) Arachidonic acid metabolites and the pathophysiology of amniotic fluid embolism. *Seminars in Reproductive Endocrinology* **3**: 253–259.

Clark, S.L., Montz, F.J., Phelan, J.P. (1985) Haemodynamic alterations associated with amniotic fluid embolism: a reappraisal. *American Journal of Obstetrics and Gynecology* **151**: 617–622.

Clark, S.L., Cotton, D.B. (1988) Clinical indications for pulmonary artery catheterization in the patient with severe preeclampsia. *American Journal of Obstetrics and Gynecology* **158**: 453–459.

Clark, S.L., Cotton, D.B., Gonik, B. et al. (1986) Central haemodynamic alterations in amniotic fluid embolism. *American Journal of Obstetrics and Gynecology* **158**: 1124–1126.

Clark, S.L., Cotton, D.B., Lee, W. et al. (1989) Central haemodynamic assessment of normal term pregnancy. *American Journal of Obstetrics and Gynecology* **161**: 1439–1442.

Cohen, G.R., O'Brien, W.F., Knuppel, R.A. (1988) ST segment depression in paired electrocardiograms and serum electrolytes in pregnant women receiving intravenous ritodrine. *Journal of Reproductive Medicine* **33**: 768–770.

Cunningham, F.G., Lindheimer, M.D. (1992) Hypertension in pregnancy. *New England Journal of Medicine* **326**: 927–932.

Cunningham, F.G., Lucas, M.J., Hankins, G.D. (1987) Pulmonary injury complicating antepartum pyelonephritis. *American Journal of Obstetrics and Gynecology* **156**: 797–807.

Davies, M.H., Wilkinson, S.P., Hamid, M.A. et al. (1980) Acute liver disease with encephalopathy and renal failure in late pregnancy and the early puerperium; a study of 14 patients. *British Journal of Obstetrics and Gynaecology* **87**: 1005–1014.

Department of Health (1989) *Report on confidential enquiries into maternal deaths in England and Wales 1982–84*. London: HMSO.

Donaldson, J.O. (1991) Neurologic emergencies in pregnancy. *Obstetrics and Gynecology Clinics of North America* **18**: 203.

Duncan, S.L. (1989) Does volume expansion in pre-eclampsia help or hinder? *British Journal of Obstetrics and Gynaecology* **96**: 631–633.

Easterling, T.R., Benedetti, T.J., Schmucker, B.C., Carlson, K.L. (1989) Antihypertensive therapy in pregnancy directed by noninvasive haemodynamic monitoring. *American Journal of Perinatology* **6**: 86–89.

Fox, H. (1988) The placenta in pregnancy hypertension. In Rubin, P.C. (ed) *Handbook of Hypertension volume 10: Hypertension in Pregnancy* pp 16–37. Amsterdam: Elsevier Science.

Gallery, E.D., Hunyor, S.N., Gyory, A.Z. (1979) Plasma volume contraction: a significant factor in both pre-eclampsia and chronic hypertension in pregnancy. *Quarterly Journal of Medicine* **48**: 593–602.

Greer, I.A., Haddad, N.G., Dawes, J. et al. (1989). Neutrophil activation in pregnancy induced hypertension. *British Journal of Obstetrics and Gynaecology* **96**: 978–982.

Hague, W.M., Fenton, D.W., Duncan, S.L., Slater, D.N. (1983) Acute fatty liver of pregnancy. *Journal of the Royal Society of Medicine* **76**: 652–661.

Hankins, G.D., Snyder, R.R., Clark, S.L. et al. (1993) Acute haemodynamic and respiratory effects of amniotic fluid embolism in the pregnant goat model. *American Journal of Obstetrics and Gynecology* **160**: 1113–1130.

Hatjis, C.G., Swain, M. (1988) Systemic tocolysis for premature labour is associated with an increased incidence of pulmonary edema in the presence of maternal infection. *American Journal of Obstetrics and Gynecology* **159**: 723–8.

Hogberg, U., Joelsson, I. (1985) Amniotic fluid embolism in Sweden, 1951–1980. *Gynecologic and Obstetric Investigation* **20**: 130–137.

Hytten, F., Chamberlain, G. (1991) *Clinical Physiology in Obstetrics*, 2nd edn. Oxford: Blackwell Scientific.

Jouppila, P., Jouppila, R., Hollmen, A., Koivula, A. (1982) Lumbar epidural analgesia to improve intervillous blood flow during labour in severe preeclampsia. *Obstetrics and Gynecology* **59**: 158–161.

Kaplan, M.M. (1985) Acute fatty liver of pregnancy. *New England Journal of Medicine* **313**: 367–372.

Katz, M., Robertson, P.A., Creasy, R.K. (1981) Cardiovascular complications associated with terbutaline treatment for preterm labour. *American Journal of Obstetrics and Gynecology* **139**: 605–608.

Katz, V.L., Dotters, D.J., Droegemeuller, W. (1986) Perimortem caesarean delivery. *Obstetrics and Gynecology* **68**: 571–576.

Kaunitz, A.M., Hughes, J.M., Grimes, D.A. et al. (1985) Causes of maternal mortality in the United States. *Obstetrics and Gynecology* **65**: 605–611.

Kerr, M.G., (1965) The mechanical effects of the gravid uterus in late pregnancy. *Journal of Obstetrics and Gynaecology of the British Commonwealth* **72**: 513–529.

Khong, T.Y., de Wolf, F., Robertson, W.B., Brosens, I. (1986). Inadequate maternal vascular response to placentation in pregnancies complicated by pre-eclampsia and by small-for-gestational-age infants. *British Journal of Obstetrics and Gynaecology* **93**: 1049–1059.

Kleinman, G., Nuwayhid, B., Rudelstorfer, R. et al. (1984) Circulatory and renal effects of beta adrenergic receptor stimulation in pregnant sheep. *American Journal of Obstetrics and Gynecology* **149**: 865–874.

Lee, W., Ginsburg, K.A., Cotton, D.B. (1986) Squamous and trophoblastic cells in the maternal pulmonary circulation identified by invasive haemodynamic monitoring during the peripartum period. *American Journal of Obstetrics and Gynecology* **155**: 999–1001.

Lipshitz, J., Vinik, A.I. (1978) The effects of hexaprenaline, a beta-2 sympathomimetic drug, on maternal glucose, insulin, glucagon, and free fatty acid levels. *American Journal of Obstetrics and Gynecology* **130**: 761–764.

Lockwood, C.J., Bach, R., Guha, A. et al. (1991) Amniotic fluid contains tissue factor, a potent initiator of coagulation. *American Journal of Obstetrics and Gynecology* **165**: 1335–1341.

Lunell, N.O., Joellson, I., Larsson, A., Persson, B. (1977) The immediate effects of a beta-adrenergic agonist (salbutamol) on carbohydrate and lipid metabolism during the third trimester of pregnancy. *Acta Obstetrica et Gynecologica Scandinavica* **56**: 475–481.

MacLennan, F.M., Thomson, M.A., Rankin, R. et al. (1985) Fatal pulmonary oedema associated with the use of ritodrine in pregnancy: case report. *British Journal of Obstetrics and Gynaecology* **92**: 703–705.

Macphail, S. (1992) Haemodynamics of hypertensive pregnancy. *Contemporary Reviews in Obstetrics and Gynaecology* **4**: 116–120.

Masson, R.G., Ruggieri, J. (1985) Pulmonary microvascular cytology, a new diagnostic application of the pulmonary artery catheter. *Chest* **88**: 908–914.

Metzger, B.E., Ravnikar, V., Veileisis, R.A., Freinkel, N. (1982) 'Accelerated starvation' and the skipped breakfast in late normal pregnancy. *Lancet* **i**:588–592.

Morgan, M. (1979) Amniotic fluid embolism. *Anaesthesia* **34**: 20–32.

Odendaal, H.J., Hall, D. (1994) Is magnesium sulphate really necessary to prevent eclampsia in patients with severe pre-eclampsia? *Abstracts of the International Congress of the International Society for the Study of Hypertension in Pregnancy:* **264**.

Oian, P., Maltau, J.M., Noddeland, H., Fadnes, H.O. (1986) Transcapillary fluid balance in pre-eclampsia. *British Journal of Obstetrics and Gynaecology* **93**: 235–239.

Parrillo, J.E. (1993) Pathogenetic mechanisms of septic shock. *New England Journal of Medicine* **328**: 1471–1477.

Philipsen, T., Eriksen, P.S., Lynggard, F. (1981) Pulmonary edema following ritodrine saline infusion in premature labour. *Obstetrics and Gynecology* **58**: 304–307.

Pisani, R.J., Rosenow, E.C. (1989) Pulmonary edema associated with tocolytic therapy. *Annals of Internal Medicine* **110**: 714–718.

Pockros, P.J., Peters, R.L., Reynolds, T.B. (1984) Idiopathic fatty liver of pregnancy: Findings in 10 cases. *Medicine* **63**: 1–14.

Pritchard, J.A., Cunningham, F.G., Pritchard, S.A. (1984) The Parkland Memorial Hospital protocol for treatment of eclampsia: Evaluation of 245 cases. *American Journal of Obstetrics and Gynecology* **148**: 951–959.

Purdie, J.M., Walters, B.N.J. (1988) Acute fatty liver of pregnancy: clinical features and diagnosis. *Australian and New Zealand Journal of Obstetrics and Gynaecology* **28**: 62–67.

Ramanathan, J., Sibai, B.M., Duggirala, V. et al. (1988) Pulmonary function in pre-eclamptic women receiving Mg_2SO_4. *Journal of Reproductive Medicine* **33**: 432–436.

Ratten, G.J. (1988) Amniotic fluid embolism – two case reports and a review of maternal deaths from this cause in Australia. *Australian and New Zealand Journal of Obstetrics and Gynaecology* **28**: 33–35.

Redman, C.W.G. (1991) Controlled trials of antihypertensive drugs in pregnancy. *American Journal of Kidney Diseases* **17**: 149–159.

Reis, R.L., Pierce, W.S., Behrendt, D.M. (1965) Hemodynamic effects of amniotic fluid embolism. *Surgery, Obstetrics and Gynecology* **129**: 45–52.

Ridgway, L.E., Martin, R.W., Hess, L.W. et al. (1991) Acute gestational pyelonephritis: the impact on colloid osmotic pressure, plasma fibronectin, and arterial oxygen saturation. *American Journal of Perinatology* **8**: 222–226.

Roberts, J.M., Taylor, R.N., Goldfien, A. (1991) Clinical and biochemical evidence of endothelial cell dysfunction in the pregnancy syndrome preeclampsia. *American Journal of Hypertension* **4**: 700–708.

Rolfes, D.B., Ishak, K.G. (1985) Acute fatty liver of pregnancy: A clinicopathologic study of 35 cases. *Hepatology* **5**: 1149–1158.

Rolfes, D.B., Ishak, K.G. (1986) Liver disease in pregnancy. *Histopathology* **10**: 555–556.

Schoeman, M.N., Batey, R.G., Wilcken, B. (1991) Recurrent acute fatty liver of pregnancy associated with a fatty-acid oxidation defect in the offspring. *Gastroenterology* **100**: 544–548.

Schwartz, M.L. (1986) Possible role for exchange plasmapheresis with fresh frozen plasma for maternal indications in selected cases of preeclampsia and eclampsia. *Obstetrics and Gynecology* **67**: 136–139.

Sheehan, H.L., Lynch, J.B. (1973) *Pathology of Toxaemia of Pregnancy*. London: Churchill Livingston.

Sibai, B.H. (1988) In Rubin, P.C. (ed.) *Handbook of Hypertension, Vol. 10: Hypertension in Pregnancy*, pp 320–340. Amsterdam: Elsevier.

Sibai, B.M., Mabie, B.C., Harvey, C.J., Gonzalez, A.R. (1987) Pulmonary edema in severe pre-eclampsia: analysis of 37 consecutive cases. *American Journal of Obstetrics and Gynecology* **156**: 1174–1179.

Slater, R.M., Wilcox, F.L., Smith W.M. et al. (1987) Phenytoin infusion in severe pre-eclampsia. *Lancet* **i**: 1417–1420.

Towers C.V., Kaminskas, C.M., Garite, T.J. et al. (1991) Pulmonary injury associated with antepartum pyelonephritis: can patients at risk be indentified? *American Journal of Obstetrics and Gynecology* **164**: 974–980.

Twickler, D.N., Lucas, M.J., Bowe, L. et al. (1994) Ultrasonographic evaluation of central and end-organ haemodynamics in antepartum pyelonephritis. *American Journal of Obstetrics and Gynecology* **170**: 814–817.

Vink, G.J., Moodley, J., Philpott, R.H. (1980) Effect of dihydralazine on the foetus in the treatment of maternal hypertension. *Obstetrics and Gynecology* **55**: 519–522.

Visser, W., Wallenburg, H.C.S. (1991) Central haemodynamic observations in untreated pre-eclamptic patients. *Hypertension* **17**: 1072–1077.

Walters, B.N.J., Redman, C.W.G. (1984) Treatment of severe pregnancy-associated hypertension with the calcium antagonist nifedipine. *British Journal of Obstetrics and Gynaecology* **91**: 330–336.

Walters, B.N.J., Walters, T. (1987) Hypertension in the puerperium. *Lancet* **ii**: 330.

Walters, B.N., Walters, T. (1991) Pre-ecalmptic angina: a characteristic symptom of severe pre-eclampsia. *Clinical and Experimental Hypertension – Hypertension in Pregnancy* **B10**: 271.

Wasserstrum, N., Cotton, D.B. (1986) Haemodynamic monitoring in severe pregnancy-induced hypertension. *Clinics in Perinatology* **13**: 781–799.

Wasserstrum, N., Kirshon, B., Willis, R.S. et al. (1989) Quantitative haemodynamic effects of acute volume expansion in severe preeclampsia. *Obstetrics and Gynecology* **73**: 546–550.

Weinstein, L. (1982) Syndrome of haemolysis, elevated liver enzymes, and low platelet count: a severe consequence of hypertension in pregnancy. *American Journal of Obstetrics and Gynecology* **142**: 159–167.

Yaffe, H., Eldor, A., Hornshtein, E., Sadovsky, E. (1977). Thromboplastin activity in amniotic fluid during pregnancy. *Obstetrics and Gynecology* **50**: 454–456.

Young, D.C., Toofanian, A., Leveno, K.J. (1983) Potassium and glucose concentrations without treatment during ritodrine tocolysis. *American Journal of Obstetrics and Gynecology* **135**: 105–106.

4

Initial Management of the Poisoned or Overdosed Patient

Francis J. De Roos, Lewis R. Goldfrank

INTRODUCTION

The initial management of the poisoned or overdosed patient is a dynamic, often empiric, and frequently controversial aspect of medical toxicology that varies with temporal, patient, and toxin specific factors. The American Association of Poison Control Centers (AAPCC) collects and publishes data regarding over two million exposures reported to United States poison centres, although it is a passive reporting system and the number of exposures is in actuality far greater (Caravati and McElwee, 1991). These data illustrate the wide variety of toxic substances as well as the particular patient demographics involved in these exposures. It is specifically this variety that limits the benefits of universal management strategies, thus giving rise to areas of controversy. This review will highlight key decisions in the initial management of the poisoned or overdosed patient and propose a rational and organized management strategy for several controversies in treatment.

CLINICAL EVALUATION

Initial History

Many critical management decisions are guided by information that can only be obtained from an accurate and thorough history. This history should focus on the specific agents involved and the factors that influence their toxicity. Clues to the agent involved such as empty pill bottles, actual pill markings and colours, odours, and biological specimens may be useful. Resources such as regional poison centres, medical toxicologists, POISINDEX, European pharmacopoeia, botanists and botanical gardens, mycologists, and herpetologists may assist in identifying toxins.

Whether the drug preparation is sustained or regular release, the quantity ingested, and duration of the exposure should be defined. The time elapsed since exposure allows application of the known pharmacokinetic and toxicokinetic principles of the specific agent to assist in the prediction of the onset and peak of toxicity. The application of these principles is a central issue in evaluating choices in gastrointestinal decontamination. Poisoning often can be excluded if the time since exposure has exceeded the longest known or predicted interval before clinically apparent toxicity. Although the diagnosis cannot be definitively made by identification of a single tablet or empty bottle, as patients routinely ingest multiple drugs and reuse prescription bottles, these pharmaceutical clues can help focus other aspects of the evaluation such as the physical and laboratory examination. Finally, the patient's underlying medical condition is one of the most important prognostic indicators in poisonings. The healthy adult tolerates physiological stress far better than one who may have multiple medical problems.

The precise history of the exposure can be extremely valuable, but is often unavailable. Suicidal patients notoriously provide inaccurate ingestion histories (Wright, 1980). Patients may be unaware of exposures from occupational or environmental poisonings, therapeutic misadventures, or attempted homicide. In addition, herbal, homoeopathic, or non-prescription preparations may not be recognized by the patient as active pharmaceutical agents, much less potential toxins. Young children or confused and combative patients may not be able to relate their exposure histories.

These limitations in the ability to obtain a definitive history necessitate clinical vigilance if potential poisonings are to be recognized. Several clinical presentations should arouse the suspicion of a poisoning such as a previously healthy person with an acute, unexplained illness, patients with suicide risk factors, a history of drug or ethanol abuse, a recent major life loss such as spouse or job, and illness temporally related to recent food or medication ingestion. Patients who present with an altered mental status or with an unexplained metabolic abnormality should also be evaluated for poisoning.

Initial Physical Examination

A directed physical examination can provide valuable clues to the agent ingested and direct subsequent management and therapeutic decisions. This physical examination should focus on vital signs, neurological status emphasizing the mental status, pupillary and occulomotor function, diaphoresis or abnormal skin colour, and evidence of abnormalities of gastrointestinal function including vomiting, peristalsis, and characteristic breath odours.

The most important aspect of the initial assessment of any poisoned patient must be the vital signs. Consequential abnormalities of pulse, blood pressure, respirations, and temperature mandate initial resuscitation and intervention including securing the airway, supporting ventilation, stabilizing any cardiovascular compromise whether from dysrhythmias or hypotension, or rapid cooling and sedation for severe hyperthermia. Once abnormalities have been assessed and management initiated, the physical examination can proceed.

The physiological heart rate is established by a balance between the adrenergic and cholinergic hormonal tone. Bradycardia is commonly caused by agents acting directly on the myocardium such as digoxin, calcium channel blockers and β-adrenergic antagonists, and antidysrhythmic agents, or indirect toxins such as cholinergic agents including organophosphates. Tachycardia can be caused by sympathomimetic agents such as cocaine, theophylline, and caffeine, anticholinergic agents including tricyclic antidepressants and antihistamines, or increased adrenergic effects due to toxin withdrawal from agents such as ethanol, sedative-hypnotics, or opioids, pain produced by caustic burns, or hypovolaemia induced by toxins including arsenic, iron, and organophosphates.

Although the blood pressure and particularly orthostatic blood pressure and pulse changes are essential in assessing a patient's clinical status, they are less helpful in defining the toxic agent involved. While hypertension is initially expected following exposure to sympathomimetic agents like cocaine and monoamine oxidase inhibitors many patients with severe overdoses progress to hypotension. Hypotension is associated with hypovolaemia resulting from exposure to agents such as iron and arsenic, myocardial dysfunction produced by digoxin, calcium channel blockers, or β-adrenergic antagonists, and decreased peripheral resistance from barbiturates or opioids.

Any alterations in a patient's respiratory status can be helpful in the assessment and differential diagnosis. Toxins can induce tachypnoea or hyperpnoea by central nervous system stimulation including salicylates and analeptic agents, the production of metabolic acidosis due to the ingestion of salicylates, methanol, or ethylene glycol, the alteration of haemoglobin's oxygen carrying abilities due to the production of methaemoblobinaemia or carbon monoxide, or direct pulmonary injury caused by hydrocarbon aspiration or phosgene. Various toxins including opiates, ethanol, barbiturates and other sedative hypnotic agents can produce hypoventilation either by bradypnoea or hypopnoea.

The assessment of the core temperature is often overlooked in the initial assessment of patients who are extremely agitated, combative, or seizing. These unfortunately are precisely the patients in whom toxin-induced life-threatening hyperthermia is a critical concern. Toxins commonly associated with hypothalamic dysfunction like phenothiazines or anticholinergic agents, with uncoupling of oxidative phosphorylation due to salicylates and dinitrophenol, with increased peripheral muscular activity caused by agents such as cocaine or phencyclidine, and decreased heat dissipation due to anticholinergic agents all can produce significant elevations in core body temperature. Hypothermia is associated with toxins that cause general central nervous system depression and predispose patients to environmental exposure; notably ethanol, opioids, sedative-hypnotic agents, and hypoglycaemic agents.

Once the vital signs have been assessed and any abnormalities addressed, a thorough neurological evaluation should focus particularly on the level of consciousness, cranial nerve function, and abnormal neuromuscular activity including agitation, seizures, and movement disorders. Numerous toxins can cause alterations in consciousness which may be due to generalized central nervous system depression as in the case of opioids or sedative hypnotic agents, impairment of cellular metabolic function notably by cyanide and salicylates, a decrease in serum glucose concentration by hypoglycaemic agents, or oxygen transport dysfunction caused by carbon monoxide. Toxic encephalopathies may manifest rostrocaudal or brainstem/cortex dissociation. This dissociation is demonstrated by the patient who is obtunded and unresponsive to painful stimuli but whose cranial nerves, reflexes, or respiratory status remains normal. Although agitated and delirious behaviour may be caused by hypoglycaemia, hypoxia, or hypotension, several agents have direct central stimulatory effects including sympathomimetic agents, phencyclidine, and anticholinergic agents while others are primarily hallucinogenic including lysergic acid diethylamide, mescaline, and psilocybin. Numerous toxins such as isoniazid, tricyclic antidepressants, theophylline, and camphor are typically associated with seizures.

Evaluation of the cranial nerves, particularly those associated with ophthalmological function can often assist in the differential diagnosis. Mydriasis can be caused by the sympathetic effects of cocaine, amphetamines, and anticholinergic agents or by direct injury to the optic nerve which impairs light perception by toxins such as methanol. Miosis may be produced by the parasympathetic stimulation of organophosphates and nicotine or by the central effects of opioids and clonidine. Alterations in ocular movements, particularly nystagmus, can be horizontal as noted following exposure to phenytoin and ethanol, vertical, or even rotatory as noted following phencyclidine use.

The cutaneous examination can also be very informative. Cyanotic or bluish-coloured skin may indicate elevated methaemoglobin levels while diffuse flushing may be suggestive of anticholinergic toxicity, scombroid intoxication or a disulfiram reaction. Profound diaphoresis may be evidence of a sympathomimetic or parasympathetic intoxication. Needle tracks, tattoos, or cutaneous abcesses suggest intravenous drug abuse particularly with agents such as heroin, amphetamines, or cocaine.

Finally, evaluation of saliva, vomitus, faeces, or urine may reveal clues to the potential toxin involved. Patients with dry mucous membranes, decreased or absent bowel sounds, and urinary retention may be exhibiting anticholinergic effects from agents such as diphenhydramine or atropine. Emesis may be non-specific evidence of gastric irritation or result from exposure to iron, theophylline, or digoxin. Toxin associated diarrhoea may be caused by increased secretory function either by cellular stimulation due to organophosphates or by cellular destruction due to arsenic and colchicine toxicity. Particular odours may be associated with exposure to specific toxins such as an acetone or fruity odour due to isopropyl alcohol, a wintergreen odour due to methyl salicylate, vinyl-like due to ethchlorovinyl, and garlic when arsenic, thallium, and organophosphates have been ingested.

After the initial clinical evaluation has been completed, a careful assessment of these data may suggest a constellation of signs and symptoms that allows the physician to refine the differential diagnosis and direct therapy. These symptom complexes have been termed toxidromes. Five major toxidromes describe cholinergic, anticholinergic, sympathomimetic, opioid, and sedative-hypnotic poisoning. Table 4.1 includes a list of the typical features and common agents associated with these toxic syndromes.

Table 4.1 Common toxic syndromes (toxidromes)

Toxidrome	Signs	Agents commonly involved
Cholinergic		
Muscarinic	Bradycardia, miosis, SLUDGE; salivation, lacrimation, urination defecation, gastrointestinal upset, emesis	Organophosphate and carbamate pesticides, physostigmine, edrophonium, pilocarpine
Nicotinic	Tachycardia, hypertension, fasciculations, weakness	
Anticholinergic	Tachycardia, hyperthermia, dry and flushed skin, mydriasis, dry mucous membranes, decreased peristalsis, urinary retention, agitation, delirium	Atropine, antihistamines, tricyclic antidepressants, scopolamine, belladonna
Sympathomimetic	Tachycardia, hypertension, hyperthermia, diaphoresis, mydriasis, normal to increased peristalsis, agitation, delirium	Cocaine, amphetamines, theophylline, caffeine, monoamine oxidase inhibitors
Opioid	Hypopnoea, miosis, lethargy, stupor, coma	Heroin, morphine, methadone, propoxyphene, diphenoxylate
Sedative-hypnotic	Relative preservation of vital signs, occasional hypopnoea, hypotension, bradycardia, hypothermia, lethargy, stupor, coma	Ethanol, barbiturates, benzodiazepines, chloral hydrate, meprobamate, ethchlorvynol

TREATMENT

The goal of the next phase of therapy is to identify and reverse any life-threatening toxicity and to prevent further absorption of ingested agents. A patient with an altered mental status should be empirically treated for hypoxia and hypoglycaemia because both are rapidly and easily reversed, and if unaddressed can lead to permanent neurological sequelae (Krauss, 1971). While most clinicians would not hesitate to administer oxygen, significant controversy surrounds the empiric administration of hypertonic dextrose (D50W) in treating these patients (Browning et al., 1990).

Hypoglycaemia can be caused by a wide variety of drugs and toxins such as oral hypoglycaemics, insulin, ethanol, and salicylates, as well as medical conditions including sepsis, hepatic failure, and adrenal insufficiency. While the actual incidence of hypoglycaemia is uncertain, several studies support the perception that it is common. Malouf and Brust (1985) identified 125 hypoglycaemic patients who presented to an emergency department over a 12-month period. Hoffman et al. (1990) identified 29 cases of hypoglycaemia in a series of 340 consecutive paramedic dispatches for patients with an altered mental status (an incidence of 8.5%).

Most clinicians would not hesitate to treat empirically for any disorder with this high an incidence if the treatment was safe, effective, and inexpensive. However, whenever any drug or 'antidote' is utilized, the agent's potential complications and adverse effects must also be considered. Several animal models have demonstrated that hyperglycaemia prior to an ischaemic cerebral insult is associated with a greater neurological morbidity and an increased mortality (Myers and Yamaguchi, 1977; Siemkowicz and Gjedde, 1980; Pulsinelli et al., 1982; D'Alecy et al., 1986).

This raised preischaemic serum glucose concentration provides cerebral tissue with greater quantities of substrate for anaerobic glycolysis during ischaemia which enhances lactate formation. High levels of lactate are known to be cytotoxic (White and Krause, 1993). Although not definitively applicable to clinical medicine, these animal models have created concern regarding empiric dextrose administration to all patients with an altered level of consciousness.

Several human studies have also examined the relationship between initial serum glucose levels and neurological outcome in patients presenting with an acute cerebral ischaemic event (Pulsinelli et al., 1983; Longstreth and Inui, 1984; Woo et al., 1988a). Interpretation of these human data is difficult for a number of reasons. The uncontrolled confounding variables such as the patients' underlying medical conditions, particularly diabetes mellitus, may increase both the admission serum glucose and the morbidity associated with any vascular event. Of great concern in most of these studies has been the use of a single serum glucose measurement not consistently analyzed with regard to nutritional status or time since the initial phase of the ischaemic event. Transient or reactive hyperglycaemia is associated with multiple physiological stressors including acute cerebral vascular accidents (Melamed, 1976; Woo et al., 1988a). Therefore greater elevations in the blood glucose may simply identify those patients with more extensive ischaemic events. When 148 patients were followed for 180 days to evaluate long-term function, the association between an initially elevated serum glucose and short-term mortality was no longer noted (Matchar et al., 1992). This finding may not be contradictory of the initial studies but may represent a methodological bias in the previously cited studies in which patients were only followed for a short period of time.

Accurate identification and treatment of only those patients with hypoglycaemia would avoid any potential risk of hypertonic dextrose. Serum glucose determinations and clinical findings have been analyzed in this regard. Any blood specimen sent to the hospital laboratory for glucose measurement even under the best of circumstances, requires far too much time to be clinically practical. Alternatively, many physicians strongly promote the utilization of rapid reagent glucose determination tests (Belsey et al., 1987, Browning et al., 1990, Hoffman et al., 1992). Unfortunately these methods are not 100% accurate. Patient variables such as age and anaemia lead to inaccurate determinations as may a specimen contaminated with isopropanol from skin preparation (Graziatis and Sexson, 1980; Perelman et al., 1982; Barreau and Buttery, 1987). Two studies in the pre-hospital setting have demonstrated a false-negative rate of 6–8% (Lavery et al., 1991; Jones et al., 1992).

Another potential problem with the rapid reagent glucose determinations is that while they enhance our ability to determine numerical hypoglycaemia quickly, physicians should not rely solely on laboratory measurements for the establishment of this diagnosis. Hypoglycaemia can be defined as a blood glucose concentration of < 60 mg/dl or as a constellation of symptoms including tachycardia, diaphoresis, visual disturbances, tremor, and alteration in cognitive function ranging from poor concentration to lethargy or coma. Boyle et al. (1988) demonstrated that patients with poorly controlled diabetes mellitis became symptomatic at a mean blood glucose concentration of 78 mg/dl, which was a significantly higher level than that noted in non-diabetic controls who became symptomatic at a mean concentration of 53 mg/dl. These data raise concern that if only laboratory glucose measurements were used in evaluating patients with an altered sensorium, several patients suffering from clinical, but not numerical, hypoglycaemia would go untreated.

This controversial issue is best addressed by utilizing both clinical skills and rapid glucose determination to create a balanced approach to empiric D50W administration. The first subset of patients to focus on is the group with an altered mental status and a focal neurological examination. Although hypoglycaemia may manifest as a focal neurological deficit, the incidence of focality in known hypoglycaemic patients is only approximately 2.5% (Malouf and Brust, 1985). Alternatively, patients with cerebral infarctions typically present with focality and rarely have an altered level of consciousness. In this subset of patients with focality and a normal level of consciousness, the administration of D50W should be guided by rapid reagent glucose measurements to minimize potential adverse effects. For reasons stated above, in obtunded patients even if the rapid glucose test demonstrates euglycaemia, D50W should be empirically given regardless of the neurological examination. This also acknowledges the fact that patients who are comatose from cerebral vascular accidents have a grave prognosis and significant lesions involving either their reticular activating system or both cortices. Conversely, patients who are comatose secondary to hypoglycaemia will show significant clinical improvement following dextrose administration and restoration to euglycaemia may prevent post-hypoglycaemic encephalopathy (Krauss, 1971). Utilizing this strategy for the administration of empiric hypertonic glucose will allow those patients with hypoglycaemia the best chance of recovering normal neurological function.

GASTROINTESTINAL DECONTAMINATION

The objective of gastrointestinal decontamination is to limit the duration of exposure to a toxin in order to minimize the potential for injury or absorption. Decontamination can be accomplished by inducing emesis, by mechanical removal either with orogastric lavage, surgery, or endoscopy, or by limiting the systemic absorption through toxin adsorption to activated charcoal or by decreasing a toxin's bowel transit time with the use of whole bowel irrigation. The following discussion will address the controversial decontamination issues by focusing upon the efficacy, safety, and indications for each of these techniques.

Syrup of Ipecac

The role of syrup of ipecac is becoming more and more limited although it remains an appropriate and valuable tool in select situations. Syrup of ipecac is a preparation derived from the Cephaelis ipecacuanha plant which contains the alkaloids emetine and cephaeline. These agents induce emesis by direct irritation of gastric mucosa and through stimulation of the medullary chemoreceptor trigger zone. Following the administration of syrup of ipecac, approximately 85–90% of patients will have three or four episodes of vomiting, the first within 30 minutes (Robertson, 1962). The obligate delay to emesis allows continued drug absorption and enhanced toxicity. This delay is of particular concern for patients who have ingested rapidly acting agents or agents known to cause seizures or depression of consciousness because of the increased risk of aspiration.

Although it is clear that ipecac effectively induces emesis, concerns remain with regard to its ability to remove ingested agents and thus decrease the potential for toxicity. Various experimental models have demonstrated the removal of 28–38% of ingested toxins (Curtis et al., 1984; Tandberg et al., 1986; Tenenbein et al., 1987a). This amount of toxin removal is directly related to the duration between ingestion and administration of syrup of ipecac. Only one clinical study has demonstrated actual efficacy with syrup of ipecac use by correlating lower serum acetaminophen levels in children with the early administration of syrup of ipecac (Amitai et al., 1987).

Syrup of ipecac should be reversed for patients older than 1 year of age who have ingested a toxin within the previous 1–2 hours, and have a normal sensorium which is expected to remain intact for the next 2 hours. The greatest benefit may be expected for those agents that bind poorly to activated charcoal or sustained release formulations that will not rapidly produce lethargy or seizures. Although experimental evidence indicates limited drug removal, this 28–38% reduction in drug burden may diminish the potential morbidity or mortality.

Whenever use of syrup of ipecac is considered the clinician must realize that a significant delay of anywhere between 2.2 to 6.0 hours in the time to administration of activated charcoal may occur (Curtis et al., 1984; Kornberg and Dolgin, 1991). This delay is of particular concern when the toxin involved is well adsorbed to activated charcoal.

The syrup of ipecac should never be given to a patient with an altered level of consciousness or seizures, or to a patient who may have ingested a toxin known to cause these effects rapidly. This approach is based upon the high risk of aspiration pneumonitis following emesis in any patient with an altered level of consciousness. In addition, caustic agents may reinjure the oesophagus and those hydrocarbons with a high aspiration potential should be considered too high a risk for removal by emesis. Other complications, although rare, related to the use of syrup of ipecac include Mallory Weiss tears, pneumomediastinum, gastric rupture, and death (Tandberg et al., 1981; Wolowodiuk et al., 1984; Knight and Doucet, 1987).

Orogastric Lavage

Orogastric lavage is an equally controversial method of gastric emptying. This technique has experimentally been shown to remove approximately 30–35% of various ingested drugs (Burton et al., 1984; Tenenbein et al., 1987a; Danel et al., 1988). As noted with ipecac-induced emesis, the earlier orogastric lavage is performed, the more successful it is (Mathew et al., 1966). Most studies have been designed to consider drug recovery and not actual clinical outcome. Kulig et al. (1985) were the first investigators actually to demonstrate an improved clinical outcome with orogastric lavage (Kulig et al., 1985). In this study a benefit was only demonstrated in obtunded patients lavaged within 1 hour of their ingestion.

Orogastric lavage should be employed when gastric emptying may be beneficial but syrup of ipecac is contraindicated – for example in patients who have or who may soon develop an altered sensorium. Orogastric lavage is particularly useful when potentially lethal ingestions of toxins such as colchicine or mercuric chloride have occurred and when any delay in the use of activated charcoal could allow further absorption.

Complications of orogastric lavage include inadvertent tracheal intubation resulting in pneumothorax and death, oesophageal perforation, and dysrhythmias (Wald et al., 1986; Thompson et al., 1987). Orogastric lavage should not be performed for ingestions involving strong alkalis or large foreign bodies, particularly those that are sharp. Since the efficacy of orogastric lavage decreases as time since ingestion increases, patients with delayed presentations and those who have already vomited should not have orogastric lavage performed.

Another controversial issue associated with orogastric lavage is airway protection. Endotracheal intubation is neither essential nor absolute in the protection against aspiration during orogastric lavage. In fact, orogastric lavage can be performed in awake and unintubated patients without complications (Mathew et al., 1966; Thomas et al., 1981; Kulig et al., 1985) and in Roy's study of 72 patients who were intubated prior to gastrointestinal lavage and activated charcoal administration 25% subsequently had activated charcoal retrieved from their airway (Roy et al., 1989). Thus the need for endotracheal intubation should be based on the assessment of the airway and not on the decision to perform gastric emptying.

UTILITY OF GASTRIC EMPTYING

For the reasons noted above, particularly the risk–benefit analysis, more and more patients are managed without gastric emptying with most medical toxicologists relying solely on activated charcoal. Two prospective studies of poisoned and overdosed patients examined the benefits of initial gastric emptying versus activated charcoal or observation alone. Kulig et al. (1985) randomized 592 patients into two treatment groups. On even-numbered days, patients received activated charcoal alone and on odd-numbered days they received gastric emptying followed by activated charcoal. Gastric emptying was performed with the syrup of ipecac if the patient was alert and orogastric lavage if they were obtunded. As previously mentioned this study revealed that early lavage (within 1 h of ingestion) in obtunded patients led to a significant improvement in outcome. No benefit was identified with orogastric lavage performed more than 1 h following ingestion or with the syrup of ipecac at any time when compared to activated charcoal alone.

While this study was actually the first to demonstrate the clinical utility of orogastric lavage, it has more frequently been misinterpreted to suggest that orogastric lavage is ineffective in patients presenting more than 1 h after ingestion and that the syrup of ipecac is never indicated. The failure of a study to demonstrate a benefit does not imply that a benefit does not exist. The conclusion can merely be that this particular study design was inadequate to demonstrate a difference.

A second study by Merigian et al. (1990) randomized 808 overdosed patients to one of two gastric decontamination treatments. On even-numbered days asymptomatic patients were treated with activated charcoal alone and symptomatic patients received the syrup of ipecac if awake and orogastric lavage if lethargic. On odd-numbered days asymptomatic patients were solely observed while those who were symptomatic were treated with activated charcoal. This study was unable to find any benefit in treating asymptomatic patients with activated charcoal and actually noted an increase in aspiration in those symptomatic patients receiving gastric emptying.

These studies were biased against demonstrating any utility of gastric emptying. Both excluded patients who ingested toxins that were poorly adsorbed by activated charcoal; precisely those patients in whom gastric emptying was likely to be the more efficacious technique. In addition, patients who ingested agents with potential delayed toxicity, sustained release preparations, monoamine oxidase inhibitors, and acetaminophen, were also excluded (Merigian et al., 1990). This further biased the study against the benefits of gastric emptying because if patients were asymptomatic at presentation, the likelihood of deterioration was remote. Furthermore, some of the most gravely ill patients were placed in the orogastric lavage group in an unrandomized fashion, presumably for the ethical concern of withholding potentially beneficial therapy (Kulig et al., 1985).

These studies do provide further definition of the role of gastric emptying in the management of the overdosed or poisoned patient. In both studies the majority of patients did well when only activated charcoal and supportive care were utilized. The studies suggest that patients who present without symptoms or with a history of low-risk exposures can be treated with activated charcoal and observation alone. Those patients who present with obtundation in the first few hours after an ingestion may benefit from orogastric lavage. None of these data, however, provide any information about the use of gastric emptying in the management of unknown ingestions, in ingestions involving sustained-release preparations, or in those involving agents poorly adsorbed to activated charcoal.

Activated Charcoal

Activated charcoal has become a mainstay of therapy in gastrointestinal decontamination due to its capacity to adsorb the vast majority of toxins and thus potentially prevent their absorption. Activated charcoal is a fine black powder produced from the burning of carbon-containing compounds such as wood that is then 'activated' by steam to increase dramatically its surface area and thus its effective adsorptive capacity. The adsorption of toxins to activated charcoal occurs rapidly due to van der Waals forces which are influenced by the law of mass action.

Activated charcoal is inert and is neither reactive nor absorbed with no inherent toxic potential. Aspiration of activated charcoal has been reported to cause pneumonitis (Menzies et al., 1988) and bowel obstruction is a potential concern following multiple dose therapy (Watson et al., 1986). The actual act of ingesting activated charcoal is unfortunately often poorly tolerated, particularly in patients who are nauseated or vomiting. Creating a slurry with fruit juice or flavourings or simply administering the activated charcoal through a nasogastic tube as a drip rather than one large bolus may increase patient tolerance. Antiemetics may be utilized in standard doses, such as 10 mg of metoclopramide in adults, but if they are ineffective higher doses of up to 1–2 mg/kg, similar to the doses used during chemotherapy, may be indicated. A new antiemetic, ondansetron, has been shown to be effective in controlling vomiting associated with theophylline poisoning (Roberts et al., 1993).

While activated charcoal has been shown to limit the absorption of many agents (Neuvonen et al., 1978, McLuckie et al., 1990), metals such as iron and lithium, simple alcohols, hydrocarbons, and strong acids and bases are poorly adsorbed to activated charcoal. All these agents tend to be small or polar compounds.

The optimal dosing for activated charcoal remains an unanswered question. Studies indicate that an activated charcoal to toxin ratio of 10:1 by weight provides optimal adsorption for those agents well-adsorbed to activated charcoal (Olkkola, 1985). While this ratio may be easily achieved in patients with ingestions of digoxin where often only milligrams of the toxin are involved, under other circumstances such as in the ingestion of salicylates and theophylline where the quantities ingested are much greater, this ratio is often not feasible. The recommended dose of activated charcoal of 1 g/kg body weight is based on ease of administration and patient tolerance, and fortunately it often also achieves this ratio. Any patient who has ingested a toxin should receive at least one dose of activated charcoal unless more valuable interventions may be impeded such as endoscopy in a caustic ingestion.

Cathartics

Cathartics such as magnesium citrate and sorbitol are often utilized during gastrointestinal decontamination particularly in conjunction with activated charcoal. They stimulate bowel evacuation by creating an intraluminal osmotic load that draws body water into the gastrointestinal tract. While intuitively, this increase in gastrointestinal motility would be beneficial in removing toxins prior to absorption, there is little data supporting this premise. Several studies have been unable to demonstrate any efficacy in cathartic use (McNamara et al., 1983; Neuvonen and Olkkola, 1986). Only one study by Keller et al., demonstrated a significant reduction in blood salicylate levels when sorbitol was used in addition to activated charcoal when compared to activated charcoal alone. No clinical outcome differences have been noted.

Adverse effects of cathartics include prolonged nausea, vomiting, and abdominal cramping and fluid and electrolyte abnormalities including hypernatraemia, hypermagnesaemia, and hypocalcaemia (Farley, 1986; Smilkstein et al., 1988). These complications are of particular concern in the elderly and in children and have resulted in death (Brett et al., 1989).

Despite the paucity of data supporting their use, most toxicologists include a cathartic with the first dose of activated charcoal to help prevent constipation (Riegel and Becker, 1981). However, they should only be given with the first dose and then only if peristalsis is noted. Several pharmaceutical companies distribute activated charcoal premixed with sorbitol. The failure to identify these preparations may lead to inadvertent repeat dosing of cathartics which may result in severe fluid and electrolyte shifts particularly in infants. Cathartics should not be given prior to adequate fluid resuscitation or in any ingestion involving a drug known to induce diarrhoea.

Whole Bowel Irrigation

Whole bowel irrigation has been used traditionally for bowel preparation prior to colonoscopy, barium enema, or gastrointestinal surgery. In toxic ingestions it is ideal for sustained release products particularly theophylline, calcium channel blockers and β-adrenergic antagonists, for toxins poorly adsorbed to activated charcoal such as iron and lithium, and for 'body packers' who smuggle within their gastrointestinal tract large quantities of carefully packaged drugs such as cocaine or heroin (Tenenbein et al., 1987b; Hoffman et al., 1990; Smith et al., 1991).

Whole bowel irrigation utilizes large volumes of a solution of polyethylene glycol to flush the bowel mechanically. Because of its isosmotic and isotonic electrolyte formulation, no fluid or electrolyte abnormalities have been observed. It is performed by administering 0.5 l/h in chidren and 2 l/h in adults usually via a nasogastric tube for 5–6 h until the rectal effluent is clear (Davis et al., 1980). Ideally the patient should be placed on a bedside commode due to the large volumes of stool produced. Common complaints include anal irritation, abdominal discomfort particularly bloating, and vomiting. Contraindications are few and include patients with intestinal ileus or perforation.

Despite the ability of whole bowel irrigation to evacuate the entire gastrointestinal tract in a few hours it cannot be recommended for use in all ingestions. Several experimental in vitro models demonstrated significant release of toxins including cocaine, salicylates, and theophylline from activated charcoal in the presence of polyethylene glycol (Kirshenbaum et al., 1990; Makosiej et al., 1990; Hoffman et al., 1991). Therefore, if any toxin is well adsorbed to activated charcoal, addition of whole bowel irrigation may decrease the activated charcoal's effectiveness in the prevention of absorption. In overdoses in which both therapies are valuable particularly in a severe sustained-release calcium channel antagonist or theophylline ingestion, alternating the activated charcoal doses with the polyethylene glycol doses, is probably the most practical approach.

CONCLUSION

The initial management of potentially poisoned patients is both a demanding and extremely rewarding experience. The importance of developing an organized and directed method of rapidly collecting both historical and clinical data cannot be overemphasized. Recognition of specific toxic syndromes and anticipation of potential manifestations of a particular agent's toxicity are critical to determine logically and effectively the most appropriate therapeutic interventions. Gastrointestinal decontamination is both a fundamental and rapidly evolving core concept in the management of potentially poisoned or overdosed patients. The choice of which decontamination modalities to use is based on the actual or potential severity of the toxicity and the consequences, risks, and contraindications associated with each method considered for each individual. Activated charcoal has been the best studied agent and due to its widespread efficacy and limited contraindications and complications it is the preferred therapy under most circumstances. The routine use of the syrup of ipecac or orogastric lavage in all ingestions is to be condemned, however they both retain their value in appropriate patients, particularly when the benefits of activated charcoal are limited.

REFERENCES

Amitai, Y., Mitchel, A.A., McGuigen, M.A. et al. (1987) Ipecac-induced emesis and reduction of plasma concentrations of drugs following accidental overdose in children. *Pediatrics* **80**: 364–370.

Barreau, P.B., Buttery, J.E. (1987) The effect of the hematocrit value on the determination of glucose levels by reagent-strip methods. *Medical Journal of Australia* **147**: 286–288.

Belsey, R., Morrison, I., Whitlow, K.J. et al. (1987) Managing beside glucose testing in the hospital. *Journal of the American Medical Association* **258**: 948–960.

Boyle, P.J., Schwartz, N.S., Shah, S.D. et al. (1988) Plasma glucose concentration at the onset of hypoglycemic symptoms in patients with poorly controlled diabetes and in nondiabetics. *New England Journal of Medicine* **318**: 1487–1492.

Brett, J., Kulig, K., Rumack, B.H. (1989) Iatrogenic death from sorbitol and magnesium sulfate during treatment for salicylism. *Veterinary and Human Toxicology 31*: 334.

Browning, R.G., Olson, D.W., Stueven, H.A., Mateer, J.R. (1990) 50% dextrose: Antidote or toxin? *Annals of Emergency Medicine* **19**: 683–687.

Burton, B.T., Bayer, M.J., Barron, L. et al. (1984) Comparison of activated charcoal and gastric lavage in the prevention of aspirin absorption. *Journal of Emergency Medicine* **1**: 411–416.

Caravati, E.M., McElwee, N.E. (1991) Use of clinical toxicology resources by emergency physicians and its impact on poison control centers. *Annals of Emergency Medicine* **20**: 147–150.

Curtis, R.A., Bartone, J., Giacona, N. (1984) Efficacy of ipecac and activated charcoal/cathartic: Prevention of salicylate absorption in a simulated overdose. *Archives of Internal Medicine* **144**: 48–52.

D'Alecy, L.G., Lundy, E.F., Barton, K.J. et al. (1986) Dextrose containing intravenous fluid impairs outcome and increases death after eight minutes of cardiac arrest and resuscitation in dogs. *Surgery* **100**: 505–511.

Danel, V., Henry, J.A., Glucksman, E. (1988) Activated charcoal, emesis, and gastric lavage in aspirin overdose. *British Medical Journal* **296**: 1507–1512.

Davis, G.R., Santa Ana, C.A., Morawski, S.G. et al. (1980) Development of a lavage solution associated with minimal water and electrolyte absorption or secretion. *Gastroenterology* **78**: 991–995.

Farley, T.A. (1986) Severe hypernatremic dehydration after use of an activated charcoal-sorbitol suspension. *Journal of Pediatrics* **109**: 719.

Graziatis, D.M., Sexson, W.R. (1980) Erroneously high Dextrostix values caused by isopropyl alcohol. *Pediatrics* **66**: 221–223.

Hoffman, R.S., Smilkstein, M.R., Goldfrank, L.R. (1990) Whole bowel irrigation and the cocaine body-packer. *American Journal of Emergency Medicine* **8**: 523–527.

Hoffman, R.S., Chiang, W.K., Howland, M.A. et al. (1991) Theophylline desorption from activated charcoal caused by whole bowel irrigation *Journal of Toxicology and Clinical Toxicology* **29**: 191–202.

Hoffman, U.R., Schriger, D.L., Votey, S.R. et al. (1992) The empiric use of hypertonic dextrose in patients with altered mental status: A reappraisal. *Annals of Emergency Medicine* **21**: 20–24.

Jones, J.L., Ray, V.G., Gough, J.E., et al. (1992) Determination of prehospital blood glucoses: A prospective controlled study. *American Journal of Emergency Medicine* **10**: 679–682.

Keller, R.E., Schwab, R.A., Krenzclok, E.P. (1990) Contribution of Sorbitol combined with activated charcoal in prevention of salicylate absorption. *Annals of Emergency Medicine* **19**: 654–656.

Kirshenbaum, L.A., Sitar, D.S., Tenebein, M. (1990) Interaction between whole bowel solution and activated charcoal. *Annals of Emergency Medicine* **19**: 1129–1132.

Knight, K.M., Doucet, H.J. (1987) Gastric rupture and death caused by ipecac syrup. *Southern Medical Journal* **80**: 786.

Kornberg, A.E., Dolgin, J. (1991) Pediatric ingestions: Charcoal alone versus ipecac and charcoal. *Annals of Emergency Medicine* **20**: 648–651.

Krauss, S. (1971) Post-hypoglycaemic encephalopathy. *British Medical Journal* **2**: 591.

Kulig, K., Bar-Or, D., Cantrill, S.V. et al. (1985) Management of acutely poisoned patients without gastric emptying. *Annals of Emergency Medicine* **14**: 562–567.

Kushner, M., Nenicni, Reivich, M. et al. (1988) Relation of hyperglycemia early in ischemic brain infarction to cerebral anatomy, metabolism and clinical outcome. *American Journal of Emergency Medicine Annals of Neurology* **28**: 129–135.

Lavery, R.F., Allegra, J.R., Cody, R.P. et al. (1991) A prospective evaluation of glucose reagent teststrips in the prehospital setting. *American Journal of Emergency Medicine* **9**: 304–308.

Longstreth, W.T. Jr., Inui, T.S. (1984) High blood glucose level on hospital admission and poor neurological recovery after cardiac arrest. *Annals of Neurology* **15**: 59–63.

McNamara, R.M., Aaron, C.K., Gemborys, M. et al. (1983) Sorbitol catharsis does not enhance efficacy of charcoal in a simulated acetaminophen overdose. *Annals of Emergency Medicine* **17**: 243–246.

McLuckie, A., Forbes, A.M., Ilett, K.F. (1990) Role of repeated doses of oral activated charcoal in the treatment of acute intoxications. *Anaesthesia and Intensive Care* **18**: 375–384.

Makosiej, F., Hoffman, R.S., Howland, M.A. (1990) Cocaine adsorption to activated charcoal: The effects of pH. (abstract) *Veterinary and Human Toxicology* **32**: 350.

Malouf, R., Brust, J.C.M. (1985) Hypoglycemia: Causes, neurologic manifestations, and outcome. *Annals of Neurology* **17**: 421–430.

Malouf, R., Brust, J.C.M. (1995) Hypoglycaemia: Causes, neurological manifestations and outcome. *Neurology* **7**: 421–430.

Matchar, D.B., Divine G.W., Heyman A. et al. (1992): The influence of hyperglycemia on outcome of cerebral infarction. *Annals of Internal Medicine* **117**: 449–456.

Mathew, H., Mackintosh, T.F., Tompsett, S.L. et al. (1966) Gastric aspiration and lavage in acute poisoning. *British Medical Journal* **1**: 1333.

Melamed, E. (1976) Reactive hyperglycemia in patients with acute stroke. *Journal of Neurological Science* **29**: 267–275.

Menzies, D.G., Busuttil, A., Prescott, L.F. (1988) Fatal pulmonary aspiration of oral activated charcoal. *British Medical Journal* **297**: 459–460.

Merigian, K.S., Woodard, M., Hedges, J.R. et al. (1990) Prospective evaluation of gastric emptying in the poisoned patient. *American Journal of Emergency Medicine* **8**: 479–483.

Myers, R.E., Yamaguchi, S. (1977) Nervous system effects of cardiac arrest in monkeys. *Archives of Neurology* **34**: 65–74.

Neuvonen, P.J., Olkkola, K.T. (1986) Effect of purgatives on antidotal efficacy of oral activated charcoal. *Human Toxicology* **5**: 255–263.

Neuvonen, P.J., Elfving, S.M., Elonen, E. (1978) Reduction of absorption of digoxin, phenytoin and aspirin by activated charcoal in man. *European Journal of Clinical Pharmacology* **13**: 213–218.

Olkkola, K.T. (1985) Effect of charcoal-drug ratio on antidotal efficacy of oral activated charcoal in man. *British Journal of Clinical Pharmacology* **19**: 767–772.

Perelman, R.H., Gutcher, G.R., Engle, M.J. et al. (1982) Comparative analysis of four methods for rapid glucose determination in neonates. *American Journal of Diseases of Children* **136**: 1051–1053.

Pulsinelli, W.A., Waldman, S., Rawlinson, D. et al. (1982) Moderate hyperglycemia augments ischemic brain damage: A neuropathic study in the rat. *Neurology* **32**: 1239–1246.

Pulsinelli, W.A., Levy, D.E., Sigsbee, B. et al. (1983) Increased damage after ischemic stroke in patients with hyperglycemia with or without established diabetis mellitus. *American Journal of Medicine* **74**: 540–544.

Riegel, J.M., Becker, C.E. (1981) Use of cathartics in toxic ingestions. *Annals of Emergency Medicine* **10**: 254–358.

Roberts, J.R., Carney, S., Boyle, S.M. et al. (1993) Ondansetron quells drug-resistant emesis in theophylline poisoning. *American Journal of Emergency Medicine* **11**: 609–610.

Robertson, W.O. (1962) Syrup of ipecac-A slow or fast emetic. *American Journal of Diseases of Children* **103**: 136–139.

Roy, T.M., Ossorio, M.A., Dipolla, L.M. et al. (1989) Pulmonary complications after tricyclic antidepressant poisoning. *Chest* **96**: 852–858.

Siemkowicz, E., Gjedde, A. (1980) Post-ischemic coma in rat: Effect of different pre-ischemic blood glocose levels on cerebral metabolic recovery after ischemia. *Acta Physiologica Scandinavica* **110**: 225–232.

Smilkstein, M.J., Steedle, D., Kulig, K.W. et al. (1988) Magnesium levels after magnesium-containing carthartics. *Clinical Toxicology* **26**: 51–65.

Smith, S.W., Ling, L.J., Halstenson, C.E. (1991) Whole bowel irrigation as a treatment for acute lithium overdose. *Annals of Emergency Medicine* **20**: 536–539.

Tandberg, D., Liechty, E.J., Fishbein, D. (1981) Mallory-Weiss syndrome: An unusual complication of ipecac-induced emesis. *Annals of Emergency Medicine* **10**: 521.

Tandberg, D., Diven, B.G., McLeod, J.W. (1986) Ipecac-induced emesis versus gastric lavage. *American Journal of Emergency Medicine* **4**: 205–209.

Tenenbein, M.D., Cohen, S., Sitar, D.S. (1987a) Efficacy of ipecac induced emesis, orogastric lavage, and activated charcoal for acute drug overdose. *Annals of Emergency Medicine* **16**: 838–841.

Tenenbein, M.D., Cohen, S., Sitar, D.S. (1987b) Whole bowel decontamination procedure after acute drug overdose. *Archives of Internal Medicine* **147**: 905–907.

Thomas, R.T., Sterling, M.L., Salness, K. et al. (1981) Absence of pulmonary aspiration in adults after gastric lavage without endotracheal intubation. *Veterinary and Human Toxicology* **23**(suppl. 1): 51.

Thompson, A.M., Robins, J.B., Prescott, L.F. (1987) Changes in cardiorespiratory function during gastric lavage for drug overdose. *Human Toxicology* **6**: 215–221.

Wald, P., Stern, J., Weiner, B. et al. (1986) Esophageal tear following forceful removal of an impacted orogastric lavage tube. *Annals of Emergency Medicine* **15**: 80–82.

Watson, P.M., Wang, R., Mercurio, M. et al. (1986) The gastrointestinal obstruction associated with multiple dose activated charcoal. *Journal of Emergency Medicine* **4**: 401–407.

White, B.C., Krause, G.S. (1993) Brain injury and repair mechanisms: The potential for pharmacologic therapy closed head trauma. *Annals of Emergency Medicine* **22**: 959–969.

Wolowodiuk, O.J., McMicken, D.B., O'Brien, P. (1984) Pneumomediastinum and retropneumoperitonium: An unusual complication of ipecac-induced emesis. *Annals of Emergency Medicine* **13**: 1148–1151.

Woo, E., Chan, Y.W., Yu, Y.L., Huang, C.Y. (1988a) Admission glucose levels in relation to mortality and morbidity outcome in 252 stroke patients. *Stroke* **19**: 185–191.

Woo, E., Ma, J.T.C., Robinson, J.D., et al. (1988b) Hyperglycemia is a stress response in acute stroke. *Stroke* **19**: 1359–1364.

Wright, N. (1980) An assessment of the unreliability of the history given by self-poisoned patients. *Journal of Toxicology and Clinical Toxicology* **16**: 381–384.

5

Treatment Limitation Decisions

J.F. Bion

BACKGROUND

The physician-surgeon who wrote what is now known as the Edwin Smith surgical papyrus was well aware of the limits to his skills. All the diseases were classified according to a simple scheme: 'a disease I will treat'; 'a disease with which I will contend'; or 'a disease not to be treated'. Few doctors would now recognize the last category. In the last 100 years medical practice has changed from clinical observation and therapeutic limitation to applied basic science and considerable therapeutic power. We can now interfere with many pathophysiological processes at genetic, molecular, cellular, whole organ, and systemic levels. Unfortunately, advances in moral and ethical development have not kept pace with those in technology. Indeed, technological developments are presenting new and unanticipated ethical dilemmas, reminding one of Bertrand Russell's dictum: '... as skill increases, wisdom fades'. These technological developments are usually more expensive than those they replace, but the benefits are often modest and limited to a small number of individuals, or may not even have been subject to proper evaluation. Remarkable reductions in mortality were produced by insulin in diabetics, penicillin in patients with pneumococcal pneumonia (Austrian and Gold, 1964), and tracheal intubation and positive pressure ventilation in patients with respiratory failure from polio (Lassen, 1953), of a degree which made statistical analysis superfluous. However, to reduce the residual mortality rate still further requires more complex studies, more complex statistics, more complex treatments, and certainly much more money, as studies of pneumococcal pneumonia (Hook et al., 1983) or the anti-endotoxin HA-1A (centoxin) trial (Schulman et al., 1991; Ziegler et al., 1991) have demonstrated in the context of Gram-negative sepsis.

At what point do these marginal costs and lost opportunity costs become unacceptable? Rising health care expenditure combined with the current international recession have made governments more aware of the importance of cost-containment and technology assessment in health care (Teres and Rapoport, 1994). Rationing is not merely an inevitable part of this exercise: it has always been present. The only difference is that whereas rationing was previously implicit or an accepted part of social inequalities, it is now becoming explicit and subject to critical examination, as in Oregon (Duggan, 1989). Doctors have tended to be reluctant to deal with the practical and ethical issues of rationing or treatment limitation, and this is unfortunate, because in the absence of informed debate decisions may be driven solely by economics. The reasons for this reluctance are complex, but in part are based on the cultural perceptions of the western world, particularly that of English libertarian tradition, which tends to interpret the needs of society in terms of those of the individual. While this helps to concentrate the mind when considering the impact of policy on real people, it makes it difficult to explore issues in the reverse direction: what is the impact on society of treating this individual? Health care professionals have generally been much more vocal in exposing the former component than in informing the latter, perhaps because determining societal issues involves sharing decision-making with many other groups, with consequent loss of territorial power.

The tension between what is possible and what is appropriate in medicine is particularly evident in the intensive care unit (ICU) where refinements in organ-system support allow the death of an individual patient to be deferred for weeks or months at considerable emotional and financial cost. The latter is easier to measure of course, and it is well recognized that it costs approximately twice as much to die in intensive care as it does to survive (Sage et al., 1986), and that when costs are expressed per survivor, certain categories consume quite disproportionate amounts of the intensive care budget (Chassin, 1982). Critical care medicine is an obvious target for health economists, particularly in the USA where 10–15% of the hospital budget and 1% of the gross national product is spent on intensive care. The reasons for the high costs of death are obvious enough, but not the solutions. Patients die despite organ-system support either because the severity of the acute illness has produced irretrievable damage, or because of pre-existing limitation to physiological reserve, or because the pathophysiological process is poorly understood and there is no specific treatment available. They die late and at greater expense because prognostic uncertainty makes medical staff reluctant to discontinue supportive treatment (Detsky et al., 1981). The wasteful use of resources on patients who subsequently die deprives other patients of treatment, and would probably not be in accordance with anyone's wishes including those of the patient, assuming that the outcome could have been determined with certainty. The problem is that death is virtually inevitable if treatment is withdrawn from a critically ill patient, whereas the same certainty does not usually apply to continuing treatment. Even more remote and uncertain are the risks and benefits to society of continuing or withdrawing treatment of an individual. To help us manage these problems we need to develop a strategy which sets specific therapeutic goals and minimizes prognostic uncertainty for individual patients, and which attempts to quantify marginal and opportunity costs in both financial and emotional terms. Treatment limitation decisions are an integral part of this strategy.

'DO NOT RESUSCITATE' ORDERS

The term commonly used to describe treatment limitation decisions in North America is the 'do not resuscitate' order, or DNR. The DNR order was a consequence of the development of cardiopulmonary resuscitation in 1960 (Kouwenhoven et al., 1960), with the growing realization that hospital cardiac arrest teams were not always called appropriately, in part because of the poor quality of documentation. Proposals to formalize such decisions were first published by the American Heart Association in 1974, with policies being published by the Beth Israel Hospital 2 years later (Rabkin et al., 1976). DNR orders in the USA are subject to professional (Quill et al., 1986) and (in certain states) legal (Kamer et al., 1990) constraints, which have improved the quality of documentation in the patients' case records, if nothing else.

In the UK a recent point-prevalence survey (Aarons and Beeching, 1991) of one hospital has shown that failure to provide written confirmation of unsuitability for resuscitation in either the medical or nursing case records would have resulted in the arrest team being called to 46 of 88 patients clearly perceived as unsuitable for such efforts. Conversely, decisions not to resuscitate patients in the event of a cardiac arrest may be documented in the notes but have been formulated without discussion with either patient or relatives: following one such incident the Health Service Commissioner (Health Service Commission 1990/1991) and the Chief Medical Officer (1991) have issued guidelines emphasizing the responsibility of consultant staff (rather than trainees) for making and transmitting information about such decisions, the need for written hospital policies, and for proper consultation with the patient or relatives. While this may not prevent all inappropriate attempts at resuscitation, hospital policies may make them less common. As only one in nine resuscitation attempts will produce a hospital survivor (Tunstall-Pedoe et al., 1992), and in one study approximately half the survivors of resuscitation did not wish to be resuscitated again were they to have sustained another cardiopulmonary arrest in the future (Bedell et al., 1983), it seems likely that a proportion of resuscitation attempts are being performed on patients who cannot benefit, and who might prefer to be allowed to die peacefully. Identifying patients who cannot benefit from resuscitation, or who would choose not to undergo it, is important for more than the immediate ethical considerations. Only one third of the 40% of patients who survive the initial resuscitation will leave hospital (Tunstall-Pedoe et al., 1992), and because many of them will have been admitted to intensive care following the initial successful resuscitation, this represents a significant allocation of resources on patients who ultimately die.

TREATMENT LIMITATION DECISIONS IN THE ICU

In ICUs the term 'DNR' is sometimes used to include treatment restriction or withdrawal (Teres, 1993), since many patients are already receiving respiratory support. However, DNR orders strictly refer to only one of several possible levels of care, while 'treatment limitation order' (TLO) is a less restrictive term than DNR, and aims to make the limitations of intensive care and the potential benefits or burdens of therapy explicit to all concerned. TLOs may be classified as unlimited therapy, therapy with specific exclusions (such as cardiac massage, mechanical ventilation, or renal dialysis), comfort care alone, or withdrawal of all support in the case of brainstem death. It could also include euthanasia, though this is not specifically considered here. It is likely that TLOs are widely employed in intensive care practice, though most of the published literature relates specifically to DNRs.

Several surveys of written DNRs in intensive care have been reported (Youngner et al., 1985; Zimmerman et al., 1986; Jayes et al., 1993; Parker et al., 1993; Koch et al., 1994), and there is evidence that in the USA their use has become more common. Jayes and colleagues (1993) surveyed 42 ICUs as part of the APACHE III study, and found that of 17 440 admissions, written DNR orders were applied to 9%; interestingly, the proportion varied between ICUs from 1.5% to 22%. Sixty per cent of all deaths were preceded by DNR orders, which were associated with patients in poorer prior health, more co-morbidities, greater severity of illness, and higher costs of care. Fifteen per cent of patients with DNR orders survived to leave hospital, which emphasizes the fact that these were treatment limitation decisions, not treatment withdrawal. This study also highlights the apparent disparity between chronic health status as an important determinant of decisions to withdraw treatment, and the very limited contribution which the same variable makes to the total APACHE III score when used to predict outcome (Knaus et al., 1991). The reason for this is perhaps that chronic ill health may only become manifest (i.e. measurable) when the individual is exposed to an acute illness. When this occurs, because physiological reserve is limited there is a proportionately greater change in acute physiology. Limited reserve then exaggerates the acute response to a given stimulus. This should be kept in mind when considering the use of physiologically-based systems for clinical decision-making outside the ICU where they have not been validated.

Several factors complicate the use of TLOs in the ICU. These are loss of autonomy on the part of the patient, prognostic uncertainty on the part of the physician, the competing demand for scarce ICU resources in some countries, and the inevitability of death if life-support is withdrawn. TLOs should therefore be based on a consensus assessment of individual risk–benefit, incorporate the opinions of the patient (if known) or close relatives, be clearly documented in the case record, and reviewable. These points are considered below.

Assessment and Measurement of Risk–benefit

This should mean measuring the differing risks and benefits to an individual patient and to society of initiating, continuing, limiting or withdrawing treatment. Risks and benefits include death and survival, the quality of living or dying, morbidity, and emotional and financial cost. It is doubtful if systems of measurement could ever be devised to accomplish this task with any degree of accuracy. We do not know how to measure quality of death or the emotional costs of care, and cannot predict outcomes at different treatment levels with any degree of certainty. Quality of life measures are available (Bowling, 1991), but our ability to predict what that quality will be is really quite limited. The most important determinant of quality of life of survivors of intensive care is pre-morbid health status (Sage, 1986; Mahul et al., 1991), but unfortunately doctors are often poor judges of their patients' perceived quality of life (Uhlmann and Pearlman, 1991). What we can do is to quantify the importance of three of the four factors which determine outcome from critical illness: severity, physiological reserve, and diagnosis. The fourth factor, therapeutic skill and specificity, is perhaps best assessed indirectly through morbidity rates and mortality ratios. Financial costs can be calculated either directly, or expressed as the proportion of bed days allocated to non-survivors. Analysis of this data in conjunction with information on deferred or refused admissions can help clinicians to identify the extent to which resources are being misapplied, as this is an important part of establishing a policy for treatment limitation orders.

Individual Risk-benefit

Severity scoring systems such as APACHE III, SAPS II and MPM II use mortality as their end-point, and have overall correct classification rates for groups of patients of around 80–85%. These systems have been validated in groups of patients admitted to the ICU, but not for other clinical areas or different levels of care. Predicting the risk of cardiopulmonary arrest outside the ICU is a less well-refined science. Sax and Charleson (1987) identified ward patients with unstable or deteriorating conditions and those with acute dyspnoea as being at particular risk, and this has been confirmed in other studies (Franklin and Mathew, 1994; Schien et al., 1990; Rubins and Moskowitz, 1988) but few scoring systems have been developed to quantify the degree of risk. One such method, the pre-arrest morbidity index (George et al., 1989), identifies hypotension, renal failure, cancer, pneumonia and a housebound lifestyle as the most important adverse factors for cardiopulmonary arrest. The same variables also predict a poor outcome from resuscitation, in particular a housebound lifestyle (Bedell et al., 1983; Urberg and Ways, 1987; Keatinge, 1989), though these reports do not state to what extent knowledge of these factors influenced the duration and intensity of therapeutic efforts at resuscitation. As mentioned above, physiologically-based predictive systems tend to underestimate the independent contribution which chronic disease makes to mortality risk, because limited physiological reserve is often occult, and tends to be expressed as an exaggerated change in acute physiology. They are therefore unlikely to be useful for the calculation of risk before an acute event. We need the equivalent of the cardiac treadmill for other organ-systems if we are to quantify limited physiological reserve with any accuracy.

Once patients have been admitted to intensive care, severity scoring systems may be helpful as an adjunct to clinical judgement; but it must be remembered that they provide continuous probabilities of risk for groups of patients, while what is needed is a dichotomous prediction of outcome for an individual: an 80% predicted mortality identifies a very sick population, but does not tell us whether this *specific* patient is one of the 80% who will die or one of the 20% who will survive. For this reason their role should be limited to confirming a clinical decision arrived at independently, or to refuting it, but they should not substitute for experienced clinical assessment. Two studies have tried to examine the impact of prognostic information on clinical practice in intensive care (Knaus et al., 1990; Murray et al., 1993). The study by Murray used the Glasgow Coma Scale to provide predictions of outcome following head injury, and found that this was associated with a reduction of 39% in the frequency of use of osmotic diuretics and intubation and ventilation in the poorest outcome group. There was no corresponding change in mortality rates or the frequency of writing DNR orders however. The authors interpreted these results as showing that, when medical staff are given access to predictions of outcome, this reduces the wasteful use of intensive care resources on patients who cannot benefit, without increasing the risks of withdrawing treatment from potential survivors. This was a 3-year study involving four neurosurgical units and 1025 patients with head injury; the difficulties of conducting such research in the more heterogeneous environment of general intensive care should not be underestimated.

One of the potential advantages of severity scoring systems in decision analysis is that they can provide an objective, broad and composite view of risk. Subjective assessments of a patient's condition are often unduly influenced by the function of specific organ systems because the clinician fails to take a wider view of previous health or the current status of other organ systems, or does not observe trends. Dynamic scoring systems are an important potential development in this respect, because they can provide an index of response to treatment. Failure to correct physiological disturbance carries an adverse prognosis while reversal of pathophysiology has a good prognosis (Wagner et al., 1986), and these changes can be quantified (Bion et al., 1988; Chang et al., 1988). Further work is needed either to refine or to simplify dynamic scoring systems and to examine their utility as an aid to clinical decision-making. Opponents of scoring systems should remember that objective estimates of risk may identify patients in whom treatment should be continued, not just those from whom it should be withdrawn. Conversely, few decisions to withdraw treatment from critically ill patients are taken without anxiety about the appropriateness of the decision or the outcome, and scoring systems may help to quantify the degree of uncertainty: the closer the predicted risk is to 50%, the greater the uncertainty about the outcome. Scoring systems do not tell us if we were right, but they may help to warn us of a wrong decision.

The third main determinant of risk which may influence the extent of treatment is diagnosis. For example, haematological malignancy and bone marrow transplantation are well recognized as having an extremely poor prognosis when complicated by respiratory failure (Denardo et al., 1989; Faber-Langendoen et al., 1993), and many clinicians would no longer refer such patients for intensive care. There are two potential problems with this approach. The first is that it assumes there will be no therapeutic advances (such as stem cell growth factors) which might improve outcome. The second is that it ignores the important contribution which intensive care can make to diagnosing the cause of respiratory failure: diagnostic bronchoscopy may be impossible unless the patient is intubated and ventilated, and a pneumococcal pneumonia may have different prognostic implications from that caused by cytomegalovirus. Diagnoses with a particularly poor prognosis should be identified early because it may be possible to formulate policies about ICU admission and duration of treatment which can then be discussed with the patient and family.

At this stage, then, we can identify patients outside the ICU who may be at high risk of cardiopulmonary arrest and a poor outcome from resuscitation, patients in the ICU with a high mortality risk, and patients whose quality of life following intensive care will be poor because it was already very limited before the acute event. Unfortunately, these are often not the 'difficult' patients. The patients who give us the greatest difficulties emotionally and ethically are relatively young with little antecedent disease, and have sustained irreversible damage to one or more organ systems. The fact that they are in a high mortality group does not solve the problem: organ-system support can be continued for weeks. The key to these very difficult decisions is identifying the fact that the disease process is irreversible. Irreversibility implies that treatment is futile. The concept of therapeutic futility has received some attention recently (Tomlinson and Brody, 1990; Hansen-Flaschen, 1991; Truog et al., 1992). Futile means useless, or producing no end result; and while this may be true in physiological terms of activities such as organ-system support for a brain-dead patient for example, it is not futile if that patient becomes an organ donor. Futility as a term is therefore not value-free, and it also depends on probabilities as does any other prediction. There are no simple solutions, but objective dynamic methods of severity measurement – if they can be developed – in conjunction with measures of therapeutic intensity, may become useful aids to clinical judgement by providing independent evidence of irreversibility of disease (Cullen, 1977; Bion et al., 1988; Chang et al., 1988).

Risks and Benefits to Society

Once individual patients or patient groups at risk of a poor outcome have been identified, the next step is to determine the financial costs of care, and contrast these with the costs of not treating other patients. The costs incurred in treating patients should ideally be expressed per year of life gained, with adjustment for quality of life. The lost opportunity costs are more complex to derive because although records of refused or delayed admissions may be kept, one rarely has information about patients who should have been referred but were not. The outcome of refused admissions also depends upon the time in the evolution of the patient's illness at which the referral was made, and the type of alternative treatment which was provided on the ward. At a practical level, I doubt that this degree of detail is achievable, or that our understanding of quality measurement is sufficiently mature. What we can do is to use information about current resource allocation to initiate wider discussion of the issues involved. The concept that useless treatment is wrong because it deprives others of the chance of cure has been given legal authority in the British Court of Appeal by Lord Justice Balcombe (Re J, 1990; Report, 1992), though a very different judgement has been made in a similar instance in the US Court of Appeal (Miller, 1994). If 20% of the ICU budget is consumed by 5% of the patients, and all of these die, it seems reasonable to ask whether this wasted expenditure was appropriate, and if not, how it could have been avoided. If clinical practice can be changed, one has the opportunity to redirect funding to alternative uses, such as high dependency care, earlier intervention, or another area of medicine altogether. Such decisions must involve wide discussion with an informed public. The Oregon 'experiment' of allowing the entire population of a State to determine health care priorities is the best recent example of this approach (Duggan, 1989), but no one knows whether rationing services rather than people produces net benefits: the consequences can be just as painful (Roberts, 1994).

MAKING DECISIONS

Autonomy

Autonomy is now a well established principle in medical decision-making. Unfortunately doctors still seem reluctant to accept that all competent patients should be empowered in this way (Stolman et al., 1990; Davies et al., 1993; Hill et al., 1994; Liddle et al., 1994). Adult patients who are competent and informed are entitled to refuse treatment which they do not wish to receive. However, as usual the issues are more complex than this bald statement suggests. Studies which show that patients' advance directives have been fulfilled may merely be demonstrating that physicians and patients have shared values (Danis et al., 1991; Orentlicher, 1992). When there is disagreement between the two, it is likely that physicians' values will take precedence (Danis et al., 1991), and while one might assume that this would take the form of an increase in the use of life-sustaining treatment, inconsistencies in the application of DNR orders between patients with different diagnoses but similar life expectancies (Wachter et al., 1989) suggests the need for caution. Moreover, the way in which doctors present information is affected by social and racial differences between them and their patients (Levy, 1985), and different presentations of the same data will influence patients' decisions (Marteau, 1989; Malloy et al., 1991).

Other questions also arise. To what extent are patients entitled to demand the converse of treatment limitation, that is, unusual or even 'futile' treatments? It has been stated that doctors are 'not obliged to offer useless interventions, and these do not need to be discussed with patients' (Doyal and Wilsher, 1994); this may be so, but it must not be used as an excuse for avoiding full discussion of therapeutic alternatives. Is attempted suicide always an expression of extreme emotional disturbance, or can it be a reasonable action, and if so, is the doctor always entitled to interfere? Could refusal to accept a treatment which offers at least some hope of cure be interpreted as suicide, as strict Judaic law implies? Is the autonomy of the physician infringed if the patient refuses such treatment? How does one determine the competence of a patient whose will to live has been undermined by a protracted but potentially reversible illness? The responses to these questions are determined in part by religion, national culture and the law.

The essential points which the physician must keep in mind are these. First, the patient and not the doctor is the best judge of that individual's quality of life (Uhlmann and Pearlman, 1991). Second, most patients want decisions about the extent of treatment to be shared with their doctor (Stolman et al., 1990; Heap et al., 1993); few wish to make such decisions in isolation. Third, the process of shared decision making takes time, and requires surrendering of traditional medical authority and a willingness to listen. Fourth, the views of family and close friends are important not just for supporting the patient but because it is they who will have to carry the emotional burden of loss. Fifth, allowance must be made for uncertainty: patients should be told that if circumstances were to change, so could their decision. This is of particular importance when discussing relatively remote risks to life; patients' preferences may change in either direction depending on changing circumstance (Bedell et al., 1983). Sixth, the patient must be properly informed both of medical fact and medical uncertainty; preferences for the extent of treatment are influenced by information about outcome. In one study the number of patients requesting active resuscitation status halved once they were informed of the current success rate (Murphy et al., 1994). Finally, decisions must be driven by compassion and a recognition that there are circumstances where the burden of treatment is greater than the probable benefits.

Surrogacy

It is comparatively unusual for critically ill patients to be able to exercise autonomy once they have been admitted to the ICU. Unanticipated life-threatening illness, the cerebral dysfunction of multiple organ failure, and sedative drugs make some degree of surrogate decision-making necessary. Legal authority for surrogates varies according to national statute; in some states in the USA the prior appointment of someone with power of attorney is sufficient, but in the UK such authority lapses once the patient becomes incompetent, and is only valid if an 'enduring' power of attorney has been granted. Close family members may be given legal authority by the courts to make surrogate decisions on behalf of adult patients in the USA (Miles, 1991; *In re* Quinlan, 1976), though other judgments have either reserved this authority to the courts (*In re* Saikewicz, 1977) or placed it within medical competence (*In re* Dinnerstein, 1978). In the UK the responsibility lies with the medical staff, or the courts in the case of disputes, not with relatives (F v West Berkshire HA, 1989). It is the doctor's legal duty to act in the best interests of the patient, and this includes not offering useless treatment. In the event of incapacity, there seems to be a preference amongst patients for allowing medical and nursing staff to make the decisions (Heap et al., 1993) but this may reflect lack of knowledge of living wills and advance directives, the use of which may be more common in the USA (Emanuel et al., 1991).

Consensus

Treatment limitation should be based on broad consensus between all health care staff as well as the patient or family. The views of relatives are of course of considerable importance to medical staff in framing surrogate decisions. It is our practice to obtain a consensus view from the family and close friends on what the patient would have wanted. A conscious effort must be made to separate this from the personal feelings of both relatives and staff. We explicitly inform relatives that the medical staff will carry the responsibility for whatever decision is made, and we do this to limit the burden of guilt which families may experience after the patient has died. The basis on which surrogates form opinions depends on many factors, as it does for competent patients. These include the manner in which information is presented to them by the medical staff, perceptions of the patient's prior quality of life and predicted quality of survival, and religious and cultural beliefs. In the USA ethics advisory committees are commonly used to help formulate TLOs for individual patients (Jayes et al., 1993), though whether this improves matters has not been subject to critical examination, and one report suggests that they may add to confusion (Edwards and Tolle, 1992). A consensus view is more likely to be obtained if the medical and nursing staff have a clear view of the medical facts of the case while at the same time retaining the ability to accept dissent. Nothing destroys consensus faster than a dogmatic and insensitive approach to moral and ethical issues. Few patients or their relatives want 'life at any cost', and the most important determinants of decisions to limit the extent of treatment seem to be loss of independence, social isolation, confusion, and constant pain (Heap et al., 1993). Age is specifically *not* a factor once co-morbidities and psychosocial limitations have been taken into account, though it does seem to influence medical decision-making (Hill et al., 1994). In cases where cultural or religious beliefs are playing an important part in forming opinion, it will be helpful to involve an appropriately skilled individual; indeed, ICU staff should form regular contacts with the ministers of the various religions represented in the community for mutual education and advice.

Disagreements

Disagreements between family and medical and nursing staff about the extent of treatment of incompetent patients can usually be resolved with adherence to the principles described above. Families must be given time. Sometimes this conflicts with the needs of other patients, for example when other patients are awaiting admission to intensive care and resources are inadequate. Using competing demand as a reason for withdrawing life support is not justified except in circumstances where the family have accepted the outcome but want support continued for days so that distant uninvolved relatives can be brought from abroad. If consensus cannot be obtained within a reasonable period, it may be necessary to reduce the intensity of nursing which the patient is receiving to allow resources to be directed to other patients. If consensus cannot be obtained at all, then the family should be offered a second opinion. Failure to resolve disputes appears to be extremely rare. Medical staff are not obliged to continue useless treatment and may take action to withdraw life-support, but it is wise to obtain legal clarification in complex cases. Most of these refer to withdrawal of either mechanical ventilation or tube feeding, two extremes of organ-system support. Other forms of support do not seem to have attracted similar attention, with the possible exception of renal dialysis. The cases which have been tested in the British courts of law have involved infants (*Re* J, 1990; *Re* C, 1989) and the persistent vegetative state in adults such as the Tony Bland case (Airedale NHS Trust v Bland, 1993; Tomkins, 1993). Judgments have broadly affirmed the right of an individual to die; that there is no absolute obligation to prolong life at all costs regardless of quality; and that the right to die is not a right to impose or hasten death. Christian traditions confirm these views (Jenkins, 1991). However, while the rigour of legal thinking can help to clarify the issues involved, the courts are not an appropriate substitute for broad consensus involving the lay public, the health care professions, religious scholars, and ethicists, as well as lawyers. The Law Lords themselves have proposed legislation and parliamentary guidelines as an alternative to the courts, and made it clear in the case of Tony Bland that specific judgments should not be seen as setting precedents for future cases, which must therefore be examined on their particular circumstances.

Clarifying the relationship between law and medicine, Lord Balcombe stated (*Re* J, 1990), 'I find it difficult to conceive of a situation where it would be a proper exercise of the jurisdiction to make an order positively requiring a doctor to adopt a particular course of treatment unless the doctor himself or herself were asking the court to make such an order.' Consensus reports have been produced in the USA (Hastings Center, 1987; ACCP/SCCM Consensus Panel, 1990) and similar discussions are taking place through the European Intensive Care Society, and the British Royal Colleges. The development of consensus statements needs to be paralled by the acquisition of accurate data on outcomes (Florin, 1993).

WITHDRAWING OR WITHHOLDING TREATMENT

Legally and ethically there is no difference between not initiating treatment and withdrawing it; but there are emotional and religious differences. The emotional distinction may be less difficult when viewed from the perspective of appropriate care, rather than that of sins of omission or commission. To implement treatment in the knowledge that it is inappropriate or useless is unkind and certainly unethical because it provides false hope; to continue it once started is cruel because it prolongs suffering either for the patient or the relatives. The aim should be to re-order priorities of care away from the medical treatment of the disease towards achievable goals such as the relief of symptoms. If death is recognized as an inevitable outcome, then it should occur without physical distress and with as much dignity as possible. The way in which this can be achieved must be a matter for discussion between staff, the patient, and the family, depending on circumstances.

Documentation

The form in which decisions are made is important. Reference has already been made to the poor quality of documentation of DNR decisions. Decisions to limit treatment must be clearly documented in the case record and the nursing notes, the reasons given, the names of those involved recorded, and the appropriateness of the decision reviewed regularly. Advance directives (living wills) are superficially attractive, but present considerable practical problems. Is the decision an informed one? Could it have been influenced by emotional pressure from other people? Is it still valid when circumstances have changed? Is it available when needed urgently? Living wills are perhaps most useful if they have been widely discussed with relatives and the family doctor (general practitioner), and avoid too much detail. What doctors need to know is the attitude of the patient to different cost–benefit–risk ratios: would he or she want life-support even if the likely outcome was a less than 5% chance of low-quality survival, or would they only request it if good quality survival was guaranteed? This approach may be more helpful than specific statements such as 'I want life-support if I have cancer or a stroke', and patients might also prefer it because it avoids the need to make unalterable decisions even though circumstances might change.

There are several items of medical information which are needed to construct an advance directive (Figure 5.1). These are the patient's current health status, the intensity and duration of treatment the patient is prepared to tolerate to achieve a given outcome, and the probability of achieving the best, most likely, and worst outcomes. The list of health states given in Figure 5.1 are not intended to be mutually exclusive, nor are they necessarily ranked in order of severity; modern medicine may have created fates worse than death. Knowledge of current health is important because it places desired outcomes in context. The patient should be asked to identify the level of treatment which he would want, given different outcomes; this information would be obtained by the doctor following a description of what the different levels of treatment involve. This would then be followed by the doctor's assessment of which specific outcomes and probabilities are applicable to the patient. Thus, a patient about to undergo bone marrow transplantation could be told that, if respiratory infection and respiratory failure were to occur, the chance of death in hospital despite mechanical ventilation is very high (> 90%); in this instance the most likely outcome is also the worst. A hypertensive diabetic with severely impaired renal function and ischaemic heart disease whose chronic health is limited to sedentary pursuits could be told that, in the event of a cardiac arrest, the best outcome would be no better than current health, the most likely outcome (> 90%) would be death in hospital, and if he survived the most likely outcome would be long-term dialysis. In this instance, 'worst' should be defined by the patient. Figure 5.1 can be adapted to local requirements for documenting such discussions, and should also include the names of those present, and the date. The medical discussant must be a senior member of staff with appropriate knowledge. The advantage of this approach is that it clarifies what prognostic information has been given to the patient and allows the

FORM OF DOCUMENTATION FOR DISCUSSING TREATMENT LIMITATION

Patient name:
Hospital Nr:
Age:
Main Diagnoses:

Date of discussion:
Persons present:

HEALTH STATES AND OUTCOMES	CURRENT HEALTH (✓)	PATIENT ATTITUDES TO TREATMENT INTENSITY FOR DIFFERENT OUTCOMES[1] (✓)							POSSIBLE OUTCOMES GIVEN FULL THERAPY[2] *Select and give % probability of:*		
		1	2	3	4	5	6	7	Best outcome	Most likely outcome	Worst outcome
Unrestricted good health											
Fatigued easily but able to do most things											
Activities restricted to sedentary pursuits											
Unable to do hobbies											
Confined to home or place of residence											
Incapable of self-care (dressing, hygeine)											
Confused requiring constant attention											
In constant pain											
Irreversible coma											
Death in hospital											

[1]**Patient attitudes**

1 = Full life-support
2 = Full support, limited period
3 = No mechanical ventilation
4 = No CPR
5 = No major intervention (eg: dialysis, major surgery)
6 = Nutrition & drugs only
7 = Comfort care only

[2]**Medical information**

Very high (>90%)
High (70%–90%)
Substantial (50%–70%)
Moderate (30%–50%)
Low (10%–30%)
Very low (<10%)

Probabilities must sum to 100%

Figure 5.1.

accuracy of this to be determined, and it also provides a measure of the intensity of treatment which the patient wishes to undergo to gain specific outcomes without excessive inflexibility.

Practical Issues

Once a decision has been made to allow a patient to die, the timing and manner of death become the most important issues. Conscious mechanically ventilated patients probably present the greatest emotional difficulties. One report demonstrates the amount of confusion which attends inexperience, excessive introspection and involvement of too many medical staff in a culture which finds the inevitability of death difficult to accept (Edwards and Tolle, 1992). In this respect it should be remembered that the main source of anxiety recalled by survivors of critical illness was concern for the welfare of their families in the event of death, rather than fear of death itself (Bion, 1988). Caring for the dying patient therefore involves caring for their relatives. Discussions should probably first take place separately with the patient and then with the family, who should then be given as much time as needed together so that they can decide how they want respiratory support withdrawn. The precise method depends on the degree of dependence. If spontaneous respiration can be maintained for several hours, extubation will probably be preferred to allow speech; careful use of opioids will relieve excessive dyspnoea. Antiemetics should be given routinely. If respiration cannot be maintained, the patient may wish to be sedated to the point of loss of consciousness and the ventilator then changed to a spontaneous mode. Sedation must be chosen with great care, and conscious patients must make the choice, not the medical staff: it is too easy to treat one's own distress by sedating the patient. If a degree of hypnosis is requested, low-dose benzodiazepines or propofol are helpful; midazolam is more amnesic, and may interfere more with communication than diazepam. Care should be taken in determining who should be present as death becomes inevitable: while the patient's wishes should be respected, a balance may need to be found between causing too much distress either by insisting on the presence of specific individuals (for example young children) or the exclusion of others who may need the opportunity to resolve past differences.

Unconscious ventilated patients may be extubated, or allowed to breathe spontaneously, and respiratory depressants or other sedatives may be used to diminish external movements which might upset the family. Hastening death is not a medical prerogative in most countries, but if this occurs as a secondary consequence of relieving distress rather than as a primary aim it is unlikely to be a cause for criticism or litigation. Tracheostomy to maintain airway patency seems an unnecessary intervention for terminal care unless time to death is likely to be measured in weeks.

The ICU is not a particularly appropriate environment for terminal care. Most open-plan units are busy and noisy, and the continuing activity at other bed spaces may add to the distress of relatives. If patients are well known to staff on the ward from which they were referred, and death is unlikely to occur immediately following treatment limitation, it may be better to continue care outside the ICU. However, usually death can be expected within hours or at most 2 days. In these circumstances, care should be continued in the ICU, as the patients are then guaranteed a high level of nursing and medical attention which may be outside the capabilities of the ordinary ward. Relatives often express a preference for continued ICU care for this reason.

SUMMARY

When formulating treatment limitation orders, the principles of beneficence, non-maleficence, autonomy, and justice must be observed. The aims of medical care should be stated explicitly, and related to the ability of different therapies to achieve goals which are acceptable to the patient. When patients are incompetent it is the responsibility of the medical staff in many countries to determine the best course of action. To discharge this responsibility properly, doctors must learn to discuss difficult issues with their patients while they are competent, and to ensure that patients are empowered to express their own views. Clear documentation is an important part of this process.

REFERENCES

Aarons, E.J., Beeching, N.J. (1991) Survey of 'do not resuscitate' orders in a district general hospital. *British Medical Journal* **303**: 1504–1506.

ACCP/SCCM consensus panel (1990) Ethical and moral guidelines for the initiation, continuation, and withdrawal of intensive care. *Chest* **97**: 949–958.

Airedale NHS Trust v Bland [1993] 1 All ER 821, HL.

American Heart Association Committee on Cardiopulmonary Resuscitation and Emergency Cardiac Care. National Academy of Sciences (1974) Standards for cardiopulmonary resuscitation (CPR) and emergency cardiac care (ECC) V: medicolegal considerations and recommendations. *Journal of the American Medical Association* **227**(suppl.) 864–866.

Austrian, R., Gold, J. (1964) Pneumococcal bacteremia with especial reference to bacteremic pneumococcal pneumonia. *Annals of Internal Medicine* **60**: 759–776.

Bedell, S.E., Delbanco, T.L. (1984) Choice about cardiopulmonary resuscitation in the hospital – when do physicians talk with patients? *New England Journal of Medicine* **310**: 1089–1093.

Bedell, S.E., Delbanco, T.L., Cook, G.F., Epstein, F.H. (1983) Survival after cardiopulmonary resuscitation in the hospital. *New England Journal of Medicine* **309**: 569–576.

Bion, J.F. (1988) Sedation and analgesia in the intensive care unit. *Hospital Update*; March: 1272–1286.

Bion, J.F., Aitchison, T.C., Edlin, S.A., Ledingham, I. McA. (1988) Sickness scoring and response to treatment as predictors of outcome from critical illness. *Intensive Care Medicine* **14**: 167–172.

Bowling, A. (1991) *Measuring Health: A Review of Quality of Life Measurement Scales*. Milton Keynes: Open University Press.

Chang, R.W.S., Jacobs, S., Lee, B. (1988) Predicting outcome among intensive care unit patients using computerised trend analysis of daily APACHE II scores corrected for organ system failure. *Intensive Care Medicine* **14**: 558–566.

Chassin, M.R. (1982) Costs and outcomes of medical intensive care. *Medical Care* **20**: 165–179.

Chief Medical Officer (1991) Letter to all consultants on resuscitation policy. 20th December 1991. PL/CMO (91) 22.

Cullen, D.J. (1977) Results and costs of intensive care. *Anesthesiology* **47**: 203–216.

Cullen, D.J., Civetta, J.M., Briggs, B.A., Ferrara, L.C. (1974) Therapeutic intervention scoring system: a method for quantitative comparison of patient care. *Critical Care Medicine* **2**: 57–60.

Danis, M., Southerland, L.I., Garrett, J.M. et al. (1991) A prospective study of advance directives for life-sustaining care. *New England Journal of Medicine* **324**: 882–8.

Davies, K.N., King, D., Silas, J.H. (1993) Professional attitudes to cardiopulmonary resuscitation in departments of geriatric and general medicine. *Journal of the Royal College of Physicians, London* **27**: 127–30.

Denardo, S.J., Oye, R.K., Bellamy, P.E. (1989) Efficacy of intensive care for bone marrow transplant patients with respiratory failure. *Critical Care Medicine* **17**: 4–6.

Detsky, A.S., Stricker, S.C., Mulley, A.G., Thibault, G.E. (1981) Prognosis, survival, and the expenditure of hospital resources for patients in an intensive-care unit. *New England Journal of Medicine* **305**: 667–672.

Doyal, L., Wilsher, D. (1994) Withholding and withdrawing life sustaining treatment from elderly people: towards formal guidelines. *British Medical Journal* **308**: 1689–92.

Duggan, J.M. (1989) Resource allocation and bioethics. *Lancet* **i**: 772–773.

Edwards, M.J., Tolle, S.W. (1992) Disconnecting a ventilator at the request of a patient who knows he will then die: the doctor's anguish. *Annals of Internal Medicine* **117**: 254–256.

Emanuel, L.L., Barry, M.J., Stoeckle, J.D., Ettelson, L.M., Emanuel, E.J. (1991) Advance directives for medical care – a case for greater use. *New England Journal of Medicine* **324**: 889–95.

F v West Berkshire HA [1989] 2 All ER 545, HL.

Faber-Langendoen, K., Caplan, A.L., McGlave, P.B. (1993) Survival of adult bone marrow transplant patients receiving mechanical ventilation: a case for restricted use. *Bone Marrow Transplanting* **12**: 501–507.

Florin, D. (1993) 'Do not resuscitate' orders: the need for a policy. *Journal of the Royal College of Physicians, London* **27**: 135–138.

Franklin, C., Mathew, J. (1994) Developing strategies to prevent inhospital cardiac arrest: analyzing responses of physicians and nurses in the hours before the event. *Critical Care Medicine* **22**: 244–247.

George, A.L., Folk, B.P., Crecelius, P.L., Cambell, W.B. (1989) Pre-arrest morbidity and other correlates of survival after in-hospital cardiopulmonary resuscitation. *American Journal of Medicine* **87**: 28–34.

Hansen-Flaschen, J.H. (1991) When life support is futile. *Chest* **100**: 1191–1192.

Hastings Center (1987) *Guidelines on the Termination of Life-sustaining Treatment and the Care of the Dying*. New York: Hastings Center.

Health Service Commission (1990/1991) Communications surrounding a decision not to resuscitate a patient – W.258/89–90. In *Report of the Health Service Commissioner*. London: The Health Service Commission.

Heap, M.J., Munglani, R., Klinck, J.R., Males, A.G. (1993) Elderly patients' preferences concerning life-support treatment. *Anaesthesia* **48**: 1027–1033.

Hill, M.E., MacQuillan, G., Forsyth, M., Heath, D.A. (1994) Cardiopulmonary resuscitation: who makes the decision? *British Medical Journal* **308**: 1677.

Hook, E.W., Horton, C.A., Schaberg, D.R. (1983) Failure of intensive care unit support to influence mortality from pneumococcal bacteremia. *Journal of the American Medical Association* **249**: 1055–1057.

In re Quinlan [1976] 355 A2d, at 669 NJ.

In re Saikewicz [1977] 370 NE2d, at 434.

In re Dinnerstein [1978] 380 NE2d, at 139.

Jayes, R.L., Zimmerman, J.E., Wagner, D.P. et al. (1993) Do-not-resuscitate orders in intensive care units. *Journal of the American Medical Association* **270**: 2213–2217.

Jenkins, D.E. (1991) Death as a fact of life. Frederick Hewitt Lecture to the Royal College of Anaesthetists, March 20th, London.

Kamer, R.S., Dieck, E.M., McClung, J.A. et al. (1990) Effect of New York State's do-not-resuscitate legislation on in-hospital cardio-pulmonary practice. *American Journal of Medicine* **88**: 108–111.

Keatinge, R.M. (1989) Exclusion from resuscitation. *Journal of the Royal Society of Medicine* **82**: 402–405.

Koch, K.A., Rodeffer, H.D., Wears, R.L. (1994) Changing pattern of terminal care management in an intensive care unit. *Critical Care Medicine* **22**: 233–243.

Kouwenhoven, W.B., Jude, J.R., Knickerboker, G.G. (1960) Closed-chest cardiac massage *Journal of the American Medical Association* **173**: 1064–1067.

Knaus, W.A., Draper, E.A., Wagner, D.P., Zimmerman, J.E. (1985) Prognosis in acute organ-system failure. *Annals of Surgery* **202**: 685–693.

Knaus, W.A., Rauss, A., Alperovitch, A., Le-Gall, J.R., Loirat, P., Patois, E., Marcus, S.E. (1990) Do objective estimates of chances for survival influence decisions to withhold or withdraw treatment? *Medical Decision-Making* **10**: 163–171.

Knaus, W.A., Wagner, D.P., Draper, E.A. et al. (1991) The APACHE III prognostic system; risk prediction of hospital mortality for critically ill hospitalized adults. *Chest* **100**: 1619–1636.

Lassen, H.C.A. (1953) A preliminary report on the 1952 epidemic of poliomyelitis in Copenhagen with special reference to the treatment of acute respiratory insufficiency. *Lancet* **i**: 37–41.

Liddle, J., Gilleard, C., Neil, A. (1994) The views of elderly patients and their relatives on cardiopulmonary resuscitation. *Journal of the Royal College of Physicians, London* **28**: 228–229.

Levy, D.R. (1985) White doctors and black patients: influence of race on the doctor patient relationship. *Pediatrics* **75**: 639–643.

Lo, B., Jonsen, A.R. (1980) Clinical decisions to limit treatment. *Annals of Internal Medicine* **93**: 764–768.

Mahul, Ph., Perrot, D., Tempelhoff, G. et al. (1991) Short and long term prognosis and functional outcome following ICU for the elderly. *Intensive Care Medicine* **17**: 7–10.

Malloy, T.R., Wigton, R.S., Meeske, J., Tape, T.G. (1991) How interventions are described affects patients decisions about life sustaining treatment. *Programme of the American Geriatric Society/American Federation for Ageing Research Annual Scientific Meeting*, Abstract A2.

Marteau, T.M. (1989) Framing of information: its influence upon decisions of doctors and patients. *British Journal of Social Psychology* **28**: 89–94.

Miles, S.H. (1991) Informed demand for 'non-beneficial' medical treatment. *New England Journal of Medicine* **325**: 512–515.

Miller, F.H. (1994) Infant resuscitation, a US/UK divide. *Lancet* **343**: 1584–1585.

Murphy, D.J., Burrows, D., Santilli, R.N. et al. (1994) The influence of the probability of survival on patients' preferences regarding cardiopulmonary resusciation. *New England Journal of Medicine* **330**: 545–549.

Murray, L.S., Teasdale, G.M., Murray, G.D. et al. (1993) Does prediction of outcome alter patient management? *Lancet* **341**: 1487–1491.

Orentlicher, D. (1992) The illusion of patient choice in end-of-life decisions. *Journal of the American Medical Association* **267**: 2101–2104.

Parker, J.M., Landry, F.J., Phillips, Y.Y. (1993) Use of do-not-resuscitate orders in an intensive care unit. *Chest* **104**: 1592–1596.

Quill, T.E., Stankatis, J.A., Krause, C.R. (1986) The effect of a community hospital resuscitation policy on elderly patients. *New York State Journal of Medicine* **86**: 622–625.

Rabkin, M.T., Gillerman, G., Rice, N.R. (1976) Orders not to resuscitate. *New England Journal of Medicine* **295**: 364–366.

Re, C. (a minor) [1989] 2 All ER 782.

Re, J. (a minor) [1990] 3 All ER 930.

Report (1992) Clinical judgement upheld by Appeal Court. *British Medical Journal* **304**: 1589.

Roberts, J. (1994) Oregon overwhelmed in its first three weeks. *British Medical Journal* **308**: 618.

Rubins, H.B., Moskowitz, M.A. (1988) Discharge decision-making in a medical intensive care unit. *American Journal of Medicine* **84**: 863–869.

Sage, W.M., Rosenthal, M.H., Silverman, J.F. (1986) Is intensive care worth it? – an assessment of input and outcome for the critically ill. *Critical Care Medicine* **14**: 777–782.

Sax, F.L., Charlson, M.E. (1987) Medical patients at high risk for catastrophic deterioration. *Critical Care Medicine* **15**: 510–515.

Schein, R.M., Hazaday, N., Pena, M. et al. (1990) Clinical antecedents to in-hospital cardiopulmonary arrest. *Chest* **98**: 1388–1392.

Schulman, K.A., Glick, H.A., Rubin, H., Eisenberg, J.M. (1991) Cost-effectiveness of HA-1A monoclonal antibody for Gram-negative sepsis. *Journal of the American Medical Association* **266**: 3466–3471.

Stolman, C.J., Gregory, J.J., Dunn, D., Levine, J.L. (1990) Evaluation of patient, physician, nurse and family attitudes toward to not resuscitate orders. *Archives of Internal Medicine* **150**: 653–658.

Teres, D. (1993) Trends from the United States with end of life decisions in the intensive care unit. *Intensive Care Medicine* **19**: 316–322.

Teres, D., Rapoport, J. (1994) (eds). Cost containment – A multicultural approach. *New Horizons* **2**: 273–274.

Tomkins, C. (1993) Lawful withdrawal of life support. *Journal of Medical Defence Union* **1**(suppl.).

Tomlinson, T., Brody, H. (1990) Futility and the ethics of resuscitation. *Journal of the American Medical Association* **264**: 1276–1280.

Truog, R.D., Brett, A.S., Frader, J. (1992) The problem with futility. *New England Journal of Medicine* **326**: 1560–1564.

Tunstall-Pedoe, H., Bailey, L., Chamberlain, D.A. et al. (1992) Survey of 3,765 cardiopulmonary resuscitations in British Hospitals (the BRESUS study): methods and overall results. *British Medical Journal* **304**: 1347–1351.

Uhlmann, R.F., Pearlman, R.A. (1991) Perceived quality of life and preferences for life sustaining treatment in older patients. *Archives of Internal Medicine* **151**: 495–497.

Urberg, M., Ways, C. (1987) Survival after cardiopulmonary resuscitation for an in-hospital cardiac arrest. *Journal of Family Practice* **25**: 41–44.

Wachter, E.M., Luce, J.M., Hearst, N., Lo, B. (1989) Decisions about resuscitation priorities among patients with different diseases but similar prognoses. *Annals of Internal Medicine* **111**: 525–532.

Wagner, D.P., Knaus, W.A., Draper, E.A. (1986) Physiologic abnormalities and outcome from acute disease. Evidence for a predictable relationship. *Archives of Internal Medicine* **146**: 1389–1396.

Youngner, S.J., Lewandowski, W., McClish, D.K., Juknialis, B.W., Coulton, C., Bartlett, E.T. (1985) 'Do not resuscitate' orders: incidence and implications in a medical intensive care unit. *Journal of the American Medical Association* **253**: 54–57.

Ziegler, E.J., Fisher, C.J., Sprung, C.L. et al. (1991) Treatment of Gram-negative bacteremia and septic shock with HA-1A human monoclonal antibody against endotoxin. *New England Journal of Medicine* **324**: 429–436.

Zimmerman, J.E., Knaus, W.A., Sharpe, S.M., Anderson, A.S., Draper, E.A., Wagner, D.P. (1986) The use and implications of Do Not Resuscitate orders in intensive care units. *Journal of the American Medical Association* **255**: 351–356.

6

Modern Techniques for Measuring Body Composition in Patients who are Critically Ill

Lindsay D. Plank, Graham L. Hill

INTRODUCTION

The quantitative assessment of the nutritionally important components of body composition, namely, protein, water and fat, provides a basic tool for research into the metabolic and nutritional disorders associated with a wide range of disease processes. Only recently has technology been available that allows for the *in vivo* determination of these three compositional variables. For many years body composition research concentrated on dividing the body into two compartments: fat and lean. The introduction of new technologies such as neutron activation analysis (NAA) and dual-energy X-ray absorptiometry (DXA) has allowed more complex modelling of the body which offers considerably more scope for the investigation of disease processes than the classical two-compartment model.

Body composition methodology may be viewed in an hierarchical manner (Table 6.1) (Heymsfield et al., 1989). At the highest level is chemical analysis of tissue. The validation of any body composition technique relies ultimately on chemical analysis of tissues from cadaver dissection or biopsies. *Level II* methods such as NAA and DXA allow semi-direct quantification of specific body constituents. *Level III* includes methods based upon experimental models requiring assumptions regarding the densities or ratios of measured components; for example, hydrodensitometry for the measurement of body fat. The methods at the lowest level require calibration against criterion measurements from a higher level method. These include skinfold anthropometry and bioimpedance analysis.

Rather than an exhaustive list of body composition techniques, the methods described below represent recent advances in the field and some of the most widely used applications.

Table 6.1 Hierarchy of body composition methodology*

I	Chemical analysis of the whole body and tissues.
II	Direct *in vivo* measurement of body constituents.
III	*In vivo* estimation of body compartments using modelling approaches.
IV	*In vivo* measurement of somatic or physical property calibrated against body constituent derived by methods at levels I–III.

* After Heymsfield et al. (1989).

NEUTRON ACTIVATION ANALYSIS (NAA)

Neutron activation techniques allow, in principle, quantitation of all the major elements of the body. *In vivo* studies require the irradiation of the subject by a beam of fast neutrons. The interaction of a neutron with an atom of a target element results in an excited nucleus which reverts to a stable condition by the emission of one or more gamma rays either immediately (within $\sim 10^{-12}$ s, called prompt gamma activation), or after a decay period characteristic of the activation product (delayed gamma activation). The gamma ray energy is characteristic of the target element and its intensity is proportional to the amount of that element. The prompt technique is able to measure most of the elements of interest for human composition studies, in particular, hydrogen, nitrogen, chlorine, carbon, oxygen, calcium, phosphorus and sodium.

The measured elements can, in principle, be used to determine the sizes of various body compartments, the principal subdivisions of which are: protoplasm, which is rich in nitrogen, potassium and phosphorus; extracellular fluid, which contains sodium and chlorine; bone, which contains calcium, phosphorus and sodium; and fat, which contains carbon and hydrogen. By virtue of the fact that nitrogen is almost exclusively confined to protein at a mean level of 16%, the measurement of total body nitrogen (TBN) makes possible valuable studies on a wide range of disease processes, including the nutritional syndromes and wasting (for example, Cohn et al., 1981, 1983a; Hill and Beddoe, 1982; Russell et al., 1983; Williams et al., 1984; Blendis et al., 1986; Preston et al., 1987; Allman et al., 1990; Hill, 1992a). The value of *in vivo* NAA over conventional nitrogen balance techniques is primarily that it affords an estimate of total body protein (TBP) at any given time, where balance techniques can only provide net changes in TBP. Moreover, NAA is logistically more suitable over long study periods and does not in principle suffer from the cumulative systematic

errors that almost inevitably occur with the nitrogen balance technique (Streat et al., 1986).

Very few centres worldwide are equipped with neutron activation equipment for the *in vivo* analysis of whole body elemental constituents. Only one or two of these are sited or constructed to enable measurement of critically ill patients. Our own unique facility comprises a prompt gamma *in vivo* neutron activation scanner situated alongside a dual-energy X-ray absorptiometer. An electrically operated hoist allows transfer of intensive care patients and incorporates a load cell for weighing during transfer. Current approaches to the measurement of TBN by the prompt gamma technique rely on hydrogen as an internal standard (Vartsky et al., 1979). The validity of this approach depends on the assumption that both elements are similarly distributed throughout the body. Critically ill patients often require massive quantities of isotonic fluids to achieve haemodynamic stability and consequently present with massive fluid overload. The assumption that nitrogen and hydrogen are similarly distributed throughout the body may not hold, not only because of whole-body fluid increase but also because of localized fluid accumulations which may occur in body cavities such as the gut, peritoneal cavity, lungs or thighs (Krishnan et al., 1990). Furthermore, in the technique of using hydrogen as the internal standard, an independent assessment of total body hydrogen is necessary. We have demonstrated, using minced meat phantoms with varying degrees of fluid overload, that our whole-body scanning approach can provide a valid, direct estimate of TBP in the intensive care situation (Hill et al., 1993; Mitra et al., 1993) with a between-measurement coefficient of variation based on phantoms of 3.5%. A single scan requires about 30 minutes and radiation exposure is 0.15 mSv.

DUAL-ENERGY X-RAY ABSORPTIOMETRY

Dual-energy X-ray absorptiometry (DXA) (Mazess et al., 1990) relies on the differential absorption of two photon energies through soft tissue and bone. Soft tissues, consisting largely of water and organic compounds, reduce photon flux to a lesser extent than bone mineral. With appropriate selection of the two photon energies body mass can therefore be subdivided into soft tissue and bone mineral (Peppler and Mazess, 1981; Gotfredsen et al., 1984). In areas where bone is not present suitable calibration allows fat and lean fractions to be resolved from soft tissue. The composition of these areas of soft tissue is extrapolated to the soft tissue overlying bone to produce total body fat and lean soft tissue. Bone mineral is the inorganic ash residue of the skeleton. Fat or triglyceride is the ether-soluble residue of the soft tissue and comprises approximately 90% of total body lipid. The remaining 10% consists largely of essential lipids such as phospholipids and sphingomyelin. Exactly how much essential lipid is measured by DXA as fat is not clear. Water and protein solids are essentially indistinguishable by absorptiometry and can be grouped together as a single 'lean' component.

Data on the use of this technique in studies of the critically ill have not yet appeared to the best of our knowledge. Concerns have been raised as to the possible confounding effects of large changes in hydration status on the accuracy with which bone mineral and fat can be determined using DXA (Roubenoff et al., 1993). Recent work by Formica et al. (1993) and Going et al. (1993) goes some way toward allaying these concerns. The former group monitored bone density and fat mass in haemodialysis patients and found these measures to be unaffected by the fluid changes, admittedly only small compared with expected shifts in ICU patients. Similarly, Going et al. (1993) found bone mass and fat to be unaffected by small changes in hydration of normal volunteers undergoing a dehydration–rehydration protocol. A study we carried out with mincemeat phantoms undergoing increasing degrees of fluid overload, comparable to those seen in ICU patients, showed a small (2–3%) dependence of total fat measurement on degree of hydration (Hill et al., 1993). The trend was significant because of the high short-term precision of this measurement (better than 2%).

With this technology the tissue content of different regions of the body can also be measured (Schlemmer et al., 1990) and quite recently the appendicular muscle mass has been estimated (Heymsfield et al., 1990) by this technique. Our group is currently applying such regional analysis in studies of intensive care patients.

COMPUTED TOMOGRAPHY

Computed tomography (CT) scanning provides detailed cross-sectional images of the body in which adipose, muscle, bone, and vascular tissues are resolved. While few computed tomography investigations of whole body composition have been conducted to date, several studies have looked at regional tissue distribution. The use of CT for measurements of body composition in intensive care patients has not been reported. Analysis of CT images provides tissue areas and, with suitable assumptions regarding changes in tissue distribution between slices, tissue volumes (Tokunaga et al., 1983; Kvist et al., 1986). Conversion to mass of tissue requires an assumption about its density. To provide fat mass with which to compare other methods of estimating fat requires knowledge of the fat content of adipose tissue, which may vary with illness and/or degree of obesity (Sjöström et al., 1986). The value of CT scanning may lie in its ability to monitor changes in fat distribution and muscularization (Termote et al., 1980; Borkan et al., 1983). The technique is capable of very high precision (better than 1% for adipose tissue) (Sjöström et al., 1986) although validation must rely ultimately on cadaver dissection (Rossner et al., 1990). Radiation dose equivalent for whole body tissue estimation is typically of the order of 2–5 mSv (Kvist et al., 1986).

MAGNETIC RESONANCE IMAGING

Magnetic resonance imaging (MRI) provides anatomical detail similar to that of CT (Ross et al., 1991; Fowler et al., 1992) and has also been used to measure total adipose tissue in the human body using multiple cross-sectional slices (Fuller et al., 1990; Fowler et al., 1991; Ross et al., 1992, 1993). As with CT, a value for the fat content of adipose tissue must be assumed in order to derive fat mass (McNeill et al., 1991; Sohlström et al., 1993). Comparison with the CT technique for adipose tissue estimation suggests that both imaging methods give similar results for subcutaneous fat but that MRI may be less accurate for visceral fat probably due to movement artifacts in the visceral area coupled with the longer acquisition time for MRI scans (Seidell et al., 1990). This technique is attractive for longitudinal studies on individuals since no radiation hazards are involved.

WHOLE BODY COUNTING

A constant small proportion of all naturally occurring potassium (0.012%) is radioactive (^{40}K) and can be measured in a whole body counter. Total body potassium is determined by extrapolating the ^{40}K measurement and is equivalent to total exchangeable potassium (K_e) (Talso et al., 1960). Over 97% of the total exchangeable potassium in the body is located within the intracellular compartment and is related to the size of the body cell mass (Moore et al., 1963). Moore's concept of the body cell mass as the central active core of the body that determines its work capacity, nutritional requirements, protein synthetic capability, oxygen consumption and carbon dioxide output has been immensely valuable and not the least in studies of patients in the intensive care unit (Moore et al., 1963). By assuming an average ratio for the intracellular K to intracellular N of 3 mmol K/g N, and that one quarter of wet cell weight is protein, Moore pointed out that the body cell mass could be derived from total exchangeable potassium as follows:

$$BCM = 6.25 \times 4 \times K_e / 3$$
$$BCM = K_e \times 8.33$$

where the small extracellular potassium compartment is neglected.

Thus, the quantification of the body cell mass is dependent on the assumptions that it has an average K:N ratio of 3 in all states of sickness and health and that protein comprises 25% of cell mass even in intensive care patients. Although Moore's description and extensive use of the 'body cell mass' has proved fundamental to our understanding of the body composition changes in intensive care patients and has aided our understanding of critical illness, the assumptions which allow total body potassium to be used to quantify body cell mass in this way cannot always be made in such patients without resort to complicated tables or nomograms (Moore, 1980).

DILUTION METHODS

Total Body Water

Undoubtedly the most important dilution method is that involved in the measurement of total body water (TBW) which can be achieved by tritium-labelled, deuterium-labelled or ^{18}O-labelled water (Schoeller et al., 1980), or by ethanol (Leoppky et al., 1977) or urea dilution (McCance and Widdowson, 1951). Measurements in human subjects of total body water by tritium dilution, the most popular technique, have been available for 60 years (von Hevesy and Hofer, 1934). Body water measurements in intensive care patients, however, are much more difficult to obtain than in normal subjects or even the vast majority of sick patients because of several factors. Firstly, such patients often have greatly expanded TBW at the end of the phase of fluid sequestration with accumulations of more than ten litres being not uncommon. Furthermore, such water expansion often includes collections of free fluid within body cavities (ascites, pleural effusions, intraluminal gut fluid, etc.) where mixing of isotope via the circulation is slow. Under these circumstances the period of isotope equilibration can be expected to be variably prolonged from the 2–3 h period sufficient in normally hydrated individuals. During this period of equilibration there will be loss of isotope in urine, nasogastric aspirates and from fluid via surgical drains and by evaporation. The patients are all receiving intravenous fluids at moderate infusion rates as well. These fluids cannot be withheld over the period of isotope equilibration and by virtue of their non-instantaneous mixing with body water lead to a dilution effect in plasma water. Finally the total body water itself may be changing during the period of isotope equilibration due to imbalance between gains and losses.

In order to study the effects of the above-mentioned factors we measured total body water in 11 critically ill intensive care patients (Streat et al., 1985a). All had major emergency surgery or severe blunt trauma and were receiving inotropic drug infusions during the measurement of TBW. Sixteen studies were performed in 11 patients. Each was given 3.7 MBq of tritiated water in 10 ml of sterile water intravenously from a syringe which was weighed before and after injection. Samples of blood were taken from indwelling arterial lines every hour for 6 h. Urine and other drain volumes were recorded and sampled for isotope each hour. The volume of fluids given IV each hour was also recorded.

At each hour (t) after injection, the volume of distribution of the isotope (TBW_t) was determined as:

$$TBW_t = \frac{\text{Isotope dose injected} - \text{Losses } (t = 0 \text{ to } t = t)}{\text{Specific activity in serum water at time } t}.$$

In order to take some account of the changes in TBW over the 6-h period, the TBW at the time of isotope injection (TBW_0) was derived from each of the six hourly results, thus:

$$TBW_0 = TBW_t - (\text{Fluid input minus output from } t = 0 \text{ to } t = t).$$

For each study there were thus a series of estimates of TBW_0 and the final value of TBW_0 chosen for the patient was usually the mean of the 4- 5- and 6-h estimates.

Table 6.2 shows the values of TBW_0 obtained at 1–6 h after injection of tritium in 16 studies in the 11 critically ill patients. It can be seen that, in general, values of TBW_0 thus obtained rise by about 6% over the first 3 h after isotope injection and are fairly stable from the fourth hour. Repeated measures analysis of variance with analysis of the differences between adjacent water measurements indicates that there are significant increases in the volume of dilution of the isotope

Table 6.2 Values of total body water in litres obtained 1–6 h after isotope injection together with the weight (kg) of each patient at the time of study

		Time after injection (h)					
Patient	Weight	1	2	3	4	5	6
RO1	89.3	48.05	50.98	50.83	51.76	51.51	51.33
WH1	70.4	44.06	47.04	48.59	50.66	49.19	49.54
FL1	81.5	48.50	50.22	51.07	49.82	50.45	51.24
FL2	79.4	48.65	49.15	49.73	49.80	48.85	49.34
PE1	89.9	51.18	51.62	52.92	52.60	54.91	52.92
PE2	93.4	50.05	53.29	54.84	53.67	54.17	53.47
PE3	96.9	53.37	54.42	55.89	56.39	56.62	57.68
MC2	71.6	39.09	41.83	42.27	43.45	42.40	42.54
NI2	89.9	48.06	49.19	49.89	49.73	48.97	49.93
MO1	83.5	46.16	50.84	50.92	51.42	50.14	52.41
MO2	88.2	56.63	58.39	55.95	57.45	57.73	57.97
HI1	72.9	39.10	42.62	42.38	43.67	43.32	43.02
BL1	68.6	40.25	42.93	44.03	44.51	44.56	43.84
TU1	93.7	55.05	60.84	59.47	63.77	63.81	64.20
RS1	117.0	70.69	74.16	75.52	76.34	75.79	76.75
RS2	122.1	71.95	75.50	78.73	78.51	77.78	82.22
Mean TBW_0		50.68	53.31	53.94	54.59	54.38	54.90

Significance of differences between 1-h values of TBW_0

Comparison	1 v 2	2 v 3	3 v 4	4 v 5	5 v 6
P value	0.00003	0.07	0.07	0.38	0.17

over the first 3 h but not thereafter in this group of patients. The extent of measured isotope losses (as urine, nasogastric fluid and surgical drain loss) at 4 h after injection varied from 0.5% to 3.3% of the administered dose with a mean value of 1.2%.

An estimate of the precision (SD) of the measurement of TBW_0 in the group of patients was obtained by analysis of the 4-, 5- and 6-h results from the table and was found to vary from 0.4% to 3.0% with a mean value of 1.2%. The experimental precision on a single estimate on the basis of counting statistics alone is approximately 0.8%. Clearly, a better estimate of the TBW at the time of isotope injection is obtained by making repeated measurements during the period 4–6 hours after injection. Because of the persistent uncertainty surrounding the size of the non-aqueous exchangeable hydrogen in humans during the 4–6 h equilibration period the systematic error that results is likely to be approximately 3% or better (Culebras and Moore, 1977).

Extracellular Water

Although extracellular water forms a fairly constant proportion of total body water in healthy adults, in sickness extracellular water invariably expands, particularly so after resuscitation where it may increase by 50% or more (Hill, 1992b; Moore, 1959). Traditionally extracellular water has been measured by radiosulfate or bromide dilution (Brodie et al., 1939; Walser et al., 1953; Shires et al., 1960; Barratt and Walser, 1969) but there are enormous difficulties in interpreting isotope dilution studies in critically ill patients (Moore and Shires, 1967). For extracellular water measurements in critically ill patients we use stable bromide dilution. Early kinetics suggests that, like tritium, bromide concentration is fairly stable after the fourth hour of equilibration. In normal subjects an allowance of 10% for bromide penetration of cells and 3% for sulfate is adequate to compensate for losses from the circulation. However, little is known of the kinetics of these substances in intensive care patients and recent work suggests that penetration of these substances into cells is quite different in the critically ill (Hannon and Boston, 1990).

Na_e/K_e Ratio

Dilution of the radioisotopes ^{42}K or ^{43}K together with ^{22}Na yields a determination of the ratio of total exchangeable sodium (Na_e) to K_e. Na_e is a measure of the extracellular supporting component of body composition and its ratio with K_e provides a sensitive index of nutritional state (Shizgal, 1976) owing to the reciprocal changes which occur in the body cell mass and the extracellular mass with malnutrition and critical illness. ^{42}K and ^{43}K possess short half-lives which makes their use expensive and logistically difficult. Whole body counting is an alternative for potassium measurement but these installations are few, particularly those able to accommodate ICU patients. Shizgal et al. (1977) has described an indirect measurement of K_e based on TBW determination (by tritium dilution) and ^{22}Na dilution entailing a radiation exposure of approximately 2.5 mSv.

BIOIMPEDANCE METHODS

Single frequency (50 kHz) impedance devices have been used to estimate fat-free mass and total body water (and its compartments) for many years in healthy populations (Lukaski et al., 1985; Kushner and Schoeller, 1986; Khaled et al., 1988; Segal et al., 1988). Recent reports indicate that the clinical usefulness of single frequency measurements on individuals who are experiencing fluid status changes is controversial (Kurtin et al., 1990; Schroeder et al., 1990; Dal Cin et al., 1991; Meguid et al., 1992; Zillikins et al., 1992). As a tool for the monitoring of nutritional status in intensive care patients, the sole study to appear thus far (Robert et al., 1993) showed strong relationships between changes in body cell mass and protein and energy intakes but independent criterion data to establish the sensitivity and specificity of the technique were not available. Multi-frequency impedance measurements which allow differential current flow through the intra- and extracellular spaces to be assessed may improve the accuracy with which hydration status and fluid distribution may be determined (Segal et al., 1991; Duerenberg and Schouten, 1992). New approaches based on bioimpedance spectroscopy and appropriate equivalent circuit models for biological tissue (Cornish et al., 1993; van Loan et al., 1993) have the potential to provide additional information of relevance to the critical care situation. Studies of intensive care patients employing this technology are currently in progress. These techniques require little operator training and are rapid, safe, inexpensive, and non-invasive.

ANTHROPOMETRIC INDICES

On the whole body level, anthropometric indices such as body weight, body volume, stature, trunk and limb circumferences, and skinfold thicknesses can be estimated directly. Our investigations of the value of measuring two anthropometric indices in intensive care patients resulted in the following conclusions:

Weight change in intensive care patients is nearly all water change

In intensive care patients weight changes cannot be used to estimate tissue changes. Changes in body mass are predominantly due to large changes in total body water greatly in excess of protein and fat and often in the opposite direction. In order to study the relationship between weight change and water change we studied the changes in body composition over a 10-day period in ten trauma and eight septic patients in our intensive care unit (see Table 6.3) (Streat and Hill, 1987). Thus, for both groups of patients the observed weight

Table 6.3 Body composition changes over 10 days in patients after severe blunt trauma and serious sepsis

	Trauma	Sepsis
Weight (kg)	$-4.2 \pm 1.2^{\dagger}$	-6.2 ± 2.9
Water (kg)	$-3.3 \pm 1.4^{*}$	$-6.8 \pm 2.6^{*}$
Protein (kg)	$-1.1 \pm 0.2^{\S}$	$-1.5 \pm 0.3^{\ddagger}$
Fat (kg)	$+0.2 \pm 0.6$	$+2.2 \pm 0.8^{*}$

All values as mean ± SEM.
Paired *t*-test: *, $p < 0.05$; †, $p < 0.01$; ‡ $p < 0.002$; § $p < 0.001$; all other changes not significant.

changes as shown in Table 6.3 were predominantly due to changes in body water.

Skinfold anthropometry cannot accurately measure fat in intensive care patients

We have shown that skinfold anthropometry is an inaccurate method of assessing total body fat in patients presenting for nutritional support in the surgical ward (Streat et al., 1985b). We found that skinfold anthropometry underestimated body fat by about 3 kg in such patients. Because of large changes in weight, use of skinfold anthropometry is even more inappropriate in the patient in intensive care. We measured total body fat by the neutron activation /tritiated water dilution method (Beddoe et al., 1984) and also derived total body fat from skinfold anthropometry in nine critically ill patients in intensive care. The results are shown in Table 6.4. The highly significant mean difference between total body fat measured by the neutron activation technique and that derived from skinfold anthropometry can be seen.

BODY COMPOSITION MODELS

Body composition research involves subdividing the body into two or more compartments. A considerable diversity of approaches to this subdivision is now possible with the advances in technology over the last three decades. At the most fundamental level is elemental analysis. *In vivo* estimation of the major elements of the body, largely by neutron activation techniques, allows the reconstruction of greater than 98% of the body mass (Wang et al., 1992). The clinical or scientific usefulness of such measurements has not yet been

Table 6.4 Total body fat (TBF) measured by IVNAA and by skinfold anthropometry

Patient	Weight	TBF (kg)	
		IVNAA	Anthropometry
1	79.4	24.0	21.7
2	81.5	14.0	23.4
3	79.4	13.5	26.3
4	83.5	15.6	26.7
5	68.6	9.8	19.3
6	65.0	12.3	16.4
7	72.9	17.4	30.8
8	59.7	20.7	22.5
9	89.9	22.0	29.6
Mean		16.6	24.1
SE		1.6	1.6
Differences			
Mean		7.5	
SE		1.8 (p = 0.003)	

demonstrated in the critical care setting although there are some theoretical bases for them becoming so in the future. For instance, changes in total body carbon may be a useful way of assessing changes in body energy stores in critically ill patients (Kinney and Moore, 1956), and measurements of total body chlorine may prove to be valuable for estimating changes in extracellular water (Yasumura et al., 1983).

The cornerstone of body composition research is the chemical (or molecular) model, primarily due to its central role in the study of energy metabolism, protein nutriture and mineral physiology (Heymsfield and Waki, 1991). This model considers the chemical compounds of the body in categories of closely related molecular species. We (Beddoe et al., 1984) and others (Wang et al., 1992) have described a five-compartment model comprising water, protein, glycogen, minerals and fat (or lipid). The combination of isotope dilution, neutron activation and dual-energy X-ray absorptiometers (DXA) makes possible the application of this model to the critical care patient. The usefulness of this model is extended by the further subdivision of water into the extra- and intracellular spaces. At present in our laboratory we are using this model in studies of patients with major blunt trauma, patients with serious sepsis, and patients after restorative panproctocolectomy. By this means we are assessing strategies for enhancing recovery which include monoclonal antibodies, nutrients acting as pharmacological agents, and growth factors.

In addition to studies of fluid balance based on the intra/extracellular division of body water, investigations into thermogenesis are aided by models based on a cellular-non-cellular compartmentalization. These are exemplified by the breakdown into body cell mass, fat, extracellular fluid and the remaining extracellular solids (Wang et al., 1992). Almost half of the body protein is an extrusion from cells and spends its life outside cells as structural protein or as soluble protein or as enzymes. These proteins form most of what is called extracellular solids; they include the fibrous supporting structures of the body, including collagen, elastin, the dermis, hair, teeth, cartilage and joint capsules. These substances probably do not contribute in any way to the active metabolic processes of the body and are usually assumed to be stable in critically ill patients. This may not be correct, however, and because of this attempts have been made to divide total body protein into that which is contained within cells and that which is present outside cells. The most widely used model was developed by Burkinshaw et al. (1979) who presented data in sick patients in which total body protein was divided into that which was contained in skeletal muscle and that which was contained in the rest of the body. Cohn et al. (1983b), extending this concept further, separated body protein into that contained within viscera and that which was extracellular. Such models are in an early stage of refinement and cannot at present cope with the changes accompanying critical illness, particularly fluctuations in cellular volumes in tissues as cell contents are consumed by the catabolic process or expanded by excess intracellular water. However, the recent availability of DXA, MRI and CT scanners makes it feasible to consider the characterization of the body in terms of tissue groupings such as skeletal muscle, adipose tissue, bone, and non-skeletal muscle soft tissue.

REFERENCES

Allman, M.A., Allen, B.J., Stewart, P.M. et al. (1990) Body protein of patients undergoing haemodialysis. *European Journal of Clinical Nutrition* **44**: 123–131.

Barratt, T.M., Walser, M. (1969) Extracellular fluid in individual tissues and in whole animals: the distribution of radiosulfate and radiobromide. *Journal of Clinical Investigation* **48**: 56–66.

Beddoe, A.H., Streat, S.J., Hill, G.L. (1984) Evaluation of an in vivo prompt gamma neutron activation facility for body composition studies in critically ill intensive care patients: results on 41 normals. *Metabolism* **33**: 270–280.

Blendis, L.M., Harrison, J.E., Russell, D.M. et al. (1986) Effects of peritoneovenous shunting on body composition. *Gastroenterology* **90**: 127–134.

Borkan, G.A., Hults, D.E., Gerzof, S.G., Burrows, B.A., Robbins, A.H. (1983) Relationships between computed tomography tissue areas, thicknesses and total body composition. *Annals of Human Biology* **10**: 537–546.

Brodie, B.B., Brand, E., Leshin, S. (1939) The use of bromide as a measure of extracellular fluid. *Journal of Biological Chemistry* **130**: 555–563.

Burkinshaw, L., Hill, G.L., Morgan, D.B. (1979) Assessment of the distribution of protein in the human body by *in vivo* neutron activation analysis. In *Nuclear activation techniques in the life sciences 1978*, pp 787–798. Vienna: International Atomic Energy Agency.

Cohn, S.H., Gartenhaus, W., Sawitsky, A. et al. (1981) Compartmental body composition of cancer patients by measurement of total body nitrogen, potassium, and water. *Metabolism* **30**: 222–229.

Cohn, S.H., Brennan, B.L., Yasumura, S. et al. (1983a) Evaluation of body composition and nitrogen content of renal patients on chronic dialysis as determined by total body neutron activation. *American Journal of Clinical Nutrition* **38**: 52–58.

Cohn, S.H., Vartsky, D., Yasumura, S., Vaswani, A.N., Ellis, K.J. (1983b) Indexes of body cell mass: nitrogen versus potassium. *American Journal of Physiology* **244**: E305–E310.

Cornish, B.H., Thomas, B.J., Ward, L.C. (1993) Improved prediction of extracellular and total body water using impedance loci generated by multiple frequency bioelectrical impedance analysis. *Physics in Medicine and Biology* **38**: 337–346.

Culebras, J.M., Moore, F.D. (1977) Total body water and the exchangeable hydrogen. Theoretical calculations of nonaqueous exchangeable hydrogen in man. *American Journal of Physiology* **232**: R54-R59.

Dal Cin, S., Braga, M., Molinari, M., Cristallo, M., Di Carlo, V. (1991) Reliability of bioelectrical impedance analysis in dehydrated subjects. *Clinical Nutrition* **10**(suppl.): 9.

Duerenberg. P., Schouten, F.J.M. (1992) Loss of total body water and extracellular water assessed by multifrequency impedance. *European Journal of Clinical Nutrition* **46**: 247–255.

Formica, C., Atkinson, M.G., Nyulasi, I. et al. (1993) Body composition following haemodialysis: Studies using dual-energy x-ray absorptiometry and bioelectrical impedance analysis. *Osteoporosis International* **3**: 192–197.

Fowler, P.A., Fuller, M.F., Glasbey, C.A. et al. (1991) Total and subcutaneous adipose tissue in women: the measurement of distribution and accurate prediction of quantity by using magnetic resonance imaging. *American Journal of Clinical Nutrition* **54**: 18–25.

Fowler, P.A., Fuller, M.F., Glasbey, C.A., Cameron, G.G., Foster, M.A. (1992) Validation of the in vivo measurement of adipose tissue by magnetic resonance imaging of lean and obese pigs. *American Journal of Clinical Nutrition* **56**: 7–13.

Fuller, M.F., Fowler, P.A., McNeill, G.M., Foster, M.A. (1990) Body composition: the precision and accuracy of new methods and their suitability for longitudinal studies. *Proceedings of Nutrition Society* **49**: 423–436.

Going, S.B., Massett, M.P., Hall, M.C. et al. (1993) Detection of small changes in body composition by dual-energy x-ray absorptiometry. *American Journal of Clinical Nutrition* **57**: 845–850.

Gotfredsen, A., Borg, J., Christiansen, C., Mazess, R.B. (1984) Total body bone mineral *in vivo* by dual photon absorptiometry. I. Measurement procedures. *Clinical Physiology* **4**: 343–355.

Hannon, R.J., Boston, V.E. (1990) Fluid and ion redistribution in skeletal muscle in an animal sepsis model. *Journal of Paediatric Surgery* **25**: 599–603.

Heymsfield, S.B., Waki, M. (1991) Body composition in humans: advances in the development of multicompartment chemical models. *Nutrition Reviews* **49**: 97–108.

Heymsfield, S.B., Wang, J., Lichtman, S. et al. (1989) Body composition in elderly subjects: a critical appraisal of clinical methodology. *American Journal of Clinical Nutrition* **50**: 1167–1175.

Heymsfield, S.B., Smith, R., Aulet, M. et al. (1990) Appendicular skeletal muscle mass: measurement by dual-photon absorptiometry. *American Journal of Clinical Nutrition* **52**: 214–218.

Hill, G.L. (1992a) Jonathan E. Rhoads Lecture. Body composition research: implications for the practice of clinical nutrition. *Journal of Parenteral and Enteral Nutrition* **16**: 197–218.

Hill, G.L. (1992b) *Disorders of nutrition and metabolism in clinical surgery: understanding and management*. Edinburgh: Churchill Livingstone.

Hill, G.L., Beddoe, A.H. (1982) *In vivo* neutron activation in metabolic and nutritional studies: II. Clinical applications. *Journal of Clinical Surgery* **1**: 333–345.

Hill, G.L., Monk, D., Plank, L.D. (1993) Measuring body composition in intensive care patients. In Wilmore, D.W. & Carpentier, Y.A. (eds.) *Metabolic Support of the Critically Ill Patient*, pp 3–18. Berlin: Springer-Verlag.

Khaled, M.A., McCutcheon, M.J., Reddy, S. et al. (1988) Electrical impedance in assessing human body composition: the BIA method. *American Journal of Clinical Nutrition* **47**: 789–792.

Kinney, J.M., Moore, F.D. (1956) Carbon balance. A clinical approach to energy exchange. *Surgery* **40**: 16–26.

Krishnan, S.S., McNeill, K.G., Mernagh, J.R., Bayley, A.J., Harrison, J.E. (1990) Improved clinical facility for in vivo nitrogen measurement. *Physics in Medicine and Biology* **35**: 489–499.

Kushner, R.F., Schoeller, D.A. (1986) Estimation of total body water by bioelectrical impedance analysis. *American Journal of Clinical Nutrition* **44**: 417–424.

Kurtin, P.S., Shapiro, A.C., Tomita, H. et al. (1990) Volume status and body composition of chronic dialysis patients: utility of bioelectric impedance plethysmography. *American Journal of Nephrology* **10**: 363–367.

Kvist, H., Sjöström, L., Tylen, U. (1986) Adipose tissue volume determinations in women by computed tomography: technical considerations. *International Journal of Obesity* **10**: 53–67.

Leoppky, J.A., Myhre, L.G., Venters, M.D. et al. (1977) Total body water and lean body mass estimated by ethanol dilution. *Journal of Applied Physiology* **42**: 803–808.

Lukaski, H.C., Johnson, P.E., Bolonchuk, W.W., Lykken, G.I. (1985) Assessment of fat-free mass using bioelectrical impedance measurements of the human body. *American Journal of Clinical Nutrition* **41**: 810–817.

McCance, R.A., Widdowson, E.M. (1951) A method of breaking down the body weights of living persons into terms of extracellular fluid, cell mass and fat, and some applications of it to physiology and medicine. *Proceedings of the Royal Society, Series B* **138**: 115–130.

McNeill, G.M., Fowler, P.A., Maughan, R.J. et al. (1991) Body fat in lean and obese women estimated by six methods. *British Journal of Nutrition* **65**: 95–103.

Mazess, R.B., Barden, H.S., Bisek, J.P., Hanson, J. (1990) Dual energy X-ray absorptiometry for total body and regional bone mineral and soft tissue composition. *American Journal of Clinical Nutrition* **51**: 1106–1121.

Meguid, M.M., Lukaski, H.C., Tripp, M.D., Rosenburg, J.M., Parker, F.B. (1992) Rapid bedside method to assess changes in postoperative fluid status with bioelectrical impedance analysis. *Surgery* **112**: 502–508.

Mitra, S., Plank, L.D., Hill, G.L. (1993) Calibration of a prompt gamma in vivo neutron activation facility for direct measurement of total body protein in intensive care patients. *Physics in Medicine and Biology* **38**: 1971–1975.

Moore, F.D. (1959) *Metabolic care of the surgical patient*. Phildelphia: W.B. Saunders.

Moore, F.D. (1980) Energy and maintenance of the body cell mass. *Journal of Parenteral and Enteral Nutrition* **4**: 228–260.

Moore, F.D., Shires, G.T. (1967) Moderation. *Annals of Surgery* **166**: 300–301.

Moore, F.D., Olesen, K.H., McMurray, J.D. et al. (1963) *The body cell mass and its supporting environment: body composition in health and disease*. Philadelphia: W.B. Saunders.

Peppler, W.W., Mazess, R.B. (1981) Total body bone mineral and lean body mass by dual-photon absorptiometry I. Theory and measurement procedure. *Calcified Tissue International* **33**: 353–359.

Preston, T., Fearon, K.C.H., Robertson, I., East, B.W., Calman, K.C. (1987) Tissue loss during severe wasting in lung cancer patients. In Ellis K.J., Yasumura S. & Morgan W.D. (eds.) *In Vivo Body Composition Studies*, pp 60–69. London: IPSM.

Robert, S., Zarowitz, B.J., Hyzy, R. et al. (1993) Bioelectrical impedance assessment of nutritional status in critically ill patients. *American Journal of Clinical Nutrition* **57**: 840–844.

Ross, R., Leger, L., Guardo, R., de Guise, J., Pike, B.G. (1991) Adipose tissue volume measured by magnetic resonance imaging and computerized tomography in rats. *Journal of Applied Physiology* **70**: 2164–2172.

Ross, R., Leger, L., Morris, D., de Guise, J., Guardo, R. (1992) Quantification of adipose tissue by MRI: relationship with anthropometric variables. *Journal of Applied Physiology* **72**: 787–795.

Ross, R., Shaw, K.D., Martel, Y., de Guise, J., Avruch, L. (1993) Adipose tissue distribution measured by magnetic resonance imaging in obese women. *American Journal of Clinical Nutrition* **57**: 470–475.

Rossner, S., Bo, W.J., Hiltbrandt, E. et al. (1990) Adipose tissue determination in cadavers – a comparison between cross-sectional planimetry and computed tomography. *International Journal of Obesity* **14**: 893–902.

Roubenoff, R., Kehayias, J.J., Dawson-Hughes, B., Heymsfield, S.B. (1993) Use of dual-energy x-ray absorptiometry in body-composition studies: not yet a 'gold standard'. *American Journal of Clinical Nutrition* **58**: 589–591.

Russell, D.M., Prendergast, P.J., Darby, P.L. et al. (1983) A comparison between muscle function and body composition in anorexia nervosa: the effect of refeeding. *American Journal of Clinical Nutrition* **38**: 229–237.

Schlemmer, A., Hassager, C., Haarbo, J., Christiansen, C. (1990) Direct measurement of abdominal fat by dual photon absorptiometry. *International Journal of Obesity* **14**: 603–611.

Schoeller, D.A., Van Senten, E., Peterson, D.W. et al. (1980) Total body water measurements in humans with ^{18}O and ^{2}H labelled water. *American Journal of Clinical Nutrition* **33**: 2686–2693.

Schroeder, D., Christie, P.M., Hill, G.L. (1990) Bioelectric impedance analysis for body composition: clinical evaluation in general surgical patients. *Journal of Parenteral and Enteral Nutrition* **14**: 129–133.

Segal, K.R., van Loan, M., Fitzgerald, P.I., Hodgdon, J.A., van Itallie, T.B. (1988) Lean body mass estimation by bioelectrical impedance analysis: a four-site cross-validation study. *American Journal of Clinical Nutrition* **47**: 7–14.

Segal, K.R., Burastero, S., Chun, A. et al. (1991) Estimation of extracellular and total body water by multiple-frequency bioelectrical-impedance measurement. *American Journal of Clinical Nutrition* **54**: 26–29.

Seidell, J.C., Bakker, C.J.G., van der Kooy, K. (1990) Imaging techniques for measuring adipose-tissue distribution-a comparison between computed tomography and 1.5-T magnetic resonance. *American Journal of Clinical Nutrition* **51**: 953–957.

Shires, G.T., Williams, J., Brown, F. (1960) Simultaneous measurement of plasma volume, extracellular fluid volume, and red blood cell mass in man utilizing I^{131}, $S^{35}O_4$, and Cr^{51}. *Journal of Laboratory and Clinical Medicine* **55**: 776–783.

Shizgal, H. (1976) Total body potassium and nutritional status. *Surgical Clinics of North America* **56**: 1185–1194.

Shizgal, H., Spanier, A.H., Humes, J., Wood, C.D. (1977) Indirect measurement of total exchangeable potassium. *American Journal of Physiology* **233**: F253-F259.

Sjöström, L., Kvist, H., Cederblad, A., Tylen, U. (1986) Determination of total adipose tissue and body fat in women by computed tomography, ^{40}K, and tritium. *American Journal of Physiology* **250**: E736–E745.

Sohlström, A., Wahlund, L.-O., Forsum, E. (1993) Adipose tissue distribution as assessed by magnetic resonance imaging and total body fat by magnetic resonance imaging, underwater weighing, and body-water dilution in healthy women. *American Journal of Clinical Nutrition* **58**: 830–838.

Streat, S.J., Hill, G.L. (1987) Nutritional support in the management of critically ill patients in surgical intensive care. *World Journal of Surgery* **11**: 194–201.

Streat, S.J., Beddoe, A.H., Hill, G.L. (1985a) Measurement of total body water in intensive care patients with fluid overload. *Metabolism* **34**: 688–694.

Streat, S.J., Beddoe, A.H., Hill, G.L. (1985b) Measurement of body fat and hydration of the fat-free body in health and disease. *Metabolism* **34**: 509–518.

Streat, S.J., Beddoe, A.H., Hill, G.L. (1986) Changes in body nitrogen – comparison of direct measurement with nitrogen balance. *Australian and New Zealand Journal of Surgery* **56**: 257.

Talso, P.J., Miller, C.E., Carballo, A.J., Yasquez, I. (1960) Exchangeable potassium as a parameter of body composition. *Metabolism* **9**: 456–471.

Termote, J.-L., Baert, A., Crolla, D., Palmers, Y., Bulcke, J.A. (1980) Computed tomography of the normal and pathologic muscular system. *Radiology* **137**: 439–444.

Tokunaga, K., Matsuzawa, Y., Ishikawa, K., Tarui, S. (1983) A novel technique for the determination of body fat by computed tomography. *International Journal of Obesity* **7**: 437–445.

Van Loan, M.D., Withers, P., Matthie, J., Mayclin, P.L. (1993) Use of bio-impedance spectroscopy to determine extracellular fluid, intracellular fluid, total body water, and fat-free mass. In Ellis, K.J. & Eastman, J.D. (eds.) *Human Body Composition. In vivo Methods, Models and Assessment*, pp 67–70. New York: Plenum.

Vartsky, D., Prestwich, W.V., Thomas, B.J. et al. (1979) The use of body hydrogen as an internal standard in the measurement of nitrogen by prompt neutron capture gamma rays. *Journal of Radioanalytical Chemistry* **48**: 243–252.

Von Hevesy, G., Hofer, E. (1934) Elimination of water from the human body. *Nature* **134**: 879.

Walser, M., Seldin, D.W., Grollman, A. (1953) An evaluation of radiosulfate for the determination of extracellular fluid in man and dogs. *Journal of Clinical Investigation* **32**: 299–311.

Wang, Z.-M., Pierson, R.N. Jr, Heymsfield, S.B. (1992) The five-level model: a new approach to organizing body composition research. *American Journal of Clinical Nutrition* **56**: 19–28.

Williams, E.D., Henderson, I.S., Boddy, K. et al. (1984).Whole-body elemental composition in patients with renal failure and after transplantation studied using total-body neutron-activation analysis. *European Journal of Clinical Investigation* **14**: 362–368.

Yasumura, S., Cohn, S.H., Ellis, K.J. (1983) Measurement of extracellular space by total body neutron activation. *American Journal of Physiology* **244**: R36-R40.

Zillikens, M.C., van den Berg, J.W.O., Wilson, J.H.P., Swart, G.R. (1992) Whole-body and segmental bioelectrical-impedance analysis in patients with cirrhosis of the liver: changes after treatment of ascites. *American Journal of Clinical Nutrition* **55**: 621–625.

7

New Developments in Specialized Nutrition Support

Thomas R. Ziegler

INTRODUCTION

The practice of nutrition support in the intensive care unit (ICU) setting has significantly evolved since the development of specialized nutrient products for enteral administration in the 1950s and modern intravenous nutrition support modalities in the late 1960s (Wilmore and Dudrick, 1969). Specialized enteral and parenteral nutrition is now routine in the clinical care of critically ill patients. Provision of adequate calories, protein and other essential nutrients is clearly beneficial in some clinical situations when adequate food intake is precluded and/or when nutrient losses are accelerated. Thus, classical nutrient deficiencies in patients receiving adequate nutritional support are uncommon, and body protein loss is attenuated compared to responses of comparable patients receiving limited or no dietary intake (Wilmore, 1991).

The risk–benefit ratio of specialized feeding in the ICU has received increased attention by clinical investigators. A number of therapeutic strategies are being studied as methods to improve the efficacy of nutrient support as a therapy to enhance recovery and rehabilitation. These include: provision of increased amounts of conditionally essential amino acids (e.g. glutamine and arginine), use of modified fat emulsions and nutrient antioxidants, administration of recombinant growth factor hormones – e.g. growth hormone (GH), insulin-like growth factor-I (IGF-I), and epidermal growth factor (EGF), and combinations of these methods. However, at present, few studies documenting beneficial clinical outcomes in critical illness with these new approaches have been published.

Recently published guidelines of the American Society for Parenteral and Enteral Nutrition (ASPEN) suggest that the major objectives of nutritional/metabolic support in critical care are: (i) to detect and correct pre-existing malnutrition; (ii) to prevent progressive protein-calorie malnutrition; (iii) to optimize the patient's metabolic state (including fluid and electrolyte status); (iv) to reduce morbidity and time to convalescence (ASPEN Board of Directors, 1993). However, nutritional support is adjunctive to primary therapies such as fluid resuscitation, oxygen delivery, abscess drainage, and provision of antibiotics. Because parenteral nutrition (PN) and tube feedings have become the standard of care in most intensive care units throughout the world, little objective data from properly designed, randomized, controlled studies are available to determine the true efficacy and the indications for nutritional support in critical illness, or when feeding should be started (Barton, 1994).

The primary focus of nutritional support has classically been to supply adequate micronutrients (vitamins, minerals, electrolytes) and to maintain or increase body protein. As body protein is critical for tissue structure and function, erosion of body protein (i.e. lean tissue or lean body mass) is clearly *associated* with worsened clinical outcomes, such as diminished immune function and increased infection rates (Scrimshaw et al., 1973), increased post-operative morbidity (Windsor and Hill, 1988), decreased tissue repair and wound healing (Haydock and Hill, 1987), and skeletal muscle dysfunction and delayed convalescence (Lopes et al., 1982; Pingleton and Harmon, 1987; Wilmore, 1991). Direct cause-and-effect relationships between nutritional status and outcomes in the ICU are difficult to prove, because malnutrition may reflect, in part, the severity or nature of the underlying illness. None the less, it is reasonable to assume that maintenance of nutritional status in general and body protein in particular is beneficial to the patient with critical illness.

Enhanced protein loss in catabolic states is manifested as negative nitrogen balance and is generally directly related to the degree of catabolic stress and quantity and quality of dietary nutrients. Net body protein loss may be due to increased rates of protein breakdown, reduced protein synthesis or a combination of these two effects. Critically ill patients generally exhibit increased protein synthetic rates which are countered by a greater rise in protein catabolic rates, leading to net loss of lean tissue. The mechanisms regulating erosion of body protein are complex, but undoubtedly involve counter-regulatory hormones (such as cortisol and catecholamines) in concert with proinflammatory cytokines, including tumour necrosis factor and the interleukins (Wilmore, 1977; Wilmore, 1991; Pomposelli et al., 1988). These signals interrelate with other mechanisms which favour net protein breakdown such as reduced nutrient intake, acidosis, and muscle disuse due to chemical neuromuscular paralysis and bedrest. In addition to effects on protein metabolism, the metabolic pattern in ICU patients is manifested by increased rates of lipolysis and gluconeogenesis, increased micronutrient losses in urine (e.g. zinc, water soluble vitamins) and alterations in the anabolic hormonal milieu (e.g. insulin resistance, diminished plasma IGF-I) (Souba and Wilmore, 1994; Ziegler et al., 1994).

A number of studies have shown that current nutritional support modalities are unable to place severely catabolic individuals into positive nitrogen balance. Nitrogen losses of 4–8 g/day (or ~ 25–50 g protein/day) are common in severely catabolic hospitalized patients despite aggressive feeding (Souba and Wilmore, 1994). In addition, body composition studies have shown that much of the observed weight gain associated with the provision of specialized nutrition is due to gain in total body fat and extracellular fluid, not lean tissue (Cerra et al., 1980; Streat et al., 1987; Warnold et al., 1988). The relative ineffectiveness of current therapy in attenuating protein breakdown is probably multifactorial. For example, ICU patients may be unable to utilize exogenously supplied nutrients effectively because of bed rest, organ dysfunction, the catabolic hormonal-cytokine environment and/or provision of imbalanced or deficient nutrient solutions (Wilmore, 1991; Ziegler et al., 1994).

Although increased flow of amino acids from skeletal muscle in catabolic stress may result in skeletal muscle weakness, acute proteolysis provides amino acids (e.g. glutamine, alanine) to be used as fuel and specific substrates for wound healing, protein synthesis, gluconeogenesis and immune cell support. Thus, the proteolytic response represents an important adaptation during critical illness. After recovery and during convalescence, standard parenteral/enteral nutrition stimulates protein synthesis and promotes nitrogen equilibrium or slight positive balance, particularly in patients with pre-existing protein-energy malnutrition, who then demonstrate protein retention.

CURRENT PRACTICES OF SPECIALIZED NUTRITION SUPPORT IN ADULT ICU PATIENTS

The overall goal of nutritional support is to maintain organ structure and function by providing adequate micronutrients, energy and amino acids to support metabolism and protein synthesis, specific tissue functions, wound healing and organ repair.

Nutritional Assessment

Nutritional assessment in the ICU involves physical examination, evaluation of the weight loss and dietary history, knowledge of the type and severity of underlying illness, organ function, fluid status, selected biochemistries, estimation of energy, protein and micronutrient needs and type of access available for nutrient delivery (Table 7.1). An integrated clinical assessment, which includes physical examination (e.g. to detect muscle and fat wasting, zinc deficiency rash, glossitis), evaluation of catabolic stress level, functional capacity, gastrointestinal function, dietary history and body weight change over time is probably the best method to assess the need for nutritional support. Using this approach, patients may be classified as normally nourished or exhibiting mild, moderate or severe protein-energy malnutrition (Baker et al., 1982). In addition, patients who are well nourished on admission may be classified at 'high risk' for subsequent significant protein wasting or protein-energy malnutrition due to the underlying illness or injury (e.g. severe trauma or burn injury).

Circulating protein concentrations (e.g. albumin, transferrin, retinol binding protein) are generally not useful indices of underlying nutritional status in ICU patients, because concentrations of these are markedly affected by non-nutritional factors, including fluid depletion or overload, capillary leak syndromes, reduced hepatic synthesis due to inflammation or infection, and body losses via the kidney or gut. Further, circulating proteins may remain low because of these non-nutritional factors despite adequate feeding.

Protein and Energy Administration

Studies on nutrient utilization efficiency in critically ill patients suggest that lower amounts of total energy (calorie) and protein should be administered than were routine in the past. Large amounts of dietary calories and protein ('hyperalimentation') can induce metabolic complications, including carbon dioxide overproduction, azotaemia, hyperglycaemia, electrolyte alterations, and hepatic dysfunction (Wolfe et al., 1979; Lowry and Brennan, 1979; Shaw et al., 1987). Energy intake should be advanced slowly over several days after initiation of specialized feeding, to provide maintenance energy intake. Energy requirements may be estimated using standard equations, such as the Harris–Benedict equation, which incorporate the patient's age, sex, weight and height to determine basal energy expenditure (BEE). The BEE is then multiplied by factors to account

Table 7.1 Nutritional assessment in the intensive care unit

1. Perform detailed physical examination
   - Skeletal muscle wasting
   - Loss of fat stores
   - Skin lesions suggestive of micronutrient deficiency
2. Obtain information on body weight pattern pre-ICU admission
   - Current body weight
   - Usual body weight
   - % Weight loss past 2 weeks and past 3 to 6 months (% weight loss)
   - Ideal body weight
3. Dietary intake pattern pre-ICU admission
   - General food intake pattern
   - Previous intravenous or enteral nutritional support
   - Use of nutritional supplements
4. Estimate overall functional status pre-ICU admission
   - Ability to perform daily activities (including ability to prepare or take meals)
   - General muscle strength and fatiguability
   - Respiratory muscle strength and fatiguability
5. Determine if gastrointestinal tract is totally or partially functional
   - Gastrointestinal symptoms (nausea, emesis, diarrhoea, steatorrhoea)
   - Delayed gastric emptying, post-operative gastroparesis
   - Ileus (small bowel or colonic)
   - Obstruction (total or partial and proximal or distal)
   - Fistulae (proximal or distal)
   - Intra-abdominal infection, bowel perforation, dehiscence, etc.
   - Acute gastrointestinal bleeding
6. Determine fluid status
   - Euvolaemic
   - Dehydrated
   - Fluid overloaded
   - Capillary leak syndrome
7. Evaluate selected serum or plasma biochemistries
   - Standard organ function indices
   - Electrolytes, including calcium, magnesium, and phosphorus
   - Triglycerides
   - Vitamins and minerals if suggested by physical examination, diet history or underlying illness(s) (serum zinc and iron status most useful)
   - Serum proteins are rarely helpful in ICU setting (especially albumin)
8. Estimate energy requirements
   - Harris–Benedict or equivalent equation for estimated basal energy needs
   - Factor in additional 20–30% to account for activity (unless paralysed)
   - Factor in stress of illness, including wound size (usually $\leq$ additional 50% above basal)

Indirect calorimetry in 'stable' ICU patient may be useful (data often vary from day to day)
Generally 25–35 kcal kg/day is adequate for maintenance energy intake

9. Estimate protein needs
   Evaluate hepatic and renal function
   Estimate stress of underlying illness
   Determine presence of unusual protein losses via kidney, gastrointestinal tract, wounds
   Generally 1.3–2.0 g protein/kg/day is adequate
   1.2 g Protein/kg/day if being dialysed
   0.6 to 1.2 g Protein/kg/day with hepatic and/or renal failure, depending on severity

10. Evaluate available intravenous and enteral access and plan route of feeding
    Dedicated central vein port for hypertonic dextrose-based parenteral nutrition
    Peripherally placed central vein access (PICC line)
    Peripheral access (peripheral vein solutions rarely indicated in ICU setting)
    Nasogastric tube or naso-small intestinal feeding tube
    Percutaneous access (e.g. PEG (percutaneous endoscopic gastrostomy tube), feeding jejunostomy tube)

---

for activity (1.2 to 1.3 times BEE unless the patient is sedated) and illness severity (usually an additional 25–50%) to arrive at the energy prescription (usually between 1.3 to 1.75 times BEE). Alternatively, energy expenditure can be determined by gas exchange using indirect calorimetry or by the Ficke equation. It is clear, however, that energy expenditure varies considerably from day-to-day in ICU patients (Van Lanschot et al., 1986). In light of complications of overfeeding, energy provision at 25–30 kcal/kg/day is a generally safe goal range for most ICU patients, keeping in mind that current body weight in the ICU may be dramatically increased due to fluid retention. Carbon dioxide overproduction (evidenced by respiratory quotients $\geqslant$ 1.0) was not uncommon in earlier decades when patients routinely received much higher energy doses (e.g. > 40 kcal/kg/day; Askanazi et al., 1980); however, this complication is now unusual as lower nutrient loads are being administered. Patients with very severe injury (e.g. large burns) may be able to utilize higher calorie doses (35–40 kcal/kg). Because of limitations in the ability of ICU patients to utilize large carbohydrate loads (Wolfe et al., 1979; Barton, 1994), dextrose in PN should be given at a dose not to exceed 4–5 mg/kg/min. Larger doses of dextrose are not efficiently oxidized for energy, and may induce hyperglycaemia and/or excessive carbon dioxide production.

Dextrose should provide ~ 70–80% of non-protein energy, unless the patient is hyperglycaemic. The dextrose load should be reduced, and/or insulin should be provided in parenteral feeding, or as a separate insulin drip, to maintain blood glucose between 100 and 200 mg/dl (Ziegler and Smith, 1993). When malnourished patients are no longer hypercatabolic (i.e. during recovery and after ICU discharge), nutritional repletion may be cautiously instituted. Energy intakes exceeding those required to maintain body weight (e.g. 35 to 45 kcal/kg) are often well tolerated at these times.

In our hospital and in many other centres, the use of an intravenous infusion port dedicated for intravenous nutrition infusion is mandatory if concentrated dextrose is to be administered. Although empiric, this protocol is designed to minimize catheter infection risk due to hypertonic dextrose infusion through ports used for blood draws, drug administration, etc. Thus, if a port is 'violated', we administer 10% dextrose as the maximal concentration in PN, until the catheter is changed over a wire or a new central line site and infusion port dedicated to PN is available. The data are mixed on whether the number of lumens in a central venous catheter contributes to risk of infection with PN. However, a recent prospective, randomized trial demonstrated a significant increase in catheter infections when PN was given via a triple-lumen catheter versus a single lumen catheter (Clark-Christoff et al., 1992).

Intravenous lipid emulsions are used to provide essential fatty acids (e.g. as 250 ml of a 20% lipid emulsion twice/weekly) or as an energy source (lipid as ≈ 20–30% of non-protein energy), generally infused over a 24 h period in patients requiring PN. The use of total nutrient admixtures (or '3 in 1') PN solutions may be helpful in fluid-restricted patients, although lipid emulsions are often given over 12 to 24 h as separate infusions in many centres. The potential immunosuppressive effects of current soybean or safflower oil-based lipid emulsions have been recently reviewed, but the significance of this potential complication is unclear, pending additional clinical investigation in humans (Carpentier et al., 1993). The maximal recommended rate of fat emulsion infusion is 1.0 to 1.5 g/kg/day (Carpentier et al., 1993; Barton, 1994). It is important to monitor serum triglyceride levels serially to assess tolerance to fat emulsion. ICU patients generally clear intravenous fat emulsions well from plasma. However, administration of fat emulsion as an energy source in ICU patients with severely diminished pulmonary diffusion capacity or hypertriglyceridemia may be contraindicated to avoid possible worsening of hypoxia or the development of pancreatitis, respectively.

Studies in ICU patients indicate that protein loads of > 2.0 g/kg/day are not efficiently utilized for protein synthesis, but may be oxidized for energy and contribute to azotaemia (Shaw J.H.F. et al., 1987). Thus, protein should be provided at ~ 1.2–2.0 g/kg/day in catabolic patients with normal renal function. A reasonable average is 1.5 g protein/kg/day (range 1.3 to 1.8 g/kg/day). The protein dose should also be lowered or raised to the target range as a direct function of degree of azotaemia and hyperbilirubinaemia. This strategy takes into account the inability of many patients to utilize exogenous nutrients efficiently during severe catabolic illness, and the knowledge that most protein and lean tissue repletion occurs over a period of several weeks during convalescence. Adequate non-protein energy is essential to allow amino acids to be utilized effectively for protein synthesis. The non-protein calorie to nitrogen ratio used in most centres ranges from 100:1 to 150:1 (nitrogen = protein/6.25). Highly catabolic patients may be given larger protein loads, assuming near normal renal and hepatic function. Branched-chain amino acid-enriched solutions have not been shown to improve clinical outcomes in critically ill patients (ASPEN Board of Directors, 1993); therefore, standard amino acid formulations should generally be used pending the results of ongoing research on newer amino acid formulations (see section on arginine and glutamine administration below).

Because fluid restrictions and/or the need for intravenous pressor, blood product or drug administration often preclude the use of large fluid volumes for intravenous or enteral feedings, peripheral vein PN solutions (which provide low concentrations of dextrose and amino acids and large proportion of energy as fat) are generally not indicated in ICU patients. Rather, central venous administration of PN often allows maintenance energy and protein intake in one-litre volumes. When fluid-restricted or dialyzed patients are able to be tube-fed, enteral solutions which provide higher concentrations of energy (e.g. 2.0 kcal/ml) and/or higher concentrations of protein may be chosen.

Micronutrient Administration

It is important to maintain blood glucose and serum electrolytes within the normal range during administration of specialized feeding. Malnourished patients frequently exhibit whole-body depletion of intracellular electrolytes (potassium, phosphorus and magnesium) and levels of these may fall rapidly to dangerously low levels during nutritional repletion (refeeding syndrome). The dosage of electrolytes required to maintain normal plasma levels appears to be directly related to the dose of administered dextrose in patients with normal renal function (phosphorus and magnesium in particular). In addition, studies indicate that maintenance of intracellular potassium, phosphorus and magnesium concentrations in muscle are essential for normal protein synthesis and the ability to achieve neutral or positive nitrogen balance (Rudman et al., 1975).

Supplemental zinc (and possibly other trace elements such as selenium) should be provided in patients with burns, large wounds, severe pancreatitis, and/or significant gastrointestinal fluid losses. Approximately 12 mg of zinc are lost per litre of small bowel fluid, and urinary excretion of zinc increases dramatically as a function of the degree of catabolic stress. Zinc is an important nutrient for immune function, wound healing and gastrointestinal mucosal regeneration, while the rate of protein synthesis and production of the endogenous anabolic peptide hormone IGF-I are both reduced in zinc deficiency (Jeejeebhoy, 1993). Thus, using serum zinc levels and/or urinary excretion as a guide to therapy, administration of 5 to 10 mg/day additional zinc intravenously, or 200 to 400 mg/day enterally during severe catabolic illness will reduce the risk of continued total body zinc depletion.

Many clinicians provide supplemental anti-oxidant nutrients during severe catabolic stress (e.g. vitamins C and E, glutamine by the intravenous or enteral route); however, blinded, controlled trials of anti-oxidant nutrient therapy in ICU patients have not been reported. Doses of oral or intravenous vitamin C in the range of 500 mg to 2 g/day and vitamin E (400 to 800 IU/day) have been used without evident untoward effects in selected ICU patients. Similarly, enteral L-glutamine powder at doses of 10 to 30 g/day appears to be well tolerated in catabolic individuals without severe renal or hepatic dysfunction.

Biochemical Monitoring

It is imperative to monitor closely plasma glucose, electrolytes (including magnesium) and triglycerides, and to assess renal, hepatic and pulmonary function on a daily basis to determine the metabolic response to specialized enteral and parenteral feeding, especially during periods of physiological instability. The nutrient mix is adjusted to maintain normal blood concentrations of standard chemistries and minimize metabolic complications. When the patient is extremely unstable, it may be necessary to provide a lowered amount of parenteral/enteral diet or to give intravenous low-dose dextrose with vitamins and minerals until organ function stabilizes.

Timing of Nutrient Administration

Little objective clinical data is available to guide timing of nutrient administration in the ICU, and clearly more work is needed in this area. The current standard of care in most units is to provide specialized PN or enteral feeding at least within 5 to 7 days after admission, although in clinical practice nutritional support is often provided several days sooner. Many specialists suggest that feeding be instituted within 48 to 72 hours after ICU admission, after standard resuscitation therapy to achieve haemodynamic stability (ASPEN Board of Directors, 1993; Barton, 1994). Recently, some clinicians have advocated provision of electrolytes, vitamins, mineral and trace elements alone during the initial 24 to 72 hours of acute ICU admission, followed by macronutrient support (dextrose, amino acids and fat) at about 50% of energy and protein needs for several days, advanced to achieve 'maintenance' energy and protein intake by days 5 to 7 of admission. This more conservative approach reflects the known metabolic complications of aggressive feeding and the lack of demonstrated improved outcomes with early nutritional support. However recent data suggests that early (within 24 h of ICU admission) institution of enteral feeding may be beneficial in terms of reducing infectious morbidity, although not hospital mortality, in ICU patients (Moore et al., 1992).

Enteral Feeding in the ICU

The increased use of enteral nutrition in the ICU setting represents the most dramatic and possibly the most beneficial change in specialized feeding since modern metabolic support was developed. A large number of animal data and some human studies support the increased use of enteral versus parenteral nutrition support. An increased rate of infection is associated with use of PN in normally nourished individuals (Veteran Affairs Total Parenteral Nutrition Cooperative Study Group, 1991). Also, PN-associated infections often involve sites distant from the intravenous catheter, such as the lung, urinary tract and wounds (ASPEN Board of Directors, 1993). The available data suggest that some component(s) of the nutrient solutions themselves, including immunosuppressive effects of lipid emulsions or other components of standard nutrient solutions, the route of feeding, and/or provision of inadequate amounts of immune-stimulating nutrients in standard PN formulations play a role in infection risk. Enteral feeding is associated with maintained gut mucosal cellularity and digestive function, reduced cholestasis, and reduced overall infection rates (Moore et al., 1992; Kudsk et al., 1992). The mechanisms for these beneficial effects remain unclear, but may be due, in part, to improved intestinal immunity and gut barrier function (Wilmore et al., 1988), stimulation of trophic intestinal hormones (e.g. gastrin, cholecystokinin, enteroglucagon, insulin-like growth factors), avoidance of hypertonic dextrose infusions and associated hyperglycaemia, or because enteral and tube feedings provide a more 'balanced' nutrient mix (e.g. amino acids are derived from whole or hydrolysed protein such as casein or whey). Enteral nutrient solutions may contain potentially important substances such as fibre, small peptides, medium chain triglycerides and increased amounts of immunomodulatory amino acids such as glutamine and arginine. In addition, lower total calorie and protein loads are usually given enterally because a degree of malabsorption may occur, and tube feedings are often intermittently withheld for various reasons unrelated to tolerance of enteral infusion.

In general, enteral feeding (even in small amounts) should be used whenever possible in light of the potential beneficial effects and its lower cost. If PN has been initiated, it should be discontinued as soon as the gut becomes functional. We have found administration of erythromycin (500 mg i.v. over 20 min) to be a useful prokinetic agent to facilitate small bowel intubation, when given just prior to bedside replacement of 10 French feeding tubes. Enteral feeds via small bore feeding-tubes are very well tolerated, and in contrast to usual impressions at the bedside, studies suggest that critically ill patients without obvious ileus often tolerate feeding into the small bowel, even when bowel sounds are diminished or even absent (ASPEN Board of Directors, 1993). Feeding may be started at low volumes and at full strength (10–20 ml/h) and advanced to the goal rate as tolerated over a 12–48 h period as PN is weaned off.

Generally, lactose-free, isotonic, liquid diets should be used in the ICU, supplemented by PN until maintenance intake is achieved. Although numerous specialized 'disease-specific' liquid diet formulas are commercially available, in general, the clinical or metabolic efficacy of most of these diets have not been directly compared in controlled, blind trials in similar groups of ICU patients. Formulae which provide amino acids as peptides or protein hydrolysates may be beneficial in patients following a period of gut disuse (and thus mucosal atrophy). Individuals with diarrhoea or constipation often

Table 7.2 General guidelines for nutritional support in the ICU

Perform detailed nutritional assessment
Use enteral feeding whenever possible
Dedicated port for central venous parenteral nutrition
Provide energy at 25–35 kcal/kg/day
Provide protein at 1.3–2.0 g/kg/day (mixed essential and non-essential amino acids)
Decrease protein load proportional to degree of renal/hepatic dysfunction
Provide dextrose at a dose not to exceed 4–5 mg/kg/min (5.8–7.2 g/kg/day)
Maintain blood glucose > 100 and < 200 mg/dl by providing adequate insulin and/or altering dextrose load (do not run insulin drip and insulin in PN at the same time)
Alter tube feeding composition as needed based on gut function, other organ-specific factors
Normalize serum electrolytes, including magnesium
Be aware of 'refeeding syndrome' in severely malnourished patients, especially when given concentrated dextrose (follow potassium, phosphorous and magnesium closely)
Administer adequate zinc

benefit from use of formulae containing fibre and/or short-chain peptides, while post-operative patients or those with gastroparesis often better tolerate formulae containing a low amount of fat, as fat inhibits gastric emptying.

Although still controversial, the use of albumin infusions to increase serum colloid osmotic pressure in adult patients receiving PN or tube feeds have not significantly improved clinical outcomes in randomized, controlled trials in ICU patients (Brown et al., 1988; Foley et al., 1990). No controlled trials have been published regarding albumin administration to improve enteral feeding tolerance; however, non-septic patients with diarrhoea (> 2 l/day) associated with enteral tube feeding intolerance and very low serum albumin (< 2.0 mg/dl) may occasionally benefit from such therapy if no other cause for diarrhoea is evident (e.g. infection, sorbitol-containing elixirs, inappropriate tube feeding formula).

General guidelines for administration of specialized feedings are summarized in Table 7.2.

USE OF SPECIFIC NUTRIENTS

Glutamine

Glutamine (GLN) is the most abundant free amino acid in the whole body as well as in the plasma (Souba and Wilmore, 1994). GLN is the major compound which facilitates the inter-organ transport of nitrogen in humans, particularly between muscle (the major site of GLN synthesis) and the splanchnic bed and kidney (the major sites of GLN uptake). GLN is physiologically important in several key metabolic processes, including nucleotide biosynthesis, skeletal muscle protein synthesis and breakdown, renal ammoniagenesis and gluconeogenesis. GLN is also utilized as a major metabolic fuel by rapidly replicating cells, such as the enterocyte (Souba et al., 1985).

The available data support the concept that GLN may become conditionally essential in catabolic states. GLN requirements increase markedly during stress, as GLN-utilizing tissues (e.g. intestinal mucosa, stimulated immune cells) consume increased amounts of GLN, and utilization exceeds endogenous production. Thus, a GLN deficiency state may develop with the fall of GLN concentrations in intracellular muscle and plasma pools, as obligatory requirements are not satisfied by adequate provision of dietary GLN. This conditional deficiency may be manifested as altered structure and function of GLN-utilizing tissues and cells. Net catabolism of skeletal muscle increases initially to provide increased quantities of GLN for the body. Evidence suggests that dietary supplementation of GLN during catabolic states may attenuate or reverse these sequelae (Ziegler et al., 1993).

L-Glutamine is generally not present in most standard parenteral nutrient solutions because of poor solubility and degradation to ammonia and pyroglutamic acid with heat sterilization. However, degradation is minimized by cold sterilization and proper storage (Ziegler et al., 1990a). Glutamine dipeptides have been also developed for parenteral use which are more soluble and may be heat-sterilized (Stehle et al., 1989).

An increasing number of clinical studies have shown that GLN administration is safe and clinically efficacious. Beneficial effects observed in trials, PN diets enriched with L-GLN or GLN analogues – ornithine α-ketoglutarate (OAK) and α-ketoglutarate (AKG) – versus standard, GLN-free or low GLN diets are shown in Table 7.3. In all of the clinical trials reported to date, GLN-enriched feeding resulted in reduced net body protein breakdown, as evidenced by improved nitrogen retention and enhanced protein synthesis when compared to results with isonitrogenous, isocaloric control diets (Hammarqvist et al., 1989; Ziegler et al., 1993).

In a recent randomized, blinded and controlled trial in adult patients undergoing allogenic bone marrow transplantation (BMT), parenteral solutions providing 0.57 g L-GLN/kg/day markedly attenuated nitrogen loss compared to patients receiving standard, GLN-free

Table 7.3 Beneficial effects of dietary supplementation with L-GLN, ALA–GLN dipeptide or GLN precursers (OAK, AKG) in patients

Maintains/restores intracellular GLN levels in skeletal muscle (L-GLN, ALA–GLN, OAK, AKG)
Maintains/increases plasma glutamine concentrations (L-GLN, ALA–GLN, OAK, AKG)
Improves nitrogen balance after operation, BMT, or burn injury (L-GLN, ALA–GLN, OAK, AKG)
Enhances post-operative skeletal muscle protein synthesis (L-GLN, ALA–GLN, OAK, AKG)
Reduces myofibrillar protein breakdown after BMT (L-GLN)
Attenuates extracellular fluid expansion after BMT (L-GLN)
Reduces clinical infection and microbial colonization after BMT (L-GLN)
Reduces hospital length of stay after BMT (L-GLN)
Enhances wound healing following burn injury (enteral OAK)
Improves growth rate and IGF-I levels in children with SBS (OAK)
Improves nutrient absorption in combination with GH and modified diet in SBS (L-GLN)
Increases D-xylose absorption in critically ill patients (ALA–GLN)

L-GLN, free L-GLN; ALA–GLN, alanine-glutamine dipeptide; OAK, ornithine-alpha-ketoglutarate; AKG, alpha-ketoglutarate, SBS, short bowel syndrome; BMT, bone marrow transplantation. Adapted from Ziegler et al. (1993).

parenteral nutrition (Figure 7.1). Additionally, significantly reduced microbial colonization and clinical infections were noted, and hospital stay was shortened by 7 days with GLN supplementation of PN (Ziegler et al., 1992a). Another recent randomized, controlled trial in a different patient population confirmed a 6-day reduction in hospital stay with use of an identical GLN-enriched PN solution in a group of patients after allogeneic and autologous BMT (Schloerb and Amare, 1993). However, the only difference in infection rates observed was a significantly reduced incidence of bacteraemia in the relatively small group of allogeneic BMT patients (Schloerb and Amare, 1993). The mechanism(s) resulting in improved clinical outcomes with GLN-supplemented nutrition are unclear, but may include improved nitrogen economy (Stehle et al., 1989; Ziegler et al., 1990a), production of the antioxidant glutathione (Hong et al., 1992), maintenance of the gut mucosal barrier function (Van der Hulst et al., 1993), attenuation of extracellular water space expansion (Scheltinga et al., 1991) and/or enhanced lymphocyte recovery (Ziegler et al., 1994). Additional studies which evaluate the metabolic, molecular and clinical mechanisms of GLN action in other catabolic states are needed to clarify the potential utility of this amino acid.

GLN administration has been well tolerated clinically, without

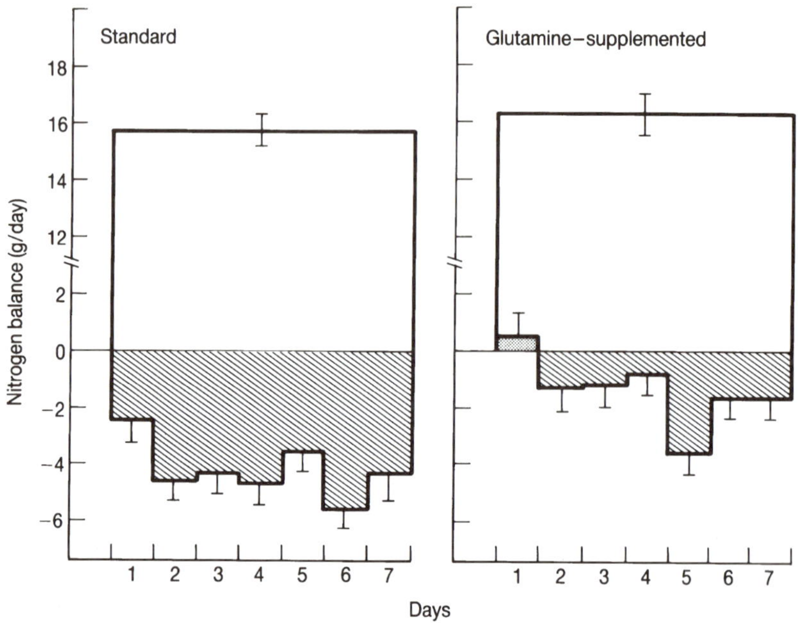

Figure 7.1. Daily nitrogen balance in adult patients receiving isonitrogenous, isocaloric PN after allogeneic bone marrow transplantation. Nitrogen intake (mean ± SE) for the week is shown by the upper horizontal line, and nitrogen balance for each 24 h period is shown by the areas in grey (positive balance) or stippled (negative balance). The patients receiving standard feeding were given no glutamine in PN, while the glutamine-supplemented group received 0.57 g/kg/day. Glutamine supplementation significantly attenuated nitrogen loss in these catabolic patients compared to standard nutritional support ($p = 0.001$ by ANOVA).

appreciable generation of end-products such as ammonia, glutamate or pyroglutamic acid in plasma, even though relatively large amounts of GLN are administered to exert beneficial effects (equivalent to 15–40 g/day, based on dose–response studies, largely done in animals). Patients with severe renal or hepatic failure or CNS dysfunction may not efficiently metabolize and utilize large protein loads, and GLN supplementation may be contraindicated in these clinical settings. However, pending ongoing research, GLN should be considered a potentially important dietary amino acid in catabolic patients, particularly those with muscle wasting, gastrointestinal dysfunction and immunodeficiency.

Intestinal effects of glutamine-enriched modified diet and GH therapy

One strategy to enhance the efficacy of metabolic support is to combine anabolic hormones with key nutrient substrates, such as GLN. We studied the combined effects of GLN (0.45 g/kg/day intravenous or enteral), parenteral GH (0.14 mg/kg/day) and a modified enteral diet (high protein, high complex carbohydrate, low to moderate fat) in adult patients with short bowel syndrome (Byrne et al., 1992, 1993).

After 3 weeks, patients receiving this combined therapy gained significantly more lean body mass (4.3 ± 0.6 kg vs. 2.0 ± 0.2; $p < 0.03$) and more protein (1.4 ± 0.3 kg vs. 0.9 ± 0.1; $p < 0.03$) than individuals treated with standard therapy (Byrne et al., 1993). Markedly improved intestinal absorption of nitrogen, calories, sodium and water occurred using GH + GLN + diet therapy (Byrne et al., 1992), suggesting that this treatment enhanced bowel function. Further work is in progress to determine the nature of this additive or synergistic effect of combined therapy on nutrient absorption in similar patients. No controlled data are available on GH + GLN therapy in ICU patients, although several studies have demonstrated that GH attenuates or abolishes glutamine release from muscle and maintains free intracellular glutamine concentrations in skeletal muscle (Hammarqvist et al., 1992). This data provides an additional rationale for combined glutamine + GH therapy as a method to maintain intracellular glutamine concentrations in stressed patients.

Arginine

Arginine is another amino acid with potentially beneficial effects in patients with critical illness, wounds and immunocompromise. Arginine has potent immunostimulatory effects when provided in amounts greater than normally present in the diet. Human data are limited; however, several studies suggest that arginine may improve immune functions, particularly when provided with adequate nutritional support (Barbul et al., 1981; Daly et al., 1988). In the first study of immune effects of supplemental arginine in injured humans, Daly et al. (1988) evaluated the immune and metabolic effects of L-arginine (25 g/day) or isonitrogenous L-glycine added to enteral feeding solutions postoperative in 30 patients with gastrointestinal malignancies requiring operation. Immune parameters were measured pre-operatively and 1 to 7 days post-operatively. The arginine-supplemented group demonstrated slightly improved nitrogen balance and significantly enhanced mean T lymphocyte responses to the mitogens PHA and Con-A vs controls on post-operative days 4 and 7. Arginine supplementation also increased the CD-4 phenotype on post-operative days 1 and 7. Arginine increased insulin-like growth factor-I (IGF-I) levels, and this hormone may have mediated the immune responses. No differences in infection rates were noted in this short-term trial (Daly et al., 1988), and effects of arginine in critical illness have not been evaluated in a randomized, double-blind trial. In our hospital, we routinely supplement enteral feedings with crystalline arginine powder (10–30 mg/day) in tube fed patients with large wounds and/or severe immunocompromise; however, no controlled data are yet available to support this approach.

Use of Modified Lipid Products

A number of new lipid products, containing medium-chain triglycerides, fish oils and 'structured lipid' products are now being tested clinically. While some evidence suggests that these may have beneficial metabolic effects compared to standard lipid products commonly administered (Carpentier et al., 1993), limited data on clinical outcomes are available. Recent studies in post-operative patients have suggested that arginine (12.5 g/l) added to enteral diets containing nucleotides and fish oil improves immune function and reduces infection rates compared to standard enteral diets without RNA or fish oil, but containing low amounts of arginine (Daly et al., 1992). Enteral diets supplemented with arginine, RNA, and fish oil improved *in vitro* lymphocyte blastogenesis and also appeared to reduce wound complications and hospital length of stay (Cerra et al., 1991). Additional studies of similar enteral formulations containing mixtures of immunomodulating nutrients are in progress in ICU patients.

ADMINISTRATION OF GROWTH FACTORS

Recombinant techniques have enabled large-scale production of peptide growth factors for clinical investigation and clinical care. The most information on adjunctive growth factor administration in ICU patients are studies on administration of human growth hormone (GH) and insulin, but ongoing studies are evaluating effects of other peptides, including recombinant insulin-like growth factor-I (IGF-I) and epidermal growth factor (EGF).

Growth Hormone

Pituitary GH administration in clinically stable non-GH deficient patients has long been known to enhance retention of nitrogen, phosphorus, potassium, sodium, magnesium and calcium. GH also diminishes urea production, induces lipolysis and increases plasma insulin levels due to insulin resistance in glucose homoeostasis (Henneman et al., 1960). A number of early studies in burn patients given adjunctive intramuscular pituitary GH (5–10 mg/day s.c. or i.m.) demonstrated improved nitrogen and mineral retention, increased appetite, and antecdotally improved wound healing (Liljedahl et al., 1961; Wilmore et al., 1974).

Recombinant GH as an adjunct to nutritional support has been extensively studied in physiologically stable patients during the post-operative period (Jiang et al., 1989; Vara-Thorbeck et al., 1993), and in patients with chronic obstructive lung disease (Pape et al., 1991), end-stage renal disease (Ziegler et al., 1991) and gastro-intestinal disease (Ziegler et al., 1988; Byrne et al., 1993). Consistent protein-anabolism, mineral retention and other metabolic effects including increased circulating IGF-I and insulin levels, enhanced fat oxidation and reduced urea generation, have been demonstrated over a wide range of calorie and nitrogen doses, underlying illnesses and GH doses (Figure 7.2; Ziegler et al., 1992b). Positive nitrogen balance occurred with GH therapy, even with *hypocaloric* PN providing only ~ 60% of maintenance energy with adequate protein (Ziegler et al., 1988). These studies in non critically ill patients demonstrate a marked improvement in enteral and parenteral nutrient utilization efficiency with recombinant GH. In addition to improved metabolic effects, a recent large Spanish study of patients given pituitary GH after cholecystectomy demonstrated improved immune function, reduced post-operative infection rates and shortened length of hospital study in the GH-treated patients (Vara-Thorbeck et al., 1993).

Fairly extensive data on recombinant GH effects in critical illness are now available. Recombinant GH therapy was given for 1 to 6 weeks in a group of severely catabolic adult patients receiving conventional enteral/parenteral nutrition support after severe burn injury (~ 60% body surface area) or vehicular trauma (Ziegler et al., 1990b). Daily GH at a range of 0.096–0.172 mg/kg/day) was administered subcutaneously after an initial control week. GH was very well tolerated in these critically ill patients, but they were selected to be without diabetus mellitus, cancer, congestive heart failure or other forms of severe fluid retention at entry into the study. Body losses of protein, potassium and phosphorus decreased markedly with GH treatment in all patients, and urea generation decreased by ~ 30% within the first few days of GH. Serum IGF-1 levels rose approximately five fold with GH, serum magnesium and alanine aminotransferase fell significantly and serum calcium and tryglycerides rose slightly but significantly, with GH over time. Serum potassium, sodium and phosphorus remained stable with GH therapy, despite significant retention of these electrolytes (Ziegler et al., 1990b; Figure 7.3). Additional studies in other groups of critically ill and septic patients have documented increased whole body and limb protein synthetic rates, improved nitrogen balance and increased fat oxidation rates with short-term GH administration compared to clinically similar patients receiving placebo injections and comparable diets (Herndon et al., 1990; Shernan et al., 1989; Douglas et al., 1990; Voerman et al., 1992). In a blinded, controlled trial in adult burn patients, 2 weeks of GH therapy (10 mg/day) was shown to attenuate expansion of the extracellular water (ECW) compartment and to minimize loss of intracellular water (ICW). These effects were opposite of control patients who demonstrated the usual expansion of ECW and contraction of ICW, suggesting a possible effect of GH on cell membrane stability or permeability (Gatzen et al., 1992). Thus, as in clinically stable patients, recombinant GH therapy appears to be a promising adjunctive therapy to improve nutrient utilization in ICU patients. GH effects on nutritional end-points, such as improved nitrogen balance and enhanced protein synthetic rates, and the ability of GH to restore IGF-I levels may represent rationales for use of GH therapy in the ICU. None the less, documentation of GH effects on important clinical outcomes such as infection rates, hospital stay and mortality in critical illness are needed to further define the ICU patients whom may benefit from GH.

We observed antecdotal improvements in wound healing and

Figure 7.2. Elemental balances of nitrogen (N), potassium (K), and phosphorus (P) in a randomized, double-blind study of clinically stable adult patients receiving isocaloric (~ 30 kcal/kg/day), isonitrogenous (≈ 1.6 g protein/kg/day) total parenteral nutrition. The patients received daily saline-placebo injections (control) or s.c. recombinant GH (10 mg/day; range 0.142–0.237 mg/kg/day). During an initial baseline week prior to the injections, N, K and P balances approached equilibrium in each group. Nutrient balances changed minimally in the control patients. In contrast, with daily s.c. GH treatment, a significant increase in N, K and P balance occurred and net nutrient retention was achieved within 1–2 days of GH administration ($p <$ 0.05). The grey area above the zero balance line represents positive nutrient balance and the black area denotes negative nutrient balance. (From Ziegler et al., 1992b, with permission.)

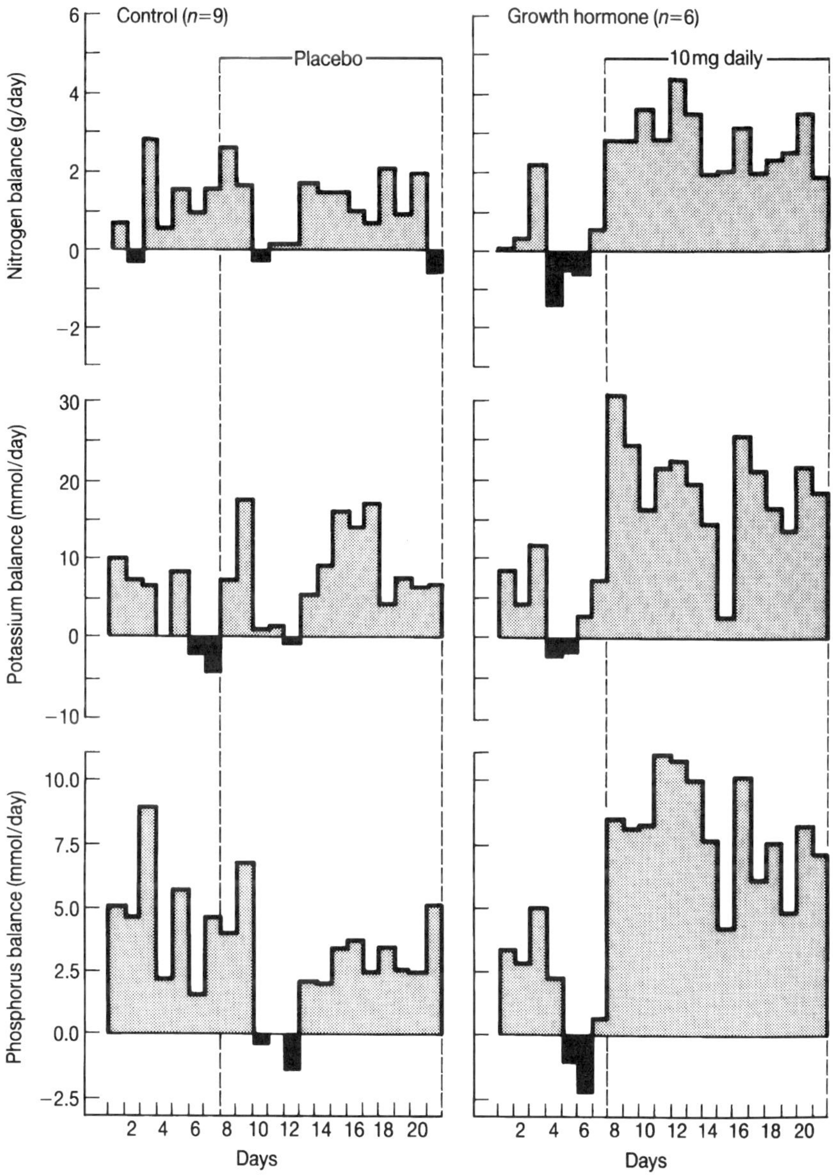
Control (n=9)
Placebo
Growth hormone (n=6)
10 mg daily
Nitrogen balance (g/day)
Potassium balance (mmol/day)
Phosphorus balance (mmol/day)
6
4
2
0
−2
30
20
10
0
−10
10.0
7.5
5.0
2.5
0.0
−2.5
2 4 6 8 10 12 14 16 18 20
Days
2 4 6 8 10 12 14 16 18 20
Days

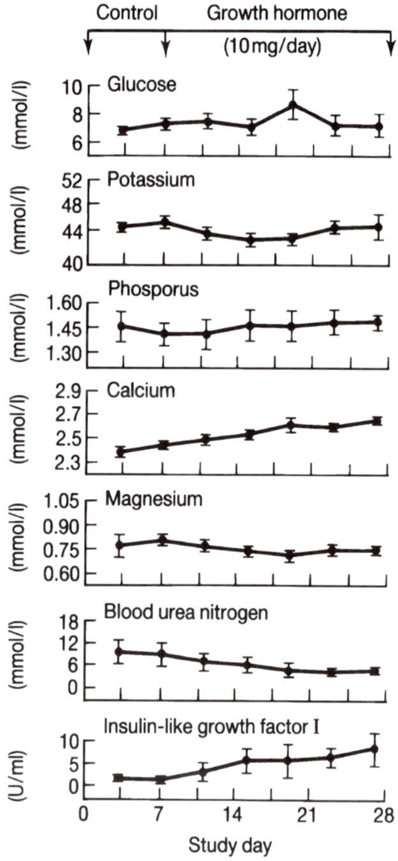

Figure 7.3. Effects of 3 weeks of GH administration on serial blood values in burn/trauma patients. Mean serum glucose and phosphorus levels remained stable over time, serum potassium and magnesium fell slightly and serum calcium values rose slightly but significantly. Circulating total ICF-I levels rose markedly and blood urea nitrogen fell markedly during GH. Data represent 4-day means over the 28-day study period. (From Ziegler et al., 1990b, with permission.)

respiratory muscle strength (Figure 7.4), a low overall rate of infectious complications and an apparent acceleration in indexes of physical rehabilitation with GH use in adult burn/trauma patients (Ziegler et al., 1990b). Improved wound healing with GH treatment in adult burn patients was subsequently confirmed utilizing skin donor site re-epithelialization as an end-point (Shernan et al., 1989). In this study, patients receiving GH (10 mg/day) after burn

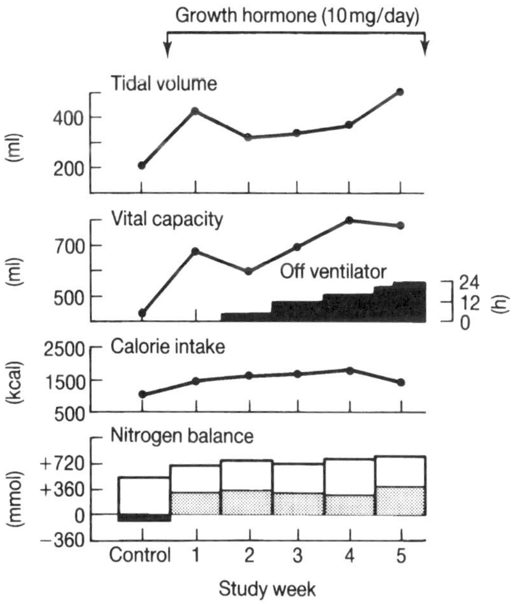

Figure 7.4. Clinical data from a 37-year-old man rendered quadraplegic after a fall. The patient had a paralyzed hemidiaphram, and had failed to wean from the ventilator for several months. Prior to GH administration, the patient was in negative nitrogen balance, despite adequate tube feedings. With GH (10 mg/day, s.c.) he exhibited net nitrogen retention, improved respiratory muscle strength and was eventually weaned from mechanical ventilation. (From Ziegler et al., 1990b, with permission.)

injury demonstrated a reduction in donor site healing time of 2–4 days when compared to clinically matched control patients receiving placebo and identical diets. In children with severe burn injury, GH (0.2 mg/kg/day) significantly decreased hospital stay and improved wound healing rates by 2–4 days compared to matched placebo control patients; however a lower dose of 0.1 mg/kg/day was ineffective (Herndon et al., 1990).

Several investigators with experience using GH in the ICU have noted improvements in respiratory muscle strength, ventilator weaning and other indices of physical rehabilitation during GH therapy in critical illness. To date, these end-points have not been well characterized. A preliminary randomized study has failed to confirm an impact of GH on ventilator weaning or peripheral skeletal muscle strength in adults with COPD (Pichard et al., 1994). In this study, 20 patients requiring mechanical ventilation were randomized to receive

GH (0.43 IU/kg/day or ~ 0.14 mg/kg/day) or saline for 12 days. Enteral feeding provided ~ 30 kcal/kg/day and 1.0 to 1.3 g protein/kg/day. Significantly improved 12-day cumulative nitrogen balance occurred with GH (control −66 g versus GH +44 g/12 day), however, no significant change in thumb muscle force or muscle fatigue indices occurred between groups. In addition, total time on mechanical ventilation did not differ between groups (control 246 h/12 days versus GH 236 h/12 days) (Pichard et al., 1994). Improved protein retention was not associated with an objective improvement in ventilator weaning during GH administration. Thus, further study is needed to determine whether skeletal muscle function is improved by GH in ICU patients.

Multiple studies in animal models and in vitro suggest that both GH and IGF-I may modulate the immune system. However, no studies have objectively documented improvements in immunity or in infection rates with GH in critically ill patients, although most studies have been short-term investigations of less than one week. In one uncontrolled study, 1.5 IU GH/kg/day (~ 0.05 mg/kg/day) was given for 5 days to severely catabolic patients with generalized sepsis with or without corresponding traumatic injury (mean APACHE II score 26) (Gottardis et al., 1991). No change in a standardized sepsis score occurred during GH treatment (between 5 to 10 days of admission) or by the end of the study at day 13 (Gottardis et al., 1991). GH did not improve wound healing or immunoglobulin number or function in burn patients when GH was given at a dose of 0.1 mg/kg/day for several days (Belcher et al., 1990). In another study, GH or placebo was given to 20 patients with a diagnosis of septic shock (mean APACHE II score 23) (Voerman et al., 1992). The patients began 24 h continuous infusions of GH (0.1 mg/kg/day) or saline after a 24–48 h of resuscitation. Despite acute and severe catabolic stress, both nitrogen and urea production decreased significantly during GH therapy. These indices of protein catabolism returned to baseline levels within 24 h after cessation of GH, and vital signs, cardiopulmonary haemodynamic parameters, haematology and other blood chemistries remained stable during GH. No changes in post-therapy infection rates or other clinical outcomes were noted between groups in this short-term trial.

Illness severity may contribute to the overall IGF-I and protein-anabolic response to exogenous GH treatment. Subcutaneous or intravenous administration of identical GH doses induced a similar increase in circulating IGF-I in critically ill patients; however, as injury severity increased, the IGF-I response to GH given by either route was significantly attenuated (Kimbrough et al., 1991). As most

Table 7.4 Metabolic and clinical effects of GH therapy in catabolic patients requiring specialized nutritional support

Metabolic effects
Improved nitrogen retention, reduced urea generation
Stimulated protein synthesis, reduced amino acid efflux
Maintained intracellular glutamine levels in skeletal muscle
Enhanced retention of potassium, phosphorus, magnesium, and sodium
Enhanced fat oxidation, increased serum glycerol and free fatty acids
Increased metabolic rate
Insulin resistance, increased plasma glucose
Variable effects on serum electrolytes, increased serum GH, IGF-I, and insulin levels
Maintained extracellular and intracellular water compartments (ICU patients)
Clinical effects
Improved wound healing (adult and paediatric burn patients)
Shortened hospital stay (paediatric burn patients, adult post-operative patients)
Increased somatic growth rate (paediatric end-stage renal failure)
Decreased infection rate, improved immune function (adult post-operative patients)
Increased hand grip strength (adult post-operative patients)
Variable effects on respiratory muscle strength (adult COPD (Chronic obstructive pulmonary Disease)

of the body's IGF-I production is thought to occur in the liver, patients with hepatic dysfunction or cirrhosis or those with multiple organ failure may exhibit an attenuated IGF-I and protein-anabolic response to GH.

GH treatment induces a number of potentially beneficial metabolic and clinical effects in catabolic and critically ill patients (Table 7.4); however, much more work is needed to define improved clinical outcomes with this peptide in randomized controlled trials. GH also has a number of potential side-effects, as reviewed recently in detail (Ziegler, 1994; Table 7.5). Given these and other unknown potential problems with GH use, careful selection and monitoring of patients is essential.

Insulin-like Growth Factor-I (IGF-I)

A number of short-term studies documented protein-anabolic effects of recombinant IGF-I (or somatomedin C) in humans (Clemmons et al., 1992; Kupfer et al., 1993). Growth hormone is the primary regulator of endogenous IGF-I synthesis and release by liver and other tissues; however, IGF-I production is also markedly reduced

Table 7.5 Potential complications of growth hormone administration in ICU patients

Insulin resistance, hyperglycaemia (may be severe)
Hypercalcaemia
Fluid retention
Arthralgias and carpel tunnel syndrome
Induction or stimulation of neoplastic growth

in malnutrition and increases with nutritional repletion (Clemmons and Underwood, 1991). In one study of normal adult men fed hypocaloric diets, combined subcutaneous GH and intravenous IGF-I therapy resulted in a significantly improved nitrogen balance over the baseline diet period compared to results with IGF-I or GH alone (Kupfer et al., 1993).

The preliminary results of one study of IGF-I use in catabolic patients have been reported (Chen et al., 1993). Recombinant IGF-I (10 μg/kg/h) or saline were infused for 14 days after severe head trauma in 24 adult patients. In saline-treated controls, daily nitrogen balance was negative (−2.9 g/day), and worsened to −5.0 g/day during the second week after injury. Nitrogen was significantly conserved during the first week post-injury in the IGF-I treated group (+ 1.3 g/day) as IGF-I levels rose significantly from 78 to 466 ng/ml. However, IGF-I levels then fell to 220 ng/ml by day 14, and the nitrogen-retaining effect of IGI-I was lost despite continued IGF-I infusion (Chen et al., 1993). Thus, IGI-I therapy may be less efficacious than GH in promoting sustained protein anabolism in other groups of ICU patients (Ziegler et al., 1990b). IGI-I may induce hypoglycaemia, which probably represents the major potential complication of this growth factor if used in patients requiring specialized enteral or parenteral nutrition. The potential metabolic and clinical utility of recombinant IGI-I in patients requiring specialized feeding requires clarification.

Other Growth Factors

In addition to GH and IGF-I, preliminary studies have been completed or are being performed using other recombinant growth factors as methods to enhance wound healing and to improve other metabolic and clinical outcomes. For example, topical recombinant epidermal growth factor (EGF) significantly enhanced wound healing in burn patients (Brown et al., 1989). Undoubtedly, additional research will determine whether these or other synthetic hormones, alone or in combination, will have roles in nutritional and metabolic support of certain groups of ICU patients in the future.

SUMMARY

Nutritional/metabolic support modalities are evolving in the ICU setting. Current practices emphasize feeding via the intestinal tract and provision of lower amounts of energy and protein than provided routinely in the recent past. These changes reflect, in part, recognition that 'more is not better', the relative inefficiency of current therapy in preventing protein wasting during severe catabolic stress, the lack of double-blind controlled trials defining which patient subgroups benefit from aggressive feeding, and appreciation of the potential complications of specialized nutritional support. However, several promising new strategies designed to improve the efficacy of nutritional care are now being investigated clinically. These approaches include use of growth factors, administration of specific nutrients, including dietary fibre, short-chain fatty acids, glutamine, arginine, dipeptides, modified lipid products, nutrient antioxidants, and combinations of these therapies (Table 7.6).

Administration of selected nutrients and hormones may reduce or alter protein-catabolic responses, influence metabolism, and provide conditionally essential substrates to cells and tissues. However, these approaches need to be evaluated in double-blind randomized, controlled clinical trials, in patients receiving an appropriate substrate/nutrient background. It is likely that nutritional and metabolic support for the critically ill patient will routinely include selected growth factors and increased amounts of certain nutrients within the next 3–5 years. Further clinical investigation is required to define the safety, clinical and metabolic efficacy and cost-effectiveness of these new approaches in specialized nutrition.

Table 7.6 New developments in nutritional support in critical illness

Emphasis on enteral feedings to maintain intestinal absorptive, immune and barrier function
Administration of growth factors (e.g. GH, IGF-I, EGF)
Administration of conditionally essential amino acids (e.g. glutamine, arginine)
Use of specialized lipid products (e.g. medium-chain tryglycerides, short-chain fatty acids)
Provision of antioxidants (e.g. vitamin E, vitamin C, glutamine)
Combination therapies (e.g. growth factors + specific nutrients)

REFERENCES

American Society for Parental and Enteral Nutrition Board of Directors. (1993) Guidelines for the use of parental and enteral nutrition in adult and pediatric patients. *Journal of Parental and Enteral Nutrition* **14**(suppl. 4): 15A–525A.

Askanazi, J., Rosenbaum, S.H., Hyman, Al. et al. (1980) Respiratory changes induced by the large glucose loads of parenteral nutrition. *Journal of the American Medical Association* **243**: 1444–1446.

Baker, J.P., Detsky, A.S., Wessen, D.E. et al. (1982) Nutritional assessment: A comparison of clinical judgement and objective measurements. *New England Journal of Medicine* **306**: 969–973.

Barbul, A., Rettura, G., Wasserkrug, H.L. et al. (1981) Arginine stimulates lymphocyte immune responses in healthy humans. *Surgery* **90**: 244–251.

Barton, R.G. (1994) Nutrition support in critical illness. *Nutrition in Clinical Practice* **9**: 127–139.

Belcher, H.J., Sheldon, J., Riches, P. (1990) An investigation of immunological subclass function in burned adults. *Burns* **16**: 286–290.

Brown, G.L., Nanney, L.B., Griffen, J. et al. (1989) Enhancement of wound healing by topical treatment with epidermal growth factor. *New England Journal of Medicine* **321**: 76–79.

Brown, R.O., Bradley, J.E., Bekemeyer, W.B., Luther, R.W. (1988) Effect of albumin supplementation during parenteral nutrition on hospital morbidity. *Critical Care Medicine* **16**: 1177–1182.

Byrne, T.A., Morrissey, T.B., Ziegler, T.R. et al. (1992) Growth hormone, glutamine and fiber enhance adaptation of remnant bowel following massive intestinal resection. *Surgical Forum* **43**: 151–153.

Byrne, T.A., Morrissey, T.B., Gatzen, C. et al. (1993) Anabolic therapy with growth hormone accelerates gain in lean tissue in surgical patients requiring nutritional rehabilitation. *Annals of Surgery* **218**: 400–418.

Carpentier, Y.A., Van Gossum, A., DuBois, D.Y. et al. (1993) Lipid metabolism in parenteral nutrition. In Rombeau, J.L., Caldwell, M.D. (eds) *Clinical Nutrition: Parenteral Nutrition*, 2nd edn, **3**: 35–74. Philadelphia: W.B. Saunders.

Cerra, F.B., Siegel, J.H., Colman, B. et al. (1980) Septic autocannibalism, a failure of exogenous nutritional support. *Annals of Surgery* **192**: 570–580.

Cerra, F.B., Lehmann, S., Konstantinides, N. et al. (1991) Improvement in immune function in ICU patients by enteral nutrition supplemented with arginine, RNA, and menhaden oil is independent of nitrogen balance. *Nutrition* **17**: 193–199.

Chen, S.A., Bukar, J.G., Mohler, M.A. et al. (1993) Recombinant human IGF-I infusion results in transient improvement in nitrogen balance: Evidence for IGF-I autoregulation. Proceedings of the 75th Annual Meeting of the Endocrinology Society, Las Vegas, NV.

Clark-Christoff, N., Watters, V., Sparks, W. et al. (1992) Use of triple-lumen subclavian catheters for administration of total parenteral nutrition. *Journal of Parenterel and Enterel Nutrition* **16**: 403–407.

Clemmons, D.R., Underwood, L.E. (1991) Nutritional regulation of IGF-I and IGF binding proteins. *Annual Review of Nutrition* **11**: 393–412.

Clemmons, D.R., Smith-Banks, A., Celniker, A.C., Underwood, L.E. (1992) Reversal of diet-induced catabolism by infusion of recombinant insulin-like growth factor-I (IGF-I) in humans. *Journal of Clinical Endocrinology and Metabolism* **75**: 1192–1197.

Daly, J.M., Reynolds, J., Thom, A. et al. (1988) Immune and metabolic effects of arginine in the surgical patient. *Annals of Surgery* **208**: 512–523.

Daly, J.M., Lieberman, M.D., Goldfine, J. et al. (1992) Enteral nutrition with supplemental arginine, RNA, and omega-3 fatty acids in patients after operation: Immunologic, metabolic, and clinical outcome. *Surgery* **112**: 56–67.

Douglas, R.G., Humberstone, D.A., Haystead, A. et al. (1990) Metabolic effects of recombinant human growth hormone: isotopic studies in the postoperative state and during total parenteral nutrition. *British Journal of Surgery* **77**: 785-790.

Foley, E.F., Borlase, B.C., Dzik, W.H., Bistrian, B.R., Benotti, P.N. (1990) Albumin supplementation in the critically ill. *Archives of Surgery* **125**: 739–742.

Gatzen, C., Scheltinga, M.R., Kimbrough, T.D. et al. (1992) Growth hormone attenuates the abnormal distribution of body water in critically ill surgical patients. *Surgery* **112**: 181–187.

Gottardis, M., Benzer, A., Koller, W. et al. (1991) Improvement of septic syndrome after administration of recombinant human growth hormone? *Journal of Trauma* **31**: 81–86.

Hammarqvist, F., Wernerman, J., Ali, R. et al. (1989) Addition of glutamine to total parenteral nutrition after elective abdominal surgery spares free glutamine in muscle, counteracts the fall in muscle protein synthesis, and improves nitrogen balance. *Annals of Surgery* **209**: 455–461.

Hammarqvist, F., Stromberg, C., Decken von der A. et al. (1992) Biosynthetic human growth hormone preserves both muscle protein synthesis and the decrease in muscle free glutamine, and improves whole-body nitrogen economy after operation. *Annals of Surgery* **216**: 184–191.

Haydock, D.A., Hill, G.L. (1987) Improved wound healing responses in surgical patients receiving intravenous nutrition. *British Journal of Surgery* **74**: 320–323.

Henneman, P.H., Forbes, A.P., Moldawer, M. et al. (1960) Effects of human growth hormone in man. *Journal of Clinical Investigation* **39**: 1223–1238.

Herndon, D.N., Barrow, R.E., Kunkle, K.R. et al. (1990) Effects of recombinant human growth hormone on donor site healing in severely burned children. *Annals of Surgery* **212**: 424–429.

Hong, R.W., Rounds, J.D., Helton, W.S. et al. (1992) Glutamine protects liver glutathione after lethal hepatic injury. *Annals of Surgery* **215**: 114–119.

Jeejeebhoy, K.N. (1993) Nutrient requirements and nutrient deficiencies in gastrointestinal diseases. In Sleisenger, M.H., Fordtran, J.S., Scharschmidt, B.E., Feldman, M. (eds) Gastrointestinal Disease: pathophysiology, diagnosis, management, 5th edn, pp. 2017–2047. Philadelphia: W.B. Saunders.

Jiang, Z.M., He, G.Z., Zhang, S.Y. et al. (1989) Low-dose growth hormone and hypocaloric nutrition attenuate the protein-catabolic response after major operation. *Annals of Surgery* **210**: 513–524.

Kimbrough, T., Shernan, S., Ziegler, T.R. et al. (1991) Insulin-like growth factor I (IGF-I) response is comparable following intravenous and subcutaneous administration of growth hormone. *Journal of Surgical Research* **51**: 472–476.

Kudsk, K.A., Croce, M.A., Fabian, A. et al. (1992) Enteral vs parenteral feeding: effects on septic morbidity following blunt and penetrating trauma. *Annals of Surgery* **215**: 503–513.

Kupfer, S.R., Underwood, L.E., Baxter, R.C., Clemmons, D.R. (1993) Enhancement of the anabolic effects of growth hormone and insulin-like growth factor I by use of both agents simultaneously. *Journal of Clinical Investigation* **91**: 391–396.

Liljedahl, S., Gemzell, C., Plantin, L. et al. (1961) Effect of human growth hormone in patients with severe burns. *Acta Chirurgica Scandinavica* **122**: 1–14.

Lopes, J., Russell, D.Mc.R., Whitwell, J., Jeejeebhoy, K.N. (1982) Skeletal muscle function in malnutrition. *American Journal of Clinical Nutrition* **36**: 602–610.

Lowry, S.F., Brennan, M.F. (1979) Abnormal liver function during parenteral nutrition: relation to infusion excess. *Journal of Surgical Research* **26**: 300–307.

Moore, F.A., Feliciano, D.V., Andrassy, R.J. et al. (1992) Early enteral feeding, compared with parenteral reduces postoperative septic complication. The results of a meta-analysis. *Annals of Surgery* **216**: 172–183.

Pape, G.S., Friedman, M., Underwood, L.E., Clemmons, D.R. (1991) The effect of growth hormone on weight gain and pulmonary function in patients with chronic obstructive lung disease. *Chest* **99**: 1495–1500.

Pichard, C., Kyle, U., Chevrolet, J.C. et al. (1994) Recombinant growth hormone (rGH) effect on muscle function in ventilated chronic obstructive pulmonary disease (COPD). *Journal of Parenterel and Enterel Nutrition* **18**(suppl. 1): 35S.

Pingleton, S.K., Harmon, G.S. (1987) Nutritional management in acute respiratory failure. *Journal of the American Medical Association* **257**: 3094–3099.

Pomposelli, J.J., Flores, E.A., Bistrian, B.R. (1988) Role of biochemical mediators in clinical nutrition and surgical metabolism. *Journal of Parenterel and Enterel Nutrition* **12**: 212–218.

Rudman, D., Millikan, W.J., Richardson, T.J. et al. (1975) Elemental balances during intravenous hyperalimentation of underweight adult subjects. *Journal of Clinical Investigation* **55**: 94–104.

Scheltinga, M., Young, L.S., Benfell, K. et al. (1991) Glutamine-enriched intravenous feedings attenuate extracellular fluid expansion after a standard stress. *Annals of Surgery* **214**: 385–395.

Schloerb, P.R., Amare, M. (1993) Total parenteral nutrition with glutamine in bone marrow transplantation and other clinical applications (A randomized, double-blind study). *Journal of Parenterel and Enterel Nutrition* **17**: 407–413.

Scrimshaw, N.S., Taylor, C.E., Gooden, J.E. (1973) Interactions of nutrition and infection. *American Journal of Medical Sciences* **237**: 367–403.

Shaw, J.H.F., Widbore, M., Wolfe, R.R. (1987) Whole body protein kinetics in severely septic patients. *Annals of Surgery* **205**: 288–294.

Shernan, S.K., Demling, R.H., LaLonde, C. et al. (1989) Growth hormone enhances re-epithelialization of human split-thickness skin graft doner sites. *Surgical Forum* **40**: 37–39.

Souba, W.W., Wilmore, D.W. (1994) Diet and nutrition in the care of the patient with surgery, trauma, and sepsis. In Shils, M.E., Olson, J.A., Shike, M. (eds) *Modern Nutrition in Health and Disease*, 8th edn, **68**: 1207–1240. Philadelphia: Lea and Febiger.

Souba, W.W., Smith, R.J., Wilmore, D.W. (1985) Glutamine metabolism by the intestinal tract. *Journal of Parenterel and Enterel Nutrition* **9**: 608–617.

Stehle, P., Mertes, N., Puchstein, Ch. et al. (1989) Effect of parenteral glutamine peptide supplements on muscle glutamine loss and nitrogen balance after major surgery. *Lancet* **i**: 231–233.

Streat, S.J., Beddoe, A.H., Hill, G.L. (1987) Aggressive nutritional support does not prevent protein loss despite fat gain in septic intensive care patients. *Journal of Trauma* **27**: 262–266.

Van der Hulst, R.R.W.J., van Kreel, B.K., von Meyenfeldt, M.F. (1993) Glutamine and the preservation of gut integrity. *Lancet* **341**: 1363–1365.

Van Lanshot, J.J.B., Feenstra, B.W.A., Vermeij, C.G. et al. (1986) Calculation versus measurement of total energy expenditure. *Critical Care Medicine* **14**: 981–985.

Vara-Thorbeck, R., Guerrero, J.A., Rosell, J. et al. (1993) Exogenous growth hormone: Effects on the catabolic response to surgically produced acute stress and on postoperative immune function. *World Journal of Surgery* **17**: 530–538.

Veteran Affairs Total Parenteral Nutrition Cooperative Study Group (1991) Perioperative total parenteral nutrition in surgical patients. *New England Journal of Medicine* **325**: 525–532.

Voerman, H.J., Strack Van Schijndel, R.J.M., Groeneveld, A.B.J. et al. (1992) Effect of recombinant human growth hormone in patients with severe sepsis. *Annals of Surgery* **216**: 648–655.

Warnold, I., Eden, E., Lundholm, K. (1988) The inefficiency of total parenteral nutrition to stimulate protein synthesis in moderately malnourished patients. *Annals of Surgery* **208**: 143–149.

Wilmore, D.W. (1977) *The Metabolic Management of the Critically Ill*. New York: Plenum Publishing.

Wilmore, D.W. (1991) Catabolic illness: Strategies for enhancing recovery. *New England Journal of Medicine* **325**: 695–702.

Wilmore, D.W., Dudrick, S.J. (1969) Growth and development of an infant receiving all nutrients exclusively by vein. *Journal of the American Medical Association* **203**: 860–863.

Wilmore, D.W., Moylan, J.A., Bristow, B.F. et al. (1974) Anabolic effects of human growth hormone and high caloric feedings following thermal injury. *Surgery Gynecology and Obstetrics* **138**: 875–84.

Wilmore, D.W., Smith, R.J., O'Dwyer, S.T. et al. (1988) The gut: A central organ after surgical stress. *Surgery* **104**: 917–923.

Windsor, J.A., Hill, G.L. (1988) Risk factors of postoperative pneumonia: The importance of protein depletion. *Annals of Surgery* **207**: 290–296.

Wolfe, R.R., Allsop, J., Burke, J. (1979) Glucose metabolism in man: responses to intravenous glucose infusion. *Metabolism* **28**: 210–220.

Ziegler, T.R. (1994) Growth hormone administration during nutritional support: What is to be gained? *New Horizons* **2**: 244–256.

Ziegler, T.R., Smith, R.J. (1993) Parenteral Nutrition in Patients with Diabetes Mellitus. In Rombeau, J.L. and Caldwell, M.D. (eds) *Clinical Nutrition, vol 2: Parenteral Nutrition*, pp. 649–666. Philadelphia: W.B. Saunders.

Ziegler, T.R., Young, L.S., Manson, J.Mck., Wilmore, D.W. (1988) Metabolic effects of recombinant human growth hormone in patients receiving parenteral nutrition. *Annals of Surgery 208*: 6–16.

Ziegler, T.R., Benfell, K., Smith, R.J. et al. (1990a) Safety and metabolic effects of L-glutamine administration in humans. *Journal of Parenterel and Enterel Nutrition* **14**: 137S–146S.

Ziegler, T.R., Young, L.S., Ferrari-Baliviera, E., Demling, R.H., Wilmore, D.W. (1990b) Use of growth hormone combined with nutritional support in a critical care unit. *Journal of Parenterel and Enterel Nutrition* **14**: 574–581.

Ziegler, T.R., Lazarus, J.M., Young, L.S. et al. (1991) Effects of recombinant human growth hormone in adults receiving maintenance hemodialysis. *Journal of the American Society of Nephrology* **2**: 1130–1135.

Ziegler, T.R., Young, L.S., Benfell, K. et al. (1992a) Clinical and metabolic efficacy of glutamine-supplemented parenteral nutrition after bone marrow transplantation. A randomized, double-blind, controlled study. *Annals of Internal Medicine* **116**: 821–828.

Ziegler, T.R., Rombeau, J., Young, L.S. et al. (1992b) Administration of recombinant human growth hormone enhances the metabolic efficacy of parenteral nutrition: A double-blind, randomized, controlled study. *Journal of Clinical Endocrinology and Metabolism* **74**: 865–873.

Ziegler, T.R., Smith, R.J., Byrne, T.A., Wilmore, D.W. (1993) Potential role of glutamine supplementation in nutrition support. *Clinical Nutrition* **12**(suppl. 1): S82–S90.

Ziegler, T.R., Gatzen, C., Wilmore, D.W. (1994) Strategies for attenuating protein-catabolic responses in the critically ill. *Annual Review of Medicine* **45**: 459–480.

8

Antioxidant Therapy

C. Deby, G. Hartstein, G. Deby-Dupont, M. Lamy

INTRODUCTION

Several of the pathological processes frequently encountered in patients hospitalized in the intensive care unit, including infections, peritonitis, septic shock, multiple trauma, hypovolaemic shock, acute pancreatitis, burns, and the acute respiratory distress syndrome, can activate the immune system and induce a systemic inflammatory response syndrome (SIRS). This can, in turn, lead to multiple organ failure (the multiple organ dysfunction syndrome, MODS). Highly active substances are released into the circulation following activation of the complement and coagulation cascades, of platelets, lymphocytes, and endothelial cells, and during the process of phagocytosis. From an evolutionary point of view, the production of these mediators aims to destroy invading microorganisms, to eliminate damaged cells and tissue, and to re-establish normal tissue and organ function. The number of mediators already described is considerable and is continually increasing. They include peptides, lipids, and polysaccharides, and range from simple molecules (prostanoids, leukotrienes, histamine, serotonin) to proteins, high molecular weight compounds, and complex structures such as receptors, expressed on the cell surface, or circulating in solution in the blood. Their actions are complex, sometimes opposing each other, often with reciprocal modulatory influences. The order with which they appear in the blood varies from one inflammatory reaction to another, and no established hierarchy exists with respect to the sequence of their production. Several of them, including the cytokines and endotoxins, have been the object of fundamental and clinical study, and have been causally associated with certain pathological processes, such as infections and septic shock.

Among these mediators are activated forms of oxygen comprising the free radicals and oxidizing substances. These are produced primarily by activated phagocytic cells and their production can be modulated by the endotoxins and cytokines (Lloyd et al., 1993;

Repine and Parsons, 1994). Normally associated with beneficial effects on host defence, such compounds, when produced to excess, can induce significant localized cell and tissue damage, and can transform a limited inflammatory reaction into a generalized response, surpassing the organism's capacity to control them. The participation of free radicals and activated oxygen species in the inflammatory reaction accompanying severe pathologies (such as ARDS, infections, and SIRS) has been proven in animal models. Their role in human pathology, while highly likely, has yet to be conclusively demonstrated (Halliwell et al., 1992; Zimmerman, 1992; Goode and Webster, 1993; Kretzschmar, 1994). Technical difficulties associated with proving the existence of free radicals and activated oxygen species (owing to their extremely short lifespan) probably explain both the failure to demonstrate a role in human pathology and the lack of in-depth knowledge concerning methods and therapeutic agents capable of modulating their production.

FREE RADICALS AND ACTIVATED OXYGEN SPECIES

Definition, Characteristics, Role of Transition Metals

In organic molecules in the ground state (that is, without application of external energy), all electrons are shared pairwise, forming covalent bonds. Homolytic rupture of a covalent bond produces molecules with an unpaired electron, called free radicals ($R^{\cdot}$). Such breaking can be caused by a pre-existing free radical, by addition of energy, or by the action of enzymes. Free radicals are highly reactive, and therefore short-lived. They often pair off their lone electron by tearing a hydrogen atom from a neighbouring molecule, producing a new free radical, and starting a chain reaction. Propagation of the radical reaction is limited by the recombination of two radicals, causing termination of the chain reaction. Recombination of radicals would be frequent if oxygen was not present in the environment (Figure 8.1). Oxygen hinders recombination and favours chain reactions. It therefore plays a crucial role in the biochemistry of free radicals (McCord, 1985; Bast et al., 1991; Deby, 1991; Deby et al., 1991; Elstner, 1991).

Transition metals (and particularly Fe^{2+} because of its abundance in biological systems), when complexed to activator ligands (adenosine diphosphate, porphyrines) play an essential role in radical reactions. They reactivate the lipoperoxidative cycle (via their action on hydroperoxides, ROOH), play a role in the production of the hydroxyl

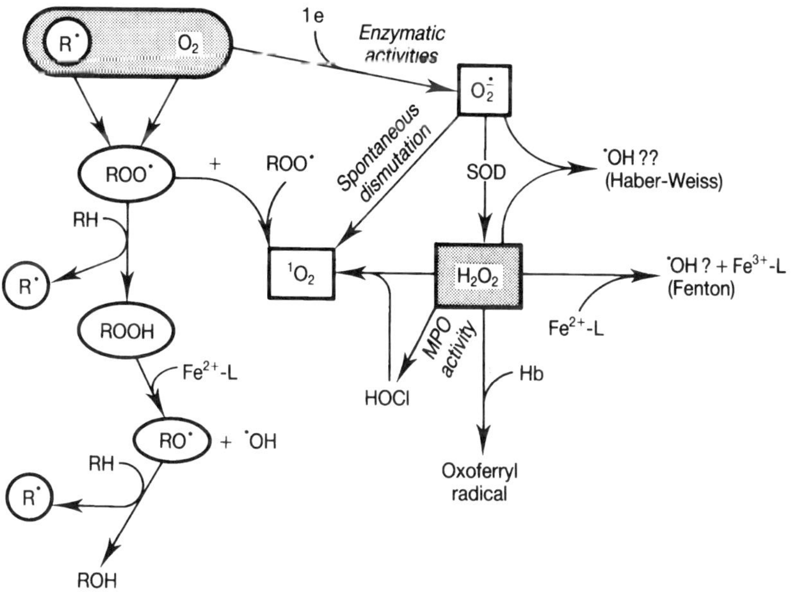

Figure 8.1. Main schematic pathways of free radicals and activated oxygen species production. ROO˙ peroxyl radical; RO˙: alkoxyl radical; ROOH: hydroperoxide; R˙, ROO˙, R˙ and ROOH are most often lipidic compounds; Fe^{2+} – L: complexed iron; Hb: haemoglobin.

radical (OH˙) via the Fenton reaction and in the formation of oxy-radical species such as the perferryl ion. This substance can generate the highly oxidizing ferryl ion (Deby et al., 1993; Halliwell, 1994). Oxygen and transition metals are thus two essential elements in the generation of free radicals and in the initiation and propagation of chain reactions leading to lipid peroxidation.

Oxygen and Activated Oxygen Species

Fundamental oxygen (O_2) contains two unpaired electrons, and is thus prohibited, by quantum mechanical rules, from reacting with most biomolecules. It is therefore relatively inert, and its participation in normal cellular respiration requires special enzymes, such as cytochrome oxidase. On the other hand, it reacts instantly with free radicals, preventing their recombination and often forming peroxyl radicals (ROO˙) (Figure 8.1); these are often liposoluble and can initiate the lipoperoxidative cycle, a typical chain reaction. Because it is incapable of reacting with most normal biomolecules, fundamental oxygen is normally devoid of toxicity. Certain enzymes, however, as well as pathological modifications of the mitochondrial respiratory chain, can lead to the occurrence of reactions which generate highly reactive and toxic oxygenated species: the superoxide anion ($O_2^{\dot{2}}$), the hydroxyl radical (OH.), hydrogen peroxide (H_2O_2), and singlet oxygen ($^1O_2$) (McCord, 1985; Bast et al., 1991; Deby, 1991).

Superoxide anion (Figure 8.1) is formed by the single electron reduction of oxygen by enzymatic action (NADPH oxidase, xanthine oxidase) (Klebanoff, 1980; Babior and Peters, 1981; Fridovich, 1984). This species is only weakly oxidizing, but in an aprotic medium (such as phospholipid membranes), it can de-esterify fatty acids, destroying membrane structure (Deby and Goutier, 1990). In a protonated medium, its lifespan is extremely short; it undergoes spontaneous dismutation to form H_2O_2 and oxygen, which can be in the singlet form.

Hydrogen peroxide has a lifespan considerably longer than that of the superoxide anion, which allows it some freedom to diffuse through the neighbouring milieu, and to act at some distance from its site of production. It can be used as a substrate by an enzyme located in the granules of polymorphonuclear neutrophiles, myeloperoxidase, to form hypochlorous acid (HOCl). This substance is a powerful oxidant, which can form, in turn, chloramines, and can oxidize thiol functions of various molecules (-SH) (Klebanoff, 1988). In the presence of ligand-bound transition metals, H_2O_2 can form the hydroxyl radical (Figure 8.1).

The hydroxyl radical is generally considered to be the most dangerous free radical species produced in vitro, capable of reacting with most biomolecules, of initiating chain reactions and the lipoperoxidative cycle. Proof of the production of $OH^{\cdot}$ only exists following radiolysis of water. The Haber-Weiss reaction (proposed in 1934) and the Fenton reaction (proposed in 1980) could also be sources of this species. In the former reaction, $O_2^{\dot{-}}$ reacts with H_2O_2 to form $OH^{\cdot}$; thermodynamic calculations have shown that this reaction is almost impossible. In the latter reaction, H_2O_2 in the presence of Fe^{2+} forms $OH^{\cdot}$ and OH^{-}, with simultaneous oxidation of Fe^{2+} to Fe^{3+} (Figure 8.1). The reaction stops unless a reductant capable of reducing iron back to Fe^{2+} is present. This reductant can be, for example, $O_2^{\dot{2}}$ or ascorbic acid (vitamin C). It must be noted that the reaction of H_2O_2 with Fe^{2+}, as well as the reduction of Fe^{3+} by $O_2^{\dot{-}}$ are slow, and are thus unlikely to exist *in vivo* (Freeman, 1994). This no doubt explains why, with the exception of the effects of ionizing radiation, the production of the hydroxyl radical *in vivo* has not yet been proven to occur using direct detection of its signal with electron paramagnetic resonance (EPR).

Singlet oxygen is an activated form wherein both normally free electrons are paired in the same orbital, after addition of 22 kcal of energy. This additional energy allows the molecule to react instantaneously with lipids, to form peroxyl radicals, in turn capable of initiating lipid peroxidation. $^1O_2$ can be formed by the spontaneous dismutation of $O_2^{\dot{-}}$ (Corey et al., 1987) or by decomposition of tetroxide bridges formed by reaction of two peroxyl functions on neighbouring phospholipid molecules (Nakano et al., 1976). It can also be produced by reaction of HOCl with H_2O_2 (Figure 8.1).

Haem-based Radicals

This group of free radicals, the oxoferryl group, is relatively poorly characterized. Oxyferryl radicals have, however, been shown to exist using EPR spectroscopy. They are formed by the reaction of methaemoglobin with H_2O_2 (Figure 8.1); the lone electron is located on a tyrosyl residue of the globin protein. The hydrogen peroxide necessary for its production could be produced by the dismutation of superoxide anion, itself resulting from the action of methaemoglobin on oxygen. This implies that the presence of deoxygenated haemoglobin in plasma, as is seen in haemolytic states, could predispose to the formation of highly reactive oxoferryl radicals, which are capable of inducing lipid peroxidation (Deby et al., 1993).

Lipid-based Radicals

Polyunsaturated fatty acids, major constituents of phospholipid membranes, are easy targets for free radical attack. After abstraction of a hydrogen atom, they form lipid radicals ($R^{\cdot}$). These react with molecular oxygen, forming peroxyl radicals, $ROO^{\cdot}$. These can react with other lipid molecules, producing new radicals, while becoming stable lipid hydroperoxides (ROOH). This chain reaction constitutes the cycle of lipid peroxidation. The lipid hydroperoxides can be reactivated by transition metals, forming $OH^{\cdot}$ and $RO^{\cdot}$, and re-initiating a new cycle of peroxidation (Figure 8.1) (Deby, 1991; Deby et al., 1991). After such peroxidative reactions, cellular membranes are altered, losing their properties as semi-permeable filters. The lipid peroxides thus formed can later decompose, forming small molecules, such as aldehydes (which are often toxic), and hydrocarbons (ethane and pentane), whose detection in the blood and/or expired gas give proof of the existence of *in vivo* lipid peroxidation (Esterbauer and Cheesman, 1990; Saran and Bors, 1991).

SOURCE OF FREE RADICALS AND ACTIVATED FORMS OF OXYGEN *IN VIVO*

The in vivo production of free radicals, under normal conditions, is generally accepted, and several types of cell participate in their formation. Because of a short lifespan, their concentration remains at a low 'steady-state' level. This attenuates their toxicity, but also renders their detection difficult. Under certain pathological circumstances, this steady state production increases, making it possible to demonstrate their existence (Bielski, 1983). The principle sources of free radicals and activated oxygen species *in vivo* are stimulated leukocytes, the mitochondrial electron transport chain, and the activity of certain intracellular enzymes. In addition to these endogenous sources, we must also consider the effects of UV, γ, and X-radiation, as well as production by xenobiotics such as paraquat or doxorubicin. These are capable of inducing continuous production of superoxide anion because they act catalytically, and are thus not consumed during the reaction (Schiller et al., 1993).

Role of Mitochondria

Normal aerobic metabolism is associated with a continuous production of free radicals and actived forms of oxygen by the mitochondrial electron transport chain. This production is usually controlled by intracellular biochemical mechanisms. The mitochondrion normally reduces oxygen directly to water, by tetravalent reduction at the level of cytochrome oxidase (Figure 8.2); none the less, 1–5% of total oxygen consumed is univalently reduced to superoxide anion. This production is rapidly converted to H_2O_2 by mitochondrial superoxide dismutase, maintaining low levels of superoxide (Loschen et al., 1974; Turrens and Boveris, 1980). Under conditions of anoxia or prolonged ischaemia, ATP production falls, followed rapidly by failure of ATP-dependent calcium pumps. This causes massive intracellular influx of calcium, with consequent cell swelling. The elevated cytoplasmic levels of calcium activate a Ca^{2+}-dependent protease, which attacks the enzyme xanthine dehydrogenase, converting it to xanthine-oxidase. Concomitantly, hypoxanthine, a substrate of this enzyme, accumulates. Upon reoxygenation, the alterations in electron

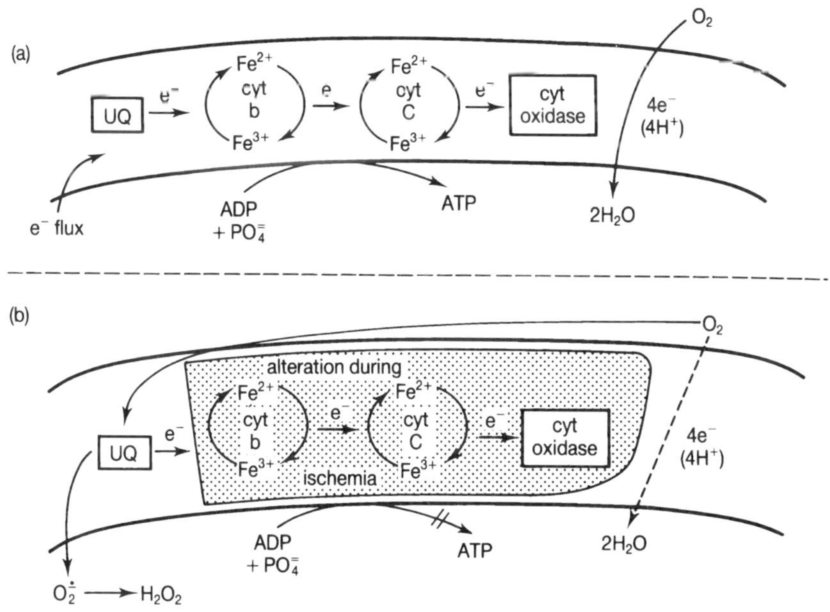

Figure 8.2. Mitochondrial electron transport chain: schematic view. A: in normal conditions: direct reduction of oxygen (O_2) to water (H_2O). B: in ischemia-reperfusion conditions. O_2 is monovalently reduced to $O_2^{\dot{-}}$ at the level of ubiquinone (UQ). Cyt: cytochrome; ATP (ADP): adenosine tri (di) phosphate.

transport render the chain incapable of reducing oxygen at the level of cytochrome oxidase (Figure 8.2). Reduction takes place at the level of ubiquinone, forming $O_2^{\dot{-}}$. Xanthine oxidase, using oxygen as an electron acceptor (instead of its usual cofactor, NADH), also produces superoxide anion, a precursor of hydrogen peroxide and other activated forms of oxygen (McCord, 1985; Granger, 1988; Haglund and Gerdin, 1991; Menger et al., 1991; Schoenberg and Beger, 1993).

Leukocyte Function

The superoxide anion is also produced by NADPH oxidase, a membrane-bound enzymatic complex found in polymorphonuclear neutrophiles (PMN) and eosinophiles, macrophages, and other cells (e.g. lymphocytes). Stimulation of PMN, and to a lesser extent monocytes/macrophages, causes an increase in the activity of NADPH oxidase, a dramatic increase in oxygen consumption (the respiratory

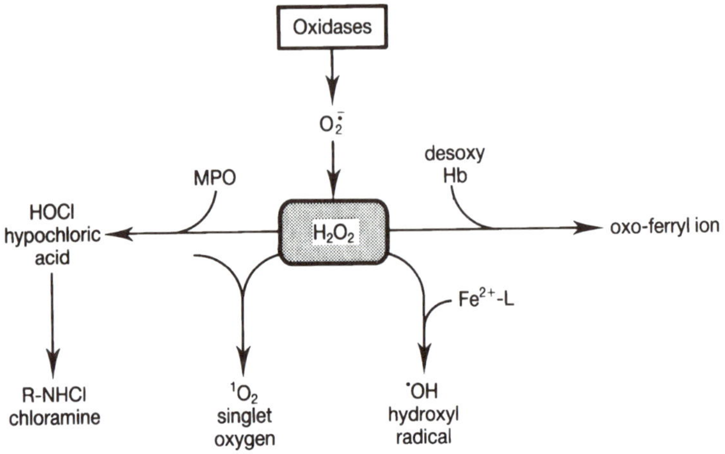

Figure 8.3. Key role of hydrogen peroxide (H_2O_2) in the production of the other active oxygen species. $O_2^{\dot{-}}$: superoxide anion; Hb: haemoglobin; MPO: myeloperoxidase; Fe^{2+} – L: ligand bound-iron.

burst), and a significant production of activated forms of oxygen (Klebanoff, 1980, 1988; Babior and Peters, 1981). These are necessary for the destruction of phagocytosed bacteria (especially to destroy their polysaccharide capsules, which are resistant to proteolytic attack), and for the 'cleaning' of necrotic areas, in conjunction with the proteases. Hydrogen peroxide is formed from the superoxide anion. Its relatively longer lifespan allows it to diffuse away from its site of production, and to become a substrate of myeloperoxidase (released from the azurophile granules of activated PMN), forming hypochlorous acid (HOCl), an aggressive oxidant capable of transforming amines into chloramines and of oxidizing -SH functions. Hydrogen peroxide can also react with HOCl to form singlet oxygen, with desoxyhaemoglobin to form oxoferryl radical, or with ligand-bound Fe^{2+} to form the hydroxyl radical, but this latter reaction is slow and unproved *in vivo* (Figure 8.3). When produced in excess, these activated forms of oxygen are cytotoxic, particularly for endothelial cells (Weiss, 1989; Cochrane, 1991; Ward, 1991; Jenkinson, 1993).

Enzymatic Activity

In addition to NADPH oxidase and xanthine oxidase, numerous intracellular enzymes have been described whose normal function leads to production of free radicals, including the oxidases, cytochrome P-450 (which can function as a peroxidase), cyclo-oxygenase (responsible for the synthesis of prostaglandins), and lipo-oxygenase (responsible for the synthesis of leukotrienes). Cyclo-oxygenase initiates co-oxygenation reactions, produces epoxides, and activates procarcinogens (Deby et al., 1991). Several oxygenases, most of which are mitochondrial, can participate in the formation of the superoxide anion.

In addition to these enzymes, the NO synthetases must also be considered. These haem enzymes are found in endothelial cells, macrophages, and several other cell lines. Endothelial cells possess a constitutive, calcium-dependent enzyme, activable (via cell surface receptors) by vasodilators (histamine, adenosine, etc.). Another form of the enzyme, non-calcium dependent, can be induced in endothelial and smooth muscle cells by infections and certain inflammatory mediators. This enzyme is not controlled by surface receptors (Kilbourn and Belloni, 1990). NO synthetases produce nitric oxide from L-arginine. This free radical has been identified as the 'endothelial-derived relaxing factor' (EDRF), and has an extremely short lifespan. It acts as a neurotransmitter and an intercellular messenger. Excessive production of NO by the inducible form of NO synthetase could explain the hypotension and myocardial depression seen in septic shock (Valance and Moncada, 1993). Many questions remain, concerning the form under which NO is liberated and transported at the cellular level (bound to -SH-containing proteins, bound to haem groups, etc.) and concerning its reactivity with other free radicals and cellular constituents. NO could react with the superoxide anion to form peroxynitrite ($ONOO^{\cdot}$), a powerful oxidant and initiator of lipid peroxidation (Moncada et al., 1991; Stamler et al., 1992; Freeman, 1994).

IN VIVO EFFECTS OF FREE RADICALS AND ACTIVATED FORMS OF OXYGEN

Free radicals and active oxygen species can attack all forms of biomolecules, but polyunsaturated lipids, proteins, and nucleic acids are especially vulnerable (Cochrane, 1991; Zimmerman, 1992; Jenkinson, 1993; Kretzschmar, 1994). De-esterification of membrane lipids by $O_2^{\dot{-}}$ acting in an aprotic milieu, and lipid peroxidation lead to changes in permeability, and are responsible for degradation products such as hydrocarbons (ethane and pentane) and aldehydes. These are toxic, can react with amino acids, and can lead to immunosuppression and mutagenesis (Deby and Goutier, 1990; Deby et al., 1991). These byproducts are more stable than the free radicals and active forms of oxygen responsible for their formation, and can diffuse considerable distances, thus enlarging the extent of damage.

The reaction of free radicals (either lipid-based, such as alkoxyl radicals, or directly derived from oxygen, such as $OH^{\cdot}$) and activated forms of oxygen with nucleic acids gives rise to hydroxylation of both bases (thymine, guanine) as well as deoxyribose. This causes chain breaks and bridging, which inhibit replication and are responsible for long-term mutagenic and carcinogenic effects. The hydroxyl radical can also attack polyoses, such as hyaluronic acid, which it depolymerizes. As for proteins, certain amino acids are particularly sensitive to free radical attack: histidine, tryptophan, and sulfated amino acids. It is, in fact, by attacking sulfhydryl (–SH) functions that free radicals and other activated forms of oxygen (especially HOCl and H_2O_2) inactivate α_1 proteinase inhibitor and α_2 macroglobulin, two important plasma antiproteinases (Weiss, 1989; Cochrane, 1991; Deby-Dupont et al., 1994a). The former neutralizes elastase, while the latter traps and eliminates several proteases. Besides neutralizing the antiproteases, these reactive oxygen species can also activate proenzymes (such as procollagenase, proelastase). This leads to unbalanced activity of proteases and antiproteases.

We should keep in mind that one of the most important roles of the free radicals and activated forms of oxygen produced by phagocytic cells is the destruction of ingested microorganisms, an indispensible function in host defence against infection. They also activate cellular functions (endothelial cells, pulmonary epithelial cells, macrophages, etc.) and act as mediators between primary and secondary inflammatory processes (Winrow et al., 1993). Only when they are produced in excess, overwhelming the organism's capacity to control them, do they become dangerous.

ENDOGENOUS PROTECTION FROM FREE RADICALS AND ACTIVATED FORMS OF OXYGEN

Natural protection against free radicals and activated forms of oxygen is the result of enzymatic activity and the activity of non-enzymatic trapping molecules. These protective agents are generally designated as antioxidants. Antioxidant protection can be expressed in two manners: (i) catalytic or anticatalytic; (ii) stoichiometric.

Catalytic protection is the result of enzymatic activity, while anti-catalytic protection is effected either by inhibitors of pro-oxidant enzymes or by chelators of transition metals. Chelation of these metals prevents them from participating in auto-oxidative cycles. In this way, one protective molecule can inhibit the production of several hundred free radicals or activated oxygen molecules. Effective concentrations are thus low compared to the situation with stoichiometric protectors. Here, one protectant molecule only protects against one deleterious species; effective concentrations are thus relatively high, near to that of the free radicals themselves (Deby et al., 1991).

The principal endogenous catalytic protectants are the three following enzyme families: the superoxide dismutases (SOD), catalase, and glutathione peroxidase (Zimmerman, 1992, 1994; Goode and Webster, 1993). The SOD are found in all living cells. They eliminate the superoxide anion by accelerating its dismutation to H_2O_2 and fundamental oxygen (Fridovich, 1984; Deby and Goutier, 1990). The cytoplasm and red blood cells contain a copper–zinc SOD, endothelial cells contain a manganese SOD, and endothelial cells express on their surface (under the mantle) an SOD activity released into the plasma by heparin (Marklund, 1984). Catalase is a haem-containing enzyme located in the peroxisomes; it catalyses the transformation of H_2O_2 into water and fundamental oxygen. The combined action of SOD and catalase prevents or inhibits the formation of hydroxyl radical and oxidizing species such as HOCl and the chloramines. Glutathione peroxidase is a cytoplasmic selenium-containing enzyme which neutralizes H_2O_2 as well as lipid peroxides. It is widely distributed throughout the organism, and acts with SOD to inhibit the initial stages of the activation of oxygen. It uses glutathione (GSH) as a cofactor, which is oxidized to dimeric GSSG. GSH is regenerated by an NADPH-dependent glutathione reductase. Those substances participating in the synthesis of GSH can indirectly be considered catalytic protectors (Bast et al., 1991).

Metal chelators are anti-catalytic non-enzymatic protectors. By chelating Fe^{2+}, which plays an essential role in the generation of free radicals, it removes a crucial participant in these reactions (Bast et al., 1991; McCord, 1993; Halliwell, 1994). Besides its presence in haemoglobin, myoglobin, and haem enzymes, iron is transported by transferrin (as Fe^{3+}) and is stored in the cell by ferritin and haemosiderin. It can also be chelated by uric acid.

Among the catalytic or anti-catalytic antioxidants, we must mention the vitamin E–vitamin C pair, as well as the polyphenol–vitamin C pair. Vitamin E, which is hydrophobic, is the principal protective agent against the toxic effects of oxygen in the hydrophobic compartment, notably within lipid membranes (Bast et al., 1991; Chow, 1991; Deby et al., 1991). It stops radical chain reactions, and inactivates hydroperoxides and alkoxyl radicals, thus preventing reactivation of the lipid peroxidation cycle. Vitamin E and the polyphenols usually act stoichiometrically. During their reactions with free radicals they themselves become radicals (vitamin E is transformed into the tocopheryl radical); these can be regenerated by vitamin C. This passes through a relatively stable radical form (the ascorbyl radical) prior to being converted to dehydroascorbate (Packer et al., 1979). Ultimately it is vitamin C which is consumed in this mechanism, which can thus be compared to a catalytic-type process. Acting alone, vitamin C is not an antioxidant; *in vitro* it can even potentiate peroxidative processes by reducing Fe^{3+} to Fe^{2+}, and deleterious *in vivo* effects have been described (Packer et al., 1979; Deby et al., 1993).

Stoichiometric protectors are 'quencher' molecules; these are capable of reacting with free radicals at least 100 times faster than neighbouring molecules. They form non-radical substances, and break chain reactions. Among these quenchers are thiol compounds (R–SH), which are transformed into thiyl radicals ($RS^{\cdot}$); the latter dimerize rapidly, thus hindering progression of the free radical reactions. In this way, amino acids and proteins containing -SH groups such as cysteine and albumin are quenchers of free radicals and activated forms of oxygen. Uric acid is also a quencher of the hydroxyl radical, but its reaction can lead to formation of alloxan, which is cytotoxic and diabetogenic. Certain amino acids, such as tryptophane and histidine, also seem to have antioxidant properties.

FREE RADICALS AND ACTIVATED FORMS OF OXYGEN IN INTENSIVE CARE MEDICINE

Infections, trauma, shock states, and, in general, situations associated with an inflammatory response stimulate leukocytes (macrophages and polymorphonuclear neutrophils [PMN]), probably via activation of mediator cascades. This leads to a respiratory burst, with production of free radicals and activated oxygen species (Figure 8.4). These substances are necessary for the destruction of microorganisms; production beyond the capacity of the system's defensive machinery can, however lead to tissue damage. The vascular endothelium is particularly sensitive to oxygen-induced damage, especially because the inflammatory response itself increases expression of

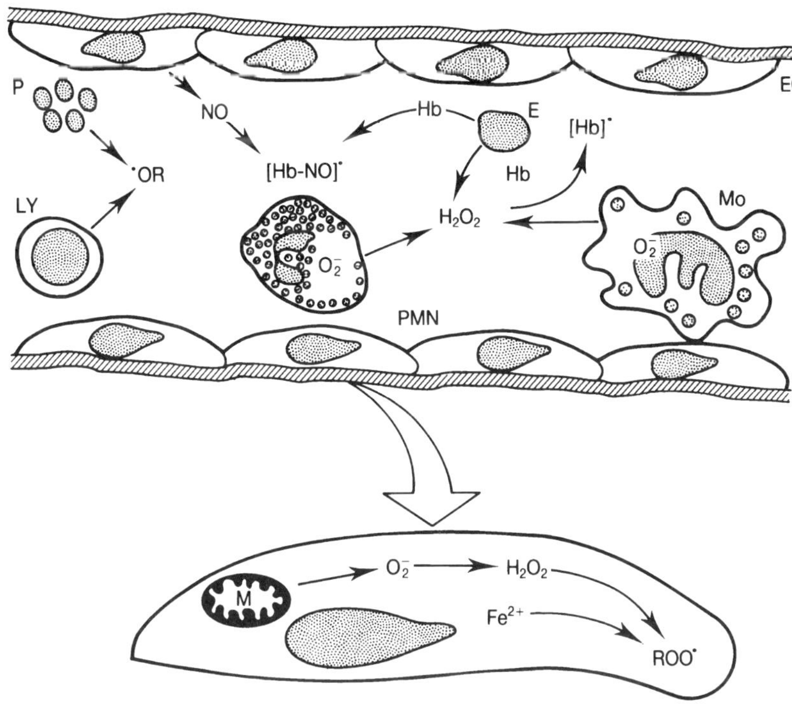

Figure 8.4. Origin of the active oxygen species in blood and endothelium. Mo: monocytes; PMN: polymorphonuclear leukocytes; LY: lymphocytes; P: platelets; E: erythrocytes; EC: endothelial cells; M: mitochondria in endothelial cells. $O_2^{\cdot-}$: superoxide anion; Hb : haemoglobin radical; NO: nitric oxide radical; ·OR and ROO·: alkoxyl and peroxyl radicals. For details, see text.

leukocyte adhesion molecules (Osborn, 1990; Cochrane, 1991; Gasic et al., 1991; Patel et al., 1991; Tagan et al., 1991; Zimmerman et al., 1992; Malik, 1993; Sellak et al., 1994). The synthesis of prostanoids and leukotrienes, which involves production of free radicals, is also increased during inflammatory states, during endotoxaemia, and during septic shock (Bernard et al., 1991; Cook et al., 1993); also increased is the production of platelet activating factor (PAF), and thus further production of free radicals (Koltai et al., 1993; Dhainaut et al., 1994). Endotoxin also activates tryptophan dioxygenase, a source of superoxide production (Hayaischi and Yoshida, 1979).

Monocytes and activated macrophages release cytokines, which have a facilitating role in the production of activated forms of oxygen (Lloyd et al., 1993). Tumour necrosis factor (TNF) induces mitochondrial production of the superoxide anion by cultured cells (Hennet et al., 1993). During inflammatory reactions, macrophages and endothelial cells also produce the NO radical (Ochoa et al., 1991; Valance and Moncada, 1993). During various shock states (hypovolaemic shock, septic shock, etc.) ischaemia followed by reperfusion leads to activation of oxygen and the production of free radicals, by both cytoplasmic (xanthine oxidase) and mitochondrial enzymes (McCord, 1985; Menger et al., 1991).

While a theoretical link between acute inflammatory states and the production of free radicals and activated forms of oxygen is clear, demonstration of the reality of such a link in man, as well as in animal models, is considerably more difficult. Most attempts to do so involve using indirect techniques to detect byproducts of lipoperoxide decomposition, such as hydrocarbons in the expired gas, conjugated dienes, or aldehydes in the bloodstream or in tissues. The most popular technique, despite numerous sources of artefacts, is measurement of thiobarbituric acid reactive substances (TBARS). These are produced by condensation of malondialdehyde with two molecules of thiobarbituric acid (Saran and Bors, 1991; Goode and Webster, 1993). Use of these techniques has provided evidence for the occurrence of lipid peroxidation in the tissues, the blood, and in bronchoalveolar lavage (BAL) fluid (Zimmerman, 1992; Goode and Webster, 1993). In BAL and in expired breath, the presence of H_2O_2 has been shown during acute respiratory distress syndrome (ARDS) (Baldwin et al., 1986; Sznajder et al., 1989). The reactivity of PMN (in terms of production of $O_2^{\cdot-}$ and H_2O_2) has also been studied in patients with sepsis and/or ARDS. These studies have shown an excessive *ex vivo* stimulability in venous blood during sepsis and in arterial blood during ARDS (Nahum et al., 1991). This is presumed to imply excessive function prior to blood sampling, with exhaustion of the cells' synthetic machinery.

Measurement of the activity of antioxidant enzymes (SOD, catalase, and glutathione peroxidase), of consumption of antioxidant compounds (vitamin E, glutathione), and assay of markers of oxidative destruction of proteins in animal models and in humans have furnished further arguments in favour of a role for free radicals and activated forms of oxygen in these pathologies. A fall in blood concentration of vitamin E has been observed in ARDS patients (Bertrand et al., 1989) and decreased GSH concentrations have been measured in BAL in ARDS and sepsis (Pacht et al., 1991). Leff et al. (1992, 1993) have shown increases in the activity of Mn–SOD and of catalase in the plasma of infected patients; this increase was more pronounced in those patients who concomitantly developed

ARDS or whose clinical course led to this complication. However, these authors could not explain the origin of these enzymatic activities in plasma. On the other hand, no change was noted in the activity of glutathione peroxidase.

High plasma concentrations of myeloperoxidase (MPO) have been found in patients with infections, with ARDS, and in those undergoing cardiac surgery with cardiopulmonary bypass (Faymonville et al., 1991). In patients with ARDS, active MPO has also been shown to be present in BAL fluid, as has oxidized a_1 proteinase inhibitor. This protein is especially sensitive to oxidation by HOCl, a product of the activity of MPO (Cochrane, 1991). Furthermore, under situations where the mechanism of ischaemia–reperfusion is likely to be operant (particularly in organ transplantation) numerous animal studies have indirectly suggested the intervention of free radicals by falls in levels of vitamin E, of glutathione, and by changes in activity of antioxidant enzymes (Defraigne et al., 1994). Endothelial dysfunction (manifested by an inability to respond to vasodilators) also occurs; this is likely a result of damage by free radicals, especially superoxide anion, produced by the endothelium itself or by activated, adherent PMN (Arndt et al., 1991; Lefer and Ma, 1993). Xanthine oxidase, a source of $O_2^{\cdot-}$, has been shown to play a role in loss of villi in the intestinal mucosa, which occurs very rapidly upon reperfusion following ischaemia (Reilly and Bulkley, 1993). Such studies are much rarer in humans.

Direct demonstration of the existence of free radicals can only be accomplished using electroparamagnetic resonance spectroscopy (EPR). When applied *in vivo*, this method is limited by the necessity to accumulate a sufficient quantity of free radicals to permit detection. Thanks to the use of spin trapping agents, which react with free radicals to form more stable radicals with both longer lifespans and characteristic resonance signals, the application of EPR to *in vivo* systems has been rendered considerably easier. Unfortunately, the number of studies published, especially about humans, remains quite limited (Novelli, 1992). To date, no EPR studies have directly demonstrated the existence of $O_2^{\cdot-}$ or $OH^{\cdot}$ *in vivo*. On the other hand, trapped radical species have been found in the liver of infected animals, and in cardiac and renal tissues during ischaemia–reperfusion in animals (Baker et al., 1988; Bolli et al., 1988; Pietri et al., 1993; Defraigne et al., 1994). During endotoxin shock in the rat, direct EPR evidence has been found for the presence of free radicals in lung and in the blood (without use of spin trapping, but working at the temperature of liquid nitrogen). An identical signal has been found in the plasma of the rat during haemorrhagic shock, and has been attributed to a haemoglobin–NO radical. Use of an inhibitor of NO synthetase, L-monomethylarginine (L-NMMA), leads to a significant fall in the signal strength of this radical, confirming the role of NO in its formation (Westenberger et al., 1990). In man, some evidence has been published concerning demonstration of free radicals by EPR during cardiac surgery with CPB; this work suggests increased production of radicals during aortic unclamping (Culcasi et al., 1993; Hartstein et al., 1993), but no similar studies exist for infections, haemorrhagic shock, ARDS, or during organ transplantation.

ANTIOXIDANT THERAPY

Normal levels of production of pro-oxidant species, due to aerobic metabolism are controlled by appropriate consumption of antioxidant agents (enzymatic and non-enzymatic). When production exceeds defensive capacities, oxidative stress occurs, implying loss of the balance between pro-oxidant and antioxidant influences. It is thus logical to consider the administration of substances which aim at bolstering the antioxidant defences of the organism. These can act at various points, occasionally intervening at steps seemingly quite distant from the free radicals themselves. It is intuitively clear that a therapeutic effect could be obtained directly by trapping the activated oxygen species themselves, or indirectly by inhibition of the enzymatic systems and/or cells responsible for their production. Reinforcement of protective enzymes and cofactors is another possible mode of action. Cells and/or tissues could also be protected by decreasing the ability of pro-oxidants to damage them, for example by antagonizing the adhesion receptors which allow PMN to bind to endothelial cells. Table 8.1 summarizes the various possibilities of therapy against oxidative stress. But many of the possibilities mentioned in the table have only been tested in animal models, or are still at the stage of hypotheses.

Current antioxidant therapies fall into four categories: trapping of free radicals and activated forms of oxygen, iron chelators, inhibitors of enzymatic and cellular systems, and reinforcement of endogenous protective enzymes (Bast et al., 1991; Zimmerman, 1992; Goode and Webster, 1993; Rangan and Bulkley, 1993; Grimble, 1994; Zimmerman, 1994). The nature of the therapeutic substance depends on both the environment in which it must function (hydro- or lipophilic), and on the species of radical to be neutralized (Deby et al., 1991). The nature of the chemical reactions by which the agent acts is also important, as it conditions the pharmacological 'efficiency' of the drug. Agents which trap free radicals or which chelate iron can act either catalytically or stoichiometrically. From a pharmacological viewpoint, preference must be given to agents active at low concentrations (less than 10^{-4} M).

Quenchers of Free Radicals and Activated Forms of Oxygen

Stoichiometric quenchers

These antioxidant substances react on a mole-for-mole basis with free radicals and activated forms of oxygen, and must thus be administered at rather high concentrations. Consideration must also be given to their solubility characteristics, to allow them access to the sites whose protection is desired (plasma, cytosol, cellular membranes). In situations where free radicals are produced continuously and in large quantities, large amounts of these substances must be used; concentrations of from 10^{-4} to 10^{-3}M must be attained. This is often impossible, both because of pharmacological considerations and because at these concentrations, many of these substances are toxic. Furthermore, these molecules must react with free radicals faster than the neighbouring molecules whose protection is desired; the kinetics necessary imply extremely rapid reactions, when one remembers that the half-life of most free radicals is between 10^{-9} and 10^{-6} seconds (Sies, 1991).

Numerous natural and synthetic antioxidants, such as mannitol, uric acid, dimethylthiourea, and dimethylsulfoxide (DMSO) have been tested, generally in animals. These substances are capable of quenching the hydroxyl radical, but either remain in the extracellular compartment, or are toxic at the required concentrations (e.g., DMSO, which is lipid soluble but toxic at the concentrations necessary to trap the hydroxyl radical, hydrogen peroxide, and HOCl) (Schiller et al., 1993). Given the special sensitivity of -SH groups to oxidative stress, albumin (which is well endowed with thiol groups) has been tested as a quencher of lipid hydroperoxides (Pirisino et al., 1988). The lazaroids, or 21-aminosteroids, molecules with a steroid nucleus but with neither mineralo- nor glucocorticoid activity, are considered to be capable of trapping free radicals and lipid hydroperoxides. They have been shown to be useful in preventing the damage induced by ischaemia/reperfusion (Johnson and Lefer, 1990).

Clinical studies are in progress, especially for cerebral ischaemia. Flavonoids are also efficient quenchers, and have been used frequently in animal models. In humans, prophylactic administration

Table 8.1 Main therapeutic possibilities against free radical and active oxygen species. DMSO: dimethylsulfoxide; DMTU: dimethylthiourea; NSAIDS: non steroidal anti-inflammatory drugs; PAF: platelet activating factor; L-NMMA: L-N-monomethylarginine; SOD: superoxide dismutase; PEG: polyethylene glycol; GSH: glutathione

Agent	Tried in	Target	Action
Mannitol, DMSO, DMTU, uric acid, albumin, lazaroids	animals	free radicals and active oxygen species	stoichiometric quenchers
Antibiotics (ceftazidime)	in vitro		
Cyclic nitrones	animals		
Vitamin E (vitamin C)	animals and humans	free radicals, hydroperoxides	catalytic type quenchers
Flavonoids			
Desferrioxamine	animals, humans	iron	chelator
Other siderophores	in vitro, animals	iron	chelator
Allopurinol, oxypurinol	animals	xanthine oxidase	inhibition of enzymatic activity
NSAIDS	animals, humans	cyclooxygenase	inhibition of enzymatic activity

NSAIDS	animals, humans	neutrophils	inhibition of excessive activation
Pentoxyfilline	animals, humans	neutrophils	inhibition of excessive activation
Adhesion molecule blockade	animals, humans	neutrophils, endothelial cells receptors	inhibition of leukocytes, adhesion to endothelium
Anti-PAF	animals, humans	PAF, PAF receptors	inhibition of platelet activation
L-NMMA	animals, humans (?)	NO-synthetase	inhibition of enzymatic activity
SOD, PEG-SOD, SOD-liposome	animals	superoxide anion	dismutation
Catalase, PEG catalase, catalase-liposome	animals	hydrogen peroxide	destruction
GSH, N-acetylcystein Organoselenium compounds	animals, humans animals, humans (?)	cofactors for GSH-peroxidase	hydroperoxide destruction
Gene therapy	in vitro, animals	SOD, catalase, GSH peroxidase	enzyme induction

of these substances decreases the production of free radicals upon reperfusion after CPB in valve replacement surgery (Culcasi et al., 1993). Cefatzidime, an antibiotic with sulfur and nitrogen groups, can protect against certain activated forms of oxygen produced by myeloperoxidase such as HOCl and $^1O_2$ (Mathy-Hartert et al., 1994; Deby-Dupont et al., 1994b). The contribution of this antioxidant activity to the reduction of morbidity seen after administration of antibiotics has not yet been evaluated. Stable cyclic nitrone compounds, used in EPR studies as spin trapping agents, have been administered to animals in models of lethal endotoxaemia, and septic and traumatic shock. In these models, they have led to decreased microvascular damage and lipoperoxidation, without acute toxicity (Novelli, 1992). Finally, coenzyme Q10 has been used successfully in animal endotoxaemia (Zimmerman, 1994).

Catalytic quenchers: vitamins E and C

Administration of vitamin E to humans and in animal models has numerous, well demonstrated beneficial effects. It improves the response of muscle submitted to transient ischaemia, protects erythrocytes from lipid peroxidation, protects from post-ischaemic injury, and reinforces the immune response (Chow, 1991; Deby et al., 1991; Tosatti et al., 1992; Grimble, 1994). However, despite its beneficial effects and its total absence of toxicity, vitamin E is almost never used in clinical practice, in severe disease processes such as ARDS or sepsis. This therapeutic hesitancy is rather difficult to understand, especially in the light of numerous multicentre trials of therapies whose toxicity and mechanism of action are much less well characterized than those of vitamin E. It has been known for more than 10 years that the administration of vitamin E to animals during endotoxin shock and/or in models of acute respiratory failure has undisputed beneficial effects, including reduced lipid peroxidation, intravascular coagulation, and mortality. More than 10 years ago, improved survival was shown in patients with ARDS who were given vitamin E (Wolf and Seegert, 1982); curiously, this preliminary trial, concerning 87 patients, was not followed by subsequent, placebo-controlled studies. In 1989, it has once again begun to appear in studies using multiple antioxidant substances simultaneously, with an aim to concomitant action on several forms of free radicals and activated oxygen (Sawyer et al., 1989). The use of vitamin E should, logically, be associated with administration of vitamin C, which acts to regenerate the former, resulting in a catalytic-type action. The beneficial role played by vitamin C in sepsis-induced ARDS is probably due to its intervention in the kinetics of vitamin E (Sawyer et al., 1989).

Transition Metal Chelators

Chelation of transition metals, of which iron is the most important (and most widespread) in biological systems may be a useful antioxidant strategy, because they intervene in the formation of the hydroxyl radical and in the reactivation of lipoperoxidative cycles. Siderophores, of which desferrioxamine is the best example, bind Fe^{3+} and prevent it being recycled as Fe^{2+}; they thus constitute anticatalytic agents of choice. While it appears to be efficacious in animal models of haemorrhagic shock and ischaemia–reperfusion, and is currently used in clinical practice, its effects in humans are less clear-cut. It has been used in cardiac surgery with cardiopulmonary bypass, to prevent formation of free radicals and lipid peroxidation; studies have shown either positive effects or no effect at all (Menasche et al., 1990). Its activity is hindered by slow penetration into cells, and it seems to have some intrinsic toxicity (Halliwell, 1994). This can, however, be diminished by binding it to hydroxyethyl starch.

Other potential chelators, such as certain antibiotics (notably ceftazidime) are being studied in cell cultures and in animal models, but have not yet had this aspect of their effects studied *in vivo*.

Inhibitors of Cellular Activation and Enzymatic Activity

The activity of a certain number of enzymes responsible for the production of free radicals can be inhibited by specific inhibitors. Allopurinol and its metabolite oxypurinol are structural analogues of hypoxanthine. They can block the production of the superoxide anion by xanthine oxidase. Their administration has led to decreased free radical induced tissue damage in animal models of ischaemia–reperfusion. The irreversible conversion of xanthine dehydrogenase to xanthine oxidase results from the activity of a protease which can itself be inhibited by antiproteases; this indirectly leads to decreased production of superoxide. This modality has been used successfully in intestinal ischaemia (McCord, 1993). On the other hand, no investigations specifically studying the effects of antiproteases or allopurinol in traumatic shock, infections, or ARDS have been published. Allopurinol has shown equivocal results in animal models of infection, suggesting that xanthine oxidase is not the principal source of free radicals during infection (Goode and Webster, 1993).

In both animals and humans, the type of severe pathological processes seen in the intensive care unit are accompanied by activation of cyclo-oxygenase and lipo-oxygenase, which can be responsible for the production of free radicals. The use of non-steroidal anti-inflammatory drugs (NSAIDS) could thus present beneficial effects; all clinical studies published to date have been inconclusive. It is also impossible, using these drugs, to differentiate between the effect of suppression of free radical production and the inhibition of inflammatory mediators (prostanoids, leukotrienes) (Bernard et al., 1991; Yu and Tomasa, 1993). Moreover, it appears that some NSAIDS such as phenylbutazone could be responsible for oxidative damages because this drug becomes itself a free radical in the presence of haemoproteins and H_2O_2 (Evans et al., 1992).

The respiratory burst of activated phagocytic cells is one of the most important sources of free radicals. Limitation of the activation of these cells, and/or of the activation of NADPH oxidase, are therapeutic modalities deserving of consideration. Certain local anaesthetics, calcium channel blockers, and NSAIDS can inhibit this enzyme, although this action is not specific (and the agents themselves are not without toxicity). For completeness, we should also mention pentoxyfilline (Mandell, 1988; Harada *et al.*, 1989; Waxman, 1990), as well as other molecules with activities on NADPH oxidase, such as adenosine, and substances capable of neutralizing leukocyte adhesion receptors (integrins and selectins) (Osborn, 1990; Zimmerman et al., 1992). Another possibility of action lies in the inhibition of PAF. This should result in decreased platelet activation, and thus reduced formation of free radicals. Clinical studies with an anti-PAF factor are underway; preliminary results suggest a beneficial effect in Gram-negative bacterial infections (Koltai et al., 1993; Dhainaut et al., 1994).

The discovery of a role for NO, particularly in infections and septic shock, opens the way for another therapeutic strategy. The hypothesis of excessive production of NO by endothelial and smooth muscle cells during septic shock leads naturally to the idea of using inhibitors of NO synthetase (for example N·-methyl-L-arginine, L-NMMA, N·-nitro-L-arginine, N·-amino-L-arginine) to treat this state. Their use in clinical practice remains controversial in view of their effects on the cardiac index and on the distribution of oxygen delivery, both in animals and in humans (Westenberger et al., 1990; Freeman, 1994). These effects can be responsible for microcirculatory problems and localized ischaemia, especially of the splanchnic bed (Lorente et al.,

1993). The therapeutic value of these non-specific inhibitors of NO synthetase, with their associated toxicity, remains to be proved; the ideal dosing regimen(s) also need to be established. A trend to use of lower doses could lead to less toxicity and more selective effects.

Reinforcement of Protective Enzymes

The control of the concentrations of antioxidant enzymes can be influenced by genetic engineering; this has been demonstrated by studies of the induction of SOD and catalase in bacteria in response to oxidant treatments (Sies, 1991). The explosive development of genetic engineering has permitted modulation of the expression of enzymes such as SOD and catalase in the lungs of mice by intravenous injection of cDNA 'packaged' in liposomes (Brigham et al., 1994). This type of treatment could be extremely useful in ARDS, but remains very experimental. On the other hand, treatment by administration of SOD (itself produced by genetic engineering) or catalase has been proposed (and attempted) in animals.

SOD has been given parenterally or by local instillation, with positive effects; among the problems with this type of therapy are the intracellular penetration of the enzyme and the short half-life in the circulation (approximately 6 min) (Koyama et al., 1992). Conjugation of the enzyme to polyethylene glycol has increased both its persistency in the bloodstream and its penetration (by active transport). Incorporation into liposomes also prolongs its half-life (4 h) and its intracellular penetration (Olson et al., 1987; Schneider et al., 1989; Suzuki et al., 1992; Schiller et al., 1993). None the less, the results obtained with these substances are controversial; their effects are diminished when administered after the inciting insult (usually in the endotoxaemia model). A similar approach uses synthetic forms of SOD (SOD 'mimics', such as copper (II) 3,5 diisopropylsalicylic acid, or CuDIPS); these low molecular weight substances reproduce the active site of the natural enzyme, and can access the intracellular compartment more easily. Unfortunately, small amounts of albumin inactivate the SOD mimics, probably by chelation of their copper (Schiller et al., 1993). Catalase has also been used, both conjugated to polyethylene glycol and encapsulated in liposomes, to improve its duration of action and its penetrability. Its beneficial effects *in vivo* are not convincing; when combined with SOD, no advantage is noted relative to SOD alone.

The use of organoselenium compounds (such as Ebselen) is another approach to increasing the activity of antioxidant enzymes. Here, glutathione peroxidase (GPx) is the target, because its active site contains a selenium atom (Sies, 1991). They have, until now, only been used in animal studies (Goode and Webster, 1993; Grimble, 1994). *N*-acetyl cysteine, which restores or increases intracellular levels of glutathione (GSH) (erythrocytes, pulmonary epithelial cells, granulocytes) can also augment the activity of GPx. It has been of some benefit in animals, but its effects are less well characterized in humans; it seems to improve oxygenation without affecting survival. Randomized, placebo-controlled multicentre studies are underway to verify initial results (Jepsen et al., 1992; Spies and Reinhart 1994; Suter et al., 1994).

Many other enzymes are implicated in antioxidant defence, including GSSG (oxidized glutathione, with dimenization of two oxidized molecules) reductase (which reduces oxidized glutathione, GSSG, back to GSH, required for the activity of GPx), but no practical suggestions as to their use in therapy have yet been made.

CONCLUSIONS

Free radicals and active forms of oxygen are produced during severe infections, septic shock, during the acute respiratory distress syndrome, and during all forms of ischaemia–reperfusion. This production is primarily caused by activation of phagocytic cells, but is difficult to demonstrate in clinical practice; this makes understanding of their exact role in these various pathological processes arduous. They are both powerful substances, capable of damaging cells and tissues, and mediators with a role in maintaining and amplifying the inflammatory response. Their deleterious effects are normally controlled by antioxidant defences, but these can be overwhelmed.

Numerous therapeutic possibilities exist; these are often efficacious when used in animal models, but few have been studied in humans by randomized, placebo-controlled investigations. Their efficiency is lessened when given separately; given the multiplicity of sources and effects of free radicals, the development of therapies using several molecules, acting both stoichiometrically and especially catalytically at different levels of the various reactions, will no doubt be the most promising path to follow.

REFERENCES

Arndt, H., Kubes, P., Granger, D.N. (1991) Involvement of neutrophils in ischemia–reperfusion injury in the small intestine. *Klinische Wochenschrift* **69**: 1056–1060.

Babior, B.M., Peters, W.A. (1981) The $O_2^{\dot{-}}$ producing enzyme of human neutrophils: further properties. *Journal of Biological Chemistry* **256**: 2321–2323.

Baker, J.E., Felix, C.C., Olinger, G.N., Kalyanaraman, K.M. (1988) Myocardial ischemia and reperfusion: direct evidence for free radical generation by electron spin resonance spectroscopy. *Proceedings of the National Academy of Sciences, USA* **85**: 2786–2789.

Baldwin, R., Grum, C.M., Boxer, L.A. et al. (1986) Oxidant activity in expired breath of patients with adult respiratory distress syndrome. *Lancet* **i**: 11–13.

Bast, A., Haenen, G.R., Doelman, C.J. (1991) Oxidants and antioxidants: state of the art. *American Journal of Medicine* **91**(suppl. 3C): 2S–13S.

Bernard, G.R., Heines, H.D., Halushka, P.V. et al. (1991) Prostacyclin and thromboxane A2 formation is increased in human sepsis syndrome: Effects of cyclo-oxygenase inhibition. *American Review of Respiratory Diseases* **144**: 1095–1101.

Bertrand, Y., Pincemail, J., Hannique, G. et al. (1989) Differences in tocopherol–lipid ratio in ARDS and no ARDS patients. *Intensive Care Medicine* **15**: 87–93.

Bielski, H.J. (1983) The chemistry of free and enzyme-bound NAD·/NADP· radicals. In Nygaard, O.F., Simic, M.G. (eds) *Radioprotection and Carcinogens*, pp 33–52. New York: Academic Press.

Bolli, R., Patel, B.S., Jerondi, M.O., Lai, E.K., McCay, P.B. (1988) Demonstration of free radical generation in 'stunned' myocardium of intact dogs with the use of the spin trap α-phenyl-*N*-tert-butyl nitrone. *Journal of Clinical Investigation* **82**: 476–485.

Brigham, K.L., Canonico, A.E., Conary, J.T., Meyrick, B.O., Schreier, H. (1994) Potential for gene therapy in the treatment of sepsis. Sepsis: Current perspectives in pathophysiology and therapy. In Reinhart, R., Eyrich, K., Sprung, S. (eds) *Update in Intensive Care and Emergency Medicine*, pp 528–535. Berlin: Springer Verlag.

Chow, C.K. (1991) Vitamin E and oxidative stress. *Free Radical Biology and Medicine* **11**: 215–232.

Cochrane, C.G. (1991) Cellular injury by oxidants. *American Journal of Medicine* **91**(suppl. 3C) : 23S–30S.

Cook, J.A., Geisel, J., Halushka, P.V., Reines, H.O. (1993) Prostaglandins, thromboxanes, leukotrienes and cytochrome P–450 metabolites of arachidonic acid. *New Horizons* **1**: 60–69.

Corey, E.J., Mehrotra, M.M., Khan, A.V. (1987) Water-induced dismutation of superoxide anion generated singlet molecular oxygen. *Biochemical and Biophysical Research Communications* **145**: 842–846.

Culcasi, M., Pietri S., Carrière, I., d'Arbigny, P., Drieu, K. (1993) Electron-spin-resonance study of the protective effects of Ginkgo biloba (EGb 761) on reperfusion-induced free-radical generation associated with plasma ascorbate consumption during open-heart surgery in man. In Ferradini, C., Droy-Lefaix, M.T., Christen, Y. (eds) *Advance in Ginkgo Biloba Extract Research*, **vol. 2**, pp 153–162. Paris: Elsevier.

Deby, C. (1991) La biochimie de l'oxygène. *La Recherche* **228**: 56–64.

Deby, C., Goutier, R. (1990) New perspectives on the biochemistry of superoxide anion and the efficiency of superoxide dimutases. *Biochemical Pharmacology* **39**: 399–405.

Deby, C., Goutier, R., Deby-Dupont, G. (1991) Rôle des radicaux libres dans le vieillissement et thérapeutique antioxygène. *Annales de Cardiologie et d'Angeiologie* **40(6)**: 341–348.

Deby, C., Deby-Dupont, G., Dister, M., Pincemail, J. (1993) Efficiency of *Ginkgo Biloba* extract (EGb 761) in neutralizing ferryl ion-induced peroxidations: therapeutic implications. In Ferradini, C., Droy-Lefaix, M.T., Christen, Y. (eds) *Advances in Ginkgo Biloba Extract Research*, vol. 2, pp 13–26. Paris: Elsevier.

Deby-Dupont, G., Croisier, J.L., Camus, G. et al. (1994a) Inactivation of a_2-macroglobulin by activated human polymorphonuclear leucocytes. *Mediators of Inflammation* **3**: 117–123.

Deby-Dupont, G., Mathy-Hastest, M., Iadoul, L. et al. (1994b) Ceftazidime – An antibiotic with a host defense spectrum interesting in cases of deletesions poly morphonuclear leukocytes activation. *34th ICAAC* **Abst G30**: 42.

Defraigne, J.O., Detry, O., Pincemail, J. et al. (1994) Direct evidence of free radical production after ischaemia and reperfusion and protective effect of desferrioxamine: ESR and vitamin E studies. *European Journal of Vascular Surgery* **8**: 537–543.

Dhainaut, J.F., Mira, J.P., Fiérobe, L. (1994) Platelet-activating factor: pathophysiological changes and therapeutic implications in sepsis. Sepsis: Current perspectives in pathophysiology and therapy. In Reinhart, K., Eyrich, K., Sprung, K. (eds) *Update in Intensive Care and Emergency Medicine*, vol. 18, pp 397–413. Berlin: Springer Verlag.

Elstner, E.F. (1991) Oxygen radicals – Biochemical basis for their efficacy. *Klinische Wochenschrift* **69**: 949–956.

Esterbauer, H., Cheesman, K.H. (1990) Determination of aldehydic lipid peroxidation products: malonedialdehyde and 4-hydroxynonenal. *Methods in Enzymology* **186**: 407–421.

Evans, P.J., Cecchini, R., Haliwell, B. (1992) Oxidative damage to lipids α_1-proteinase inhibitor by phenylbutazone in the presence of haem proteins: protection by ascorbic acid. *Biochemical Pharmacology* **44**: 981–984.

Faymonville, M.E., Pincemail, J., Duchateau, J. et al. (1991) Myeloperoxidase and elastase as markers of leukocyte activation during cardiopulmonary bypass in humans. *Journal of Thoracic Cardiovascular Surgery* **102**: 309–317.

Freeman, B. (1994) Free radical chemistry of nitric oxide. Looking at the dark side. *Chest* **105(3)**: 79S–84S.

Fridovich, I. (1984) Overview: Biological sources of $O_2^{\dot{-}}$. *Methods in Enzymology* **105:** 56–61.

Gasic, A.C., McGuize, G., Krater, S. et al. (1991) Hydrogen peroxide pretreatment of perfused canine vessels induces ICAM–1 and CD18-dependent neutrophil adherence. *Circulation* **84**: 2154–2166.

Goode, H.F., Webster, N.R. (1993) Free radicals and antioxidants in sepsis. *Critical Care Medicine* **21(11)**: 1770–1776.

Granger, D.N. (1988) Role of xanthine oxidase and granulocytes in ischemia-reperfusion injury. *American Journal of Physiology* **255**: H1269–H1275.

Grimble, R.F. (1994) Nutritional antioxidants and the modulation of inflammation: theory and practice. *New Horizons* **2:** 175–185.

Haglund, U., Gerdin, B. (1991) Oxygen-free radicals (OFR) and circulatory shock. *Circulatory Shock* **34**: 405–411.

Halliwell, B. (1994) Iron, oxidative damage and chelating agents. In Bergeron, R.J., Brittenham, G.M. (eds) *The Development of Iron Chelators for Clinical Use*, pp 33–56. Boca Raton: CRC Press.

Halliwell, B., Gutteridge, J.M.C., Cross, C.E. (1992) Free radicals, antioxidants, and human disease: where are we now? *Journal of Laboratory and Clinical Medicine* **119**: 598–620.

Harada, H., Ishizaka, A., Yonemaru, M. et al. (1989) The effects of aminophylline and pentoxifylline on multiple organ damage after Escherichia coli sepsis. *American Review of Respiratory Diseases* **140**: 974–980.

Hartstein, G., Pincemail, J., Deby-Dupont, G. et al. (1993) Evidence for free radical formation during cardiopulmonary bypass in man. *Anesthesiology* **79**: 3A.

Hayaischi, O., Yoshida, R. (1979) Specific induction of pulmonary indoleamine 2,3-dioxygenase by bacterial lipopolysaccharide. In *Oxygen Free Radicals and Tissue Damage*, pp 199–203. Amsterdam: Ciba Foundation Symposium 65, Excerpta Medica.

Hennet, T., Richter, C., Peterhans, E. (1993) Tumour necrosis factor-a induces superoxide anion generation in mitochondria of L929 cells. *Biochemical Journal* **289**: 587–592.

Jenkinson, S.G. (1993) Oxygen toxicity. *New Horizons* **1:** 504–511, 1993.

Jepsen, S., Herlevsen, P., Knudsen, P., Bud, M.I., Klausen, N.O. (1992) Antioxidant treatment with N-acetylcysteine during adult respiratory distress syndrome: a prospective, randomized, placebo-controlled study. *Critical Care Medicine* **20(7)**: 918–923.

Johnson, G., Lefer, A.M. (1990) Protective effects of a novel 21-aminosteroid during splanchnic artery occlusion shock. *Circulatory Shock* **30**: 155–164.

Kilbourn, R.G., Belloni, P. (1990) Endothelial cell production of nitrogen oxides in response to interferon gamma in combination with tumor necrosis factor, interleukin–1, or endotoxin. *Journal of the National Cancer Institute* **82**: 772–776.

Klebanoff, S.J. (1980) Oxygen metabolism and the toxic properties of phagocytes. *Annals of Internal Medicine* **93**: 480–489.

Klebanoff, S.J. (1988) Phagocytic cells: products of oxygen metabolism. In Gallin, J.I., Goldstein, J.M., Snyderman, R. (eds) *Inflammation*: basic principles and clinical correlates, pp 391–444. Raven Press, New York.

Koltai, M., Hosford, D., Braquet, P. (1993) Platelet-activating factor in septic shock. *New Horizons* **1**: 87–95.

Koyama, S., Kobayashi, T., Kubo, K., Sekiguchi, M., Ueda, G. (1992) Recombinant-human superoxide dismutase attenuates endotoxin-induced lung injury in awake sheep. *American Review of Respiratory Diseases* **145**: 1404–1409.

Kretzschmar, M. (1994) Role of oxygen free radicals in the pathophysiology of sepsis. Sepsis: Current perspectives in pathophysiology and therapy. In Reinhart, K., Eyrich, K., Sprung, C. (eds) *Update in Intensive Care and Emergency Medicine*, vol. 18, pp 122–135. Berlin: Springer Verlag.

Lefer, A.M., Ma, X.L. (1993) Cytokines and growth factors in endothelial dysfunction. *Critical Care Medicine* **21**: S9–S14.

Leff, J.A., Parsons, P.E., Day, C.E. et al (1992) Increased serum catalase activity in septic patient with the adult respiratory distress syndrome. *Americal Review of Respiratory Diseases* **146**: 985–989.

Leff, J.A., Parsons, P.E., Day, C.E. et al. (1993) Serum antioxidants as predictors of adult respiratory distress syndrome in patients with sepsis. *Lancet* **341**: 777–780.

Lloyd, S.S., Chang, A.K., Taylor, F.B., Janzen, E.G., McCay, P.B. (1993) Free radicals and septic shock in primates: the role of tumor necrosis factor. *Free Radicals in Biology and Medicine* **14**: 233–242.

Lorente, J.A., Landin, L., De Pablo, R. et al (1993) L-arginine pathway in the sepsis syndrome. *Critical Care Medicine* **21**: 1287–1295.

Loschen, G., Azzi, A.A., Richter, C., Flohé, L. (1974) Superoxide radicals as precursors of mitochondrial hydrogen peroxide. *FEBS Letters* **42**: 68–72, 1974.

McCord, J.M. (1985) Oxygen-derived free radicals in postischemic tissue injury. *New England Journal of Medicine* **312**: 159–163.

McCord, J.M. (1993) Oxygen-derived free radicals. *New Horizons* **1**: 70–76.

Malik, A.B. (1993) Endothelial cell interactions and integrins. *New Horizons* **1**: 37–51, 1993.

Mandell, G. (1988) ARDS, neutrophils and pentoxifylline. *American Review of Respiratory Diseases* **138**: 1103–1105.

Marklund, S.L. (1984) Extracellular superoxide dismutase and other superoxide dismutase isoenzymes in tissues from nine mammalian species. *Biochemical Journal* **222**: 649–655, 1984.

Mathy-Hartert, M., Deby, C., Deby-Dupont, G., Vandenberghe, A., Jadoul, L., Lamy, M. (1994) Mechanisms of antioxidant protection of endothelial cells against polymorphonuclear leucocyte oxidant stress by ceftazidime. *Clinics in Intensive Care* **5**(suppl): 74.

Menasche, P., Grousset, C., Movas, C., Piwnica, A. (1990) A promising approach for improving the recovery of heart transplants. Prevention of free radical injury through iron chelation by deferoxamine. *Journal of Thoracic and Cardiovascular Surgery* **100**: 13–31.

Menger, M.D., Lehr, H.A., Messmer, K. (1991) Role of oxygen radicals in the microcirculatory manifestations of postischemic injury. *Klinische Wochenschrift* **69**: 1050–1055.

Moncada, S., Palmer, R., Higgs, E. (1991) Nitric oxide:physiology, pathophysiology and pharmacology. *Pharmacology Reviews* **43**: 109–142.

Nahum, A., Chamberlin, W., Sznajder, J.I. (1991) Differential activation of mixed venous and arterial neutrophils in patients with sepsis syndrome and acute lung injury. *American Review of Respiratory Diseases* **143**: 1083–1087.

Nakano, M., Takayama, K., Shimizu, Y., Tsuji, Y., Inaba, H., Migita, T. (1976) Spectroscopic evidence for the generation of singlet oxygen in self-reaction of sec-peroxy-radicals. *Journal of the American Chemical Society* **98**: 1974–1975.

Novelli, G.P. (1992) Oxygen radicals in experimental shock : effects of spin-trapping nitrones in ameliorating shock pathophysiology. *Critical Care Medicine* **20**: 499–507.

Ochoa, J.B., Udekura, A.O., Billiar, T.R. et al. (1991) Nitrogen oxide levels in patients following trauma and during sepsis. *Annals of Surgery* **214**: 621–626.

Olson, N., Grizzle, M., Anderson, D. (1987) Effect of polyethylene glycol superoxide dismutase and catalase on endotoxemia in pigs. *Journal of Applied Physiology* **63**: 1526–1532.

Osborn, L. (1990) Leukocyte adhesion to endothelium in inflammation. *Cells* **62**: 3–6.

Pacht, E.R., Timerman, A.P., Lykens, M.G., Merola, A.J. (1991) Deficiency of alveolar fluid glutathione in patients with sepsis and the adult respiratory distress syndrome. *Chest* **100(5)**: 1397–1403.

Packer, J.E., Slater, T.F. Willson, R.L. (1979) Direct observation of a free radical interaction between vitamin E and vitamin C. *Nature* **278**: 737–738.

Patel, K.D., Zimmerman, G.A., Prescott, S.M., McEver, R.P., McIntyre, T.M. (1991) Oxygen radicals induce human endothelial cells to express GMP-140 and bind neutrophils. *Journal of Cell Biology* **112(4)**: 749–759.

Pietri, S., Culcasi, M., Vernière, E., d'Arbigny, P., Drieu, K. (1993). Effect of Ginkgo biloba (EGb 761) on free radical-induced ischemia-reperfusion injury in isolated rat hearts: a hemodynamic and electron-spin-resonance investigation. In Ferradini C, Droy-Lefaix MT, Christen Y (eds.) *Advance in Ginkgo Biloba Extract Research*, **vol 2**, pp 164–171. Paris: Elsevier.

Pirisino, R., Di Simplicio, P., Ignesti, G. et al. (1988) Sulfhydryl groups and peroxidase-like activity of albumin as scavenger of organic peroxides. *Pharmacological Research Communications* **20**: 545–552.

Rangan, U., Bulkley, G.B. (1993) Prospects for treatment of free radical-mediated tissue injury. *British Medical Bulletin* **49(3)**: 700–718.

Reilly, R.M., Bulkley, C.B. (1993) Vasoactive mediators and splanchnic perfusion. *Critical Care Medicine* **21**: S55–S68.

Repine, J.E., Parsons, P.E. (1994) Oxidant-antioxidant balance in endotoxin-induced oxidative injury and tolerance to oxidative injury. In Brigham K.L. (ed.) *Endotoxin and the Lungs*, pp 207–227. New York, Marcel Dekker.

Saran, M., Bors, W. (1991) Direct and indirect measurement of oxygen radicals. *Klinische Wochenschrift* **69**: 957–694.

Sawyer, M.A., Mike, J.J., Charvin, K. et al. (1989) Antioxidant therapy and survival in ARDS. *Critical Care Medicine* **17**: S153.

Schiller, H.J., Reilly, P.M., Bulkley, G.B. (1993) Antioxidant therapy. *Critical Care Medicine* **21(2)**: S92–S102.

Schneider, J., Friderichs, E., Giertz, H. (1989) Protection by recombinant human superoxide dismutase in lethal rat endotoxemia. *Progressin Clinical Biological Research* **308**: 913–917.

Schoenberg, M.H., Beger, H.G. (1993) Reperfusion injury after intestinal ischemia. *Critical Care Medicine* **21(9)**: 1376–1386.

Sellak, H., Franzini, E., Hakin, J., Pasquier, C. (1994) Reactive oxygen species rapidly increase endothelial ICAM–1 ability to bind neutrophils without detectable upregulation. *Blood* **83(9)**: 2669.

Sies, H. (1991) Oxidative stress: from basic research to clinical application. *American Journal of Medicine* **91**(suppl. 3C): 31S–38S.

Spies, C., Reinhart, K. (1994) N-Acetylcysteine in sepsis. Sepsis: Current perspectives in pathophysiology and therapy. In Reinhart, K., Eyrich, K., Sprung, C. (eds) *Update in Intensive Care and Emergency Medicine*, vol. 18, pp 425–442. Berlin: Springer Verlag.

Stamler, J.S., Singel, D.J., Loscalzo, J. (1992) Biochemistry of nitric oxide and its redox-activated forms. *Science* **258**: 1898–1902.

Suter, P.M., Domenighetti, G., Schaller, M.-D. et al. (1994) N-Acetylcysteine enhances recovery from acute lung injury in man. A randomized, double-blind, placebo-controlled clinical study. *Chest* **105**: 190–194.

Suzuki, Y., Tanigaki, T., Heimer, D. et al. (1992) Polyethylene glycol-conjugated superoxide dismutase attenuates septic lung injury in guinea pigs. *American Review of Respiratory Diseases* **145**: 388–393.

Sznajder, J.L., Fraiman, A., Hall, J.B. et al. (1989) Increased hydrogen peroxide in the expired breath of patients with acute hypoxemic respiratory failure. *Chest* **96**: 606–612.

Tagan, M., Markert, M., Schaller, M. et al. (1991) Oxidative metabolism of circulating granulocytes in adult respiratory distress syndrome. *American Journal of Medicine* **91**(suppl. 3c): 72S–78S.

Tosatti, Righini, E.R., Chieregato, A. et al. (1992) Protection from postischaemic renal pathology by a-tocoferol administration. *Acta Anaesthesiologica Italica* **43**(suppl. 2): 99–110.

Turrens, J.F., Boveris, A. (1980) Generation of superoxide anion by the NADH deshydrogenase of bovine heart mitochondria. *Biochemical Journal* **191**: 421–427.

Vallance, P., Moncada, S. (1993) Role of endogenous nitric oxide in septic shock. *New Horizons* **1**: 77–86.

Ward, P.A. (1991) Mechanisms of endothelial cell killing by H_2O_2 or products of activated neutrophils. *American Journal of Medicine* **91**(suppl. 3c): 89S–94S.

Waxman, K. (1990) Pentoxifylline in septic shock. *Critical Care Medicine* **18(2)**: 243–244.

Weiss, S.J. (1989) Tissue destruction by neutrophils. *New England Journal of Medicine* **320**: 365–375.

Westenberger, U., Thanner, S., Ruf, H.H., Gersonde, K., Sutter, G., Trentz, O. (1990) Formation of free radicals and nitric oxide derivative of hemoglobin in rats during shock syndrome. *Free Radical Research Communications* **11(1**–3): 167–178.

Winrow, V.R., Winyard, P.G., Morris, C.J., Blake, D.R. (1993) Free radicals in inflammation: second messengers and mediators of tissue destruction. *British Medical Bulletin* **49(3)**: 506–522.

Wolf, H.R., Seegert, H.W. (1982) Experimental and clinical results in shock lung treatment with vitamin E. In Lubin B., Machin L.J. (eds) Vitamin E: biochemical, hematological and clinical aspects. *Annals of the New York Academy of Sciences* **393**: 392–409.

Yu, M., Tomasa, G. (1993) A double-blind, prospective, randomized trial of ketoconazole, a thromboxane synthetase inhibitor, in the prophylaxis of the adult respiratory distress syndrome. *Critical Care Medicine* **21(11)**: 1635–1644.

Zimmerman, G.A., Prescott, S.M., McIntyre, T.M. (1992) Endothelial cell interactions with granulocytes : tethering and signaling molecules. *Immunology Today* **13**: 93–99.

Zimmerman, J.J. (1992) Oxyradical pathogenesis in sepsis. 'Mediators of sepsis'. In Lamy, M., Thys, L.G. (eds) *Update in Intensive Care and Emergency Medicine*, vol. 16, pp 136–151. Berlin: Springer Verlag.

Zimmerman, J.J. (1994) Potential of oxyradical scavengers in the therapy of sepsis. 'Sepsis: Current perspectives in pathophysiology and therapy'. In Reinhart, K., Eyrich, K., Sprung, C. (eds) *Update in Intensive Care and Emergency Medicine*, vol. 18, pp 414–424. Berlin: Springer Verlag.

9

Growth Factors in Tissue Healing

Malcolm R. Alison

INTRODUCTION

Peptide growth factors and their cell surface-associated receptors are multifunctional molecules involved in inflammation, angiogenesis and cancer as well as tissue healing. Through signal transduction pathways, receptor occupancy triggers the production of intracellular downstream effector molecules which ultimately cause cell proliferation. Changes in ion channels, a rise in cytosolic calcium, phosphatidyl inositol hydrolysis and protein phosphorylation are amongst the most common intracellular events triggered by growth factors. Almost all peptide growth factors are 'misnamed' in that their biological functions extend far beyond the original context of their discovery, and whereas cell biologists have historically called this set of molecules 'growth factors', immunologists have called some of them 'interleukins', and haematologists have used the term 'colony stimulating factors' (CSFs).

Cell proliferation in wound healing is dependent upon both the availability of peptide growth factors, and the expression of receptors for these peptides on the surface of the target cells. Cells can communicate with each other over very great distances, while others have their cellular targets only a very short distance away. The receptors have a similar overall design and can be viewed as rivets straddling the plasma membrane, and many of these are essentially allosteric enzymes, often tyrosine kinases, whose catalytic activity is stimulated by ligand binding. Some of the enzymes which produce downstream effector molecules have a common binding motif which allows them to bind to tyrosine-phosphorylated receptors and thus be in close contact with their membrane-associated substrates. Since growth factors are critical determinants of almost every aspect of the response of all tissues to injury, they clearly have enormous therapeutic potential, and now almost every one is being made by recombinant DNA techniques. Experimental studies indicate that recombinant growth factors will be widely used in clinical practice, although presently their widespread use is restricted largely to CSFs for the reduction of neutropenia after chemotherapy or bone marrow transplantation, and erythropoietin for the promotion of red blood cell production in renal failure. This chapter therefore concentrates on the potential therapeutic uses of growth factors in the very near future. Let us first examine the basic components of the healing response in a variety of tissues, since each is a potential target for therapeutic manipulation.

WOUND HEALING

The living body is subject to injury, whether accidental or deliberately inflicted as in surgical operations. To return it to its pristine condition, or at least to a state commensurate with survival, the process of healing needs to occur. When an organ is injured, a set of events follows which obviously depends on the nature and magnitude of the injury and the ability of the various surviving cell types to proliferate and repopulate the damaged area (Figure 9.1). With regard to the latter point, there are three major categories of tissues: (i) static cell populations; (ii) continually renewing cell populations and (iii) conditionally renewing cell populations.

Static cell populations such as neurones in the central nervous system (CNS) and cardiac muscle cells have lost the ability to divide by adulthood. Healing in the CNS is brought about by specialized supportive elements, and is called *reactive gliosis*, while damaged myocardium (often as a result of myocardial infarction in humans) is replaced by connective tissue, with the loss of functional muscle that this involves. Most other tissue types are capable of repopulating damaged areas and on the basis of their normal proliferative activity can be classified as either continually renewing or conditionally renewing cell populations.

Continually renewing cell populations such as stratified squamous and gastric epithelia are characterized by constant proliferative activity throughout adult life to replace routinely exfoliated, post-mitotic, terminally differentiated cells. Also in this category are haemopoietic cells, where pluripotential stem cells, committed precursor cells and maturing cells continue to divide to satisfy the peripheral demand for mature blood cells. Conditionally renewing populations ordinarily exhibit a very low rate of cell division, but they, too, are capable of rapid proliferation after loss of 'like' cells because they retain full proliferative potential. The epithelial cells of virtually all glandular organs are included in this category, e.g.

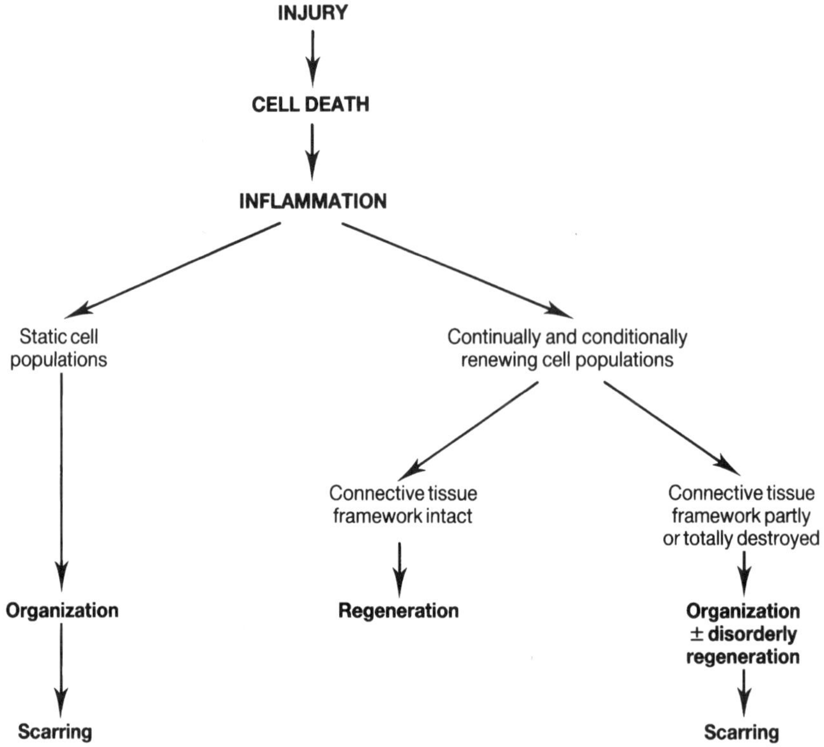

Figure 9.1. The sequelae of cellular events leading to a healing response in various tissues.

prostatic and pancreatic acinar cells, thyroid follicular cells, renal tubule cells and hepatocytes. The proliferative response of hepatocytes to partial hepatectomy is the classical example of healing in conditionally renewing cell populations. Connective tissue cells (fibroblasts, chondrocytes and osteocytes), vascular endothelial cells, and smooth muscle cells of visceral walls and blood vessels also belong to this group. Skeletal muscle is also classified as a conditionally renewing system because myogenic stem cells (satellite cells) are able to divide in response to injury.

The restitution of normal structure and function of a damaged organ depends not only on the replicative ability of the surviving cells but also on their orderly replacement, under the control of the supporting stroma. The preservation of an intact basement membrane is probably critical in this respect as it provides the physical scaffolding for the progressive replacement of lost parenchymal cells.

Disruption of the basement membrane can result in haphazard epithelial regeneration, while permanent ischaemia results in the gradual replacement of dead tissue by granulation tissue with its subsequent maturation into scar tissue.

Conventionally, healing is divided into two categories – *regeneration* and *repair*. Regeneration is the process in which lost cells are replaced by cells of the same type, and the tissue can in many instances, return to its native state; it is usually applicable to epithelial tissues. Repair involves the synthesis of connective tissue which results in the development of a scar. Often both processes contribute to the healing response and the healing of easily accessible linear skin wounds is commonly described in textbooks since both regeneration and repair are involved.

Tissue Differences in Healing

Skin

Healing of a wound of the skin and subcutaneous tissue, particularly after a surgical operation, is considered the prototype of wound healing as the formation of scar tissue is allied with epidermal regeneration (Alison, 1992). Healing of a cleanly incised wound where the edges are in close apposition (held together by surgical tapes or sutures) occurs with a minimal loss of tissue and without significant bacterial contamination. This is referred to as *primary union* or *healing by first intention*. Where there has been a large tissue defect, making it impossible for the edges to be stitched together, then this more open type of wound is referred to as *secondary union* or *healing by second intention*. The formation of granulation tissue, fibrosis and scarring are florid features of secondary rather than primary union, but the basic mechanism is the same for both; differences are thus quantitative rather than qualitative.

The response of the marginal epidermis involves *cell migration, cell proliferation* and post-wounding *remodelling*. The onset of cell migration is one of the earliest signs of epithelial activity and occurs between 18 and 24 hours post-wounding in man. The stimulus for the initiation of cell movement is, perhaps, related to the release from contact-inhibition by neighbouring cells; re-establishment of contact would provide a mechanism for the cessation of migration. Increased numbers of mitotic figures are found in marginal epidermis from 24–36 h after wounding, and tongues of epithelium, consisting of a sheet of flattened epithelial cells, infiltrate down from the margins of the wound, cleaving a path between dead and living collagen fibres thus displacing the remnants of the scab towards the surface. These cells only migrate over viable tissue, and are aided in this process both by the secretion of collagenase and plasminogen activators which facilitate opening of a pathway through the extracellular matrix (Grondahl-Hansen et al., 1988). The presence of fibronectin promotes the adhesion of cells to collagen and other substrates; in turn the trailing cells not only divide but secrete epidermal basement membrane components so that its continuity is gradually restored. The epithelial response can be very rapid and within 48 h the whole epithelial defect can be covered by a continuous, though thin, epithelial layer.

Both basal and supra-basal epithelial cells participate in the proliferative response, but the migrating cells which initially cover the wound are essentially *non-dividing.* DNA synthesis and mitosis are very low or absent in the advancing epithelial tongue, and only become more prominent at a distance of around 15–20 cell diameters behind the protruding tip. Peak mitotic activity occurs between two and five days after wounding (Maibach and Rovee, 1972), and the cell-cycle time of the stimulus-responsive cells is much shorter than that of controls. Advancing cells in the encroaching margin either roll or slide over the ones previously laid down, either as in the movement of a caterpillar track, or alternatively by amoeboid action by pushing out pseudopodia: the speed of migration in pig epidermis is 7 μm/h. Initially the 'healed' epidermis may be thicker than normal (acanthotic) due to an increased number of suprabasal cells; rete ridges are absent in the regenerated epidermis.

Repair of the dermis and subcutaneous tissue is accomplished through the formation of *granulation tissue* composed of newly proliferated blood vessels and fibroblasts. The term derives from its pink, granular appearance on the surface of a large tissue defect, where the tiny 'granules' are, in fact, loops of fragile new capillaries. Vascular proliferation begins two to three days after injury, with solid cords of endothelial cells growing out as buds or sprouts from the surviving capillaries at the wound edge, a process called *neovascularization* or *angiogenesis.* The sprouts are solid at first but rapidly become canalized. Proliferation occurs just behind the growing tips and tip advancement can be as much as 0.6 mm/day. The growth of new blood vessels also involves the local degradation of the parent basement membrane at positions from which the vascular sprouts arise, and also changes to the extracellular matrix through which the capillaries must grow. Such changes are largely due to the development of extracellular proteolytic activity by the endothelial cells themselves. The endothelial cells can produce two metalloproteinases, *collagenase*, which is capable of degrading the interstitial collagens, and *stromelysin* which can digest a broad range of matrix molecules including proteoglycans, fibronectin, laminin and type IV collagen. There is coordinated secretion of the metalloproteinases and a *tissue inhibitor of metalloproteinase* (TIMP) so that degradation is limited to the path of capillary endothelial cell migration during angiogenesis (Herron et al., 1986a, 1986b). Endothelial cells can also produce *plasminogen activators* responsible for the conversion of *plasminogen* to plasmin. This proteolytic activity also, can be limited by specific inhibitors; endothelial cells can produce a potent *plasminogen activator inhibitor* called PAI-1 (Moscatelli and Rifkin, 1988).

The wounding of connective tissue also causes fibroblasts to migrate into the wound and undergo a brief period of intense mitotic activity. The chief function of the fibroblast in this context is to synthesize extracellular matrix components, particularly *glycosaminoglycans* (GAGs), fibronectin and *collagen types I and III.* The synthesis of collagen by fibroblasts begins within 24 h of wounding, but no significant collagen deposition occurs before the third or fourth day; this corresponds with the first real increase in the breaking strength of the wound. Both type I and type III collagens are produced, although type III is the principal one synthesized in the wound. Collagen fibres orientate to lie across the incision line and thus help to unite the severed edges; this happens from about the end of the first week after injury. At this time the rate of extracellular degradation of collagen at the healing site is greatly elevated, and this activity remains abnormally high for some months. Over this period a process of remodelling occurs; much of the type III collagen is replaced by type I collagen and the new fibres are orientated according to the new lines of mechanical stress. Although the collagen content of the wound reaches a maximum by about the third week after injury, the development of maximum tensile strength takes many months and never reaches the strength of unwounded tissue.

The gastrointestinal tract

Healing in the gastrointestinal tract can also be divided into two parts: regeneration, the replacement of the mucosal epithelial component; and repair, the healing of the connective tissue including the smooth muscle. Regeneration is vital, for example, to the healing of ulcers and mucosae damaged by intensive cytotoxic chemotherapy and abdominal irradiation, while the rate of repair of connective tissue is of major concern to the surgeon, since it largely determines the strength of gastrointestinal anastomoses.

Injuries such as erosions involving small, circumscribed losses of less than the full thickness of the mucosa, so that some basal gland elements remain, probably occur fairly frequently in the gastric mucosa due to substances like alcohol or aspirin, and studies in animals suggest that the process of re-epithelialization can be remarkably rapid with totally desquamated surfaces re-establishing epithelial integrity within 1–2 h. This process is called *restitution* and occurs through the migration of cells *before* any increased rate of cell production. On the other hand, ulcers are circumscribed lesions involving loss of the full thickness of the mucosa with a variable degree of penetration into the underlying tissues, and as such healing includes the production of scar tissue. Peptic and duodenal ulceration result from a breakdown of the mucosal defence barrier (mucous and bicarbonate) by endogenous aggressors, acid and pepsin, in the gastric juice. The currently used anti-ulcer drugs do not actually heal ulcers but they alter the local environment so that healing can take place. The most effective medical therapy is to reduce acid secretion either by blocking the promoting action of histamine on parietal (acid-secreting) cells by *H_2-receptor antagonists* (e.g. Zantac® and Tagamet®) or by using proton-pump inhibitors (e.g. Losec®). In the future, growth factors such as epidermal growth factor (EGF) and transforming growth factor alpha (TGF-α) may have a role to play (see below). In humans, most ulcers occur in the pyloric mucosa and re-epithelialization can occur, although the regenerated mucous glands are probably more irregular and fewer in number. As with excised skin wounds, the granulation tissue in the ulcer base contracts which can cause marked distortion leading to pyloric stenosis or the formation of an 'hour glass' stomach.

Most cytotoxic chemotherapeutic drugs are designed to cause the death of proliferative cells, thus gastrointestinal side-effects can be a limiting factor when chemotherapy is used to treat tumours elsewhere in the body. In rats at least, such damage can promote enhanced crypt cell production through the more rapid cycling of the basally-situated (stem) cells (Wright and Alison, 1984). Ionizing radiation also causes the death of proliferative cells, and in severe cases can lead to the *gastrointestinal radiation syndrome*, i.e. intestinal haemorrhage, bacterial infection and fluid loss. Rapid regeneration can be achieved through the production of large hyperplastic crypts whose cells show initially a reduced commitment towards terminal differentiation, and a propensity for the spawning of new crypts through a budding process (Potten et al., 1983; Alison, 1992).

The liver

The rodent liver has been a popular model for studying regeneration, usually after a two-thirds partial hepatectomy (Alison, 1986). The restoration of pre-operative liver mass is achieved within 10 days, and involves hyperplasia of all cell types in the liver, not just the hepatocytes (Wright and Alison, 1984). Complete regeneration is also seen in the rodent liver after exposure to xenobiotics such as carbon tetrachloride and paracetamol. In man too, liver regeneration is vital after such poisoning, and is also necessary in virally-induced diseases (both the hepatitis viruses and cytopathic viruses) and in conditions such as fulminant hepatic failure (Alison and Sarraf, 1994a).

Other tissues

The kidney is reasonably able to compensate for loss of renal parenchyma, although after unilateral nephrectomy the mass of the remaining kidney increases (by as much as 50%), largely through hypertrophy of the tubular cells (Harris et al., 1986). The regenerative capabilities of the adrenal gland are well seen in the response to *enucleation*, a procedure in which the medulla and most of the cortex are 'shelled out' from under the capsule, leaving behind a fibrous covering with an irregular lining of glomerulosa cells. Following enucleation in the rat, cords of cells begin to grow inwards and can be 30 cells in length within a week, with the normal cortical architecture restored after about a month; there is no regeneration of the medulla (Dallman, 1985). When there is excess TSH, usually caused by thyroid dyshormonogenesis, the thyroid gland shows prodigious growth (Wynford-Thomas et al., 1982). The major salivary glands such as the submaxillary and parotid can undergo a prominent growth response to treatment with β-sympathomimetic agents such as isoproterenol, with hypertrophy and hyperplasia of acinar cells. The response of these paired glands to unilateral extirpation is much more modest, and can, in fact, be completely abolished if the activity of the autonomic innervation to the residual gland is reduced by switching to a liquid diet. Thus, functional demand seems to play a pivotal role in regenerative growth. In the male, accessory sex glands (prostate, seminal vesicles, etc.) are almost wholly dependent upon androgenic stimulation for the maintenance of normal function. If androgen levels are severely depleted, then these tissues atrophy but the tissue loss alone is not sufficient to elicit a compensatory response. However, if such atrophic tissues are presented with a functional demand in the shape of renewed androgenic stimulation, then all the regressive changes can be reversed by a wave of hypertrophy and hyperplasia (Alison and Wright, 1979).

Pneumonectomy causes diffuse pulmonary proliferation (Thurlbeck, 1983), and local wounds of the trachea heal by the migration of cells across the wound floor, with increased proliferation of marginal cells. Agents such as NO_2 cause the destruction of bronchiolar epithelium and alveolar lining cells, eliciting a regenerative response from Clara cells and type 2 pneumocytes, respectively. Bleomycin also stimulates the proliferation of type 2 pneumocytes (the supposed stem cells of the alveoli) by causing diffuse alveolar damage. Neurones in the CNS are very sensitive to insults such as hypoxia, and in the post-natal human brain they are irreplaceable, although some limited regrowth of neuronal processes is possible (Weller et al., 1983); in the peripheral nervous system axonal regeneration is more successful.

GROWTH FACTORS: STRUCTURES, FUNCTIONS AND APPLICATIONS

Strategies of Chemical Signalling

Growth factors are among the most potent of biological substances, being biologically active at concentrations of picograms per millilitre (1 pg = 10^{-12} g), while the specificity and magnitude of the response is believed to be mainly due to the type and abundance of membrane-bound receptor rather than the availability of the growth factor. Operationally *in vivo*, it is possible to distinguish at least three principal types of growth factor secretion, dependent upon the distance between the secreting cell(s) and the cellular target (Alison and Wright, 1993). In *endocrine secretion* the effector cells are typically in groups surrounded by a rich vascular network, and secrete a hormone directly into blood vessels; the hormone acts on target cells with the necessary receptive machinery, at some distance from the source. Androgens or oestrogens from the gonads induce growth in the prostate or endometrium through this means. The immune system too can be regarded as an endocrine system, albeit a mobile one, since the whole range of cellular functions is controlled by an intricate *cytokine* network (see below). *Paracrine* secretion on the other hand, involves growth factors only acting within the immediate vicinity of the effector cells, perhaps within a millimetre or so. This mode of action undoubtedly occurs in the alimentary tract where several families of neuro-endocrine cells produce multiple locally acting peptides, some of which influence growth.

The relative autonomous nature of malignant cells in culture has been appreciated for many years; i.e. they require fewer exogenous growth factors for optimal growth than do their normal counterparts. One explanation was that the malignant cells had the ability to produce their own growth factors, and the same cells had functional receptors for them – a mechanism termed *autocrine* secretion (reviewed by Sporn and Roberts, 1985). Such a mechanism could clearly bestow a growth advantage to cancer cells who would be under less strong external growth control than neighbouring normal cells. Autocrine secretion was first described by DeLarco and Todaro (1978) in rodent cells transformed by sarcoma viruses, where the mixture of secreted polypeptides (originally called 'sarcoma growth factor') contained a factor structurally related to (but distinct from) EGF and now called TGF-α. Autocrine secretion of TGF-α plays an important role in the malignant behaviour of many cell types, and may also be operative during hepatocyte regeneration (Mead and Fausto, 1989). Other peptides which function in this way include platelet-derived growth factor (PDGF) produced by osteosarcoma and glioma cells, and bombesin, the tetradecapeptide secreted by human small cell ('oat cell') lung cancer cells. In these examples it has been possible to inhibit cell growth by antibodies to the peptides, leaving no doubt that antibody therapy can interfere with an essential autocrine pathway intimately associated with aberrant growth of tumour cells.

Growth Factors

Table 9.1 summarizes the major growth factor families which probably influence wound healing.

The EGF family

EGF is the prototypic member of a family of growth factors which includes TGF-α, amphiregulin, heparin-binding EGF, pox virus growth factors and cripto. EGF was first isolated from male mouse submaxillary glands by Stanley Cohen in 1962, and like almost every other growth factor it has a spectrum of biological activities far

Table 9.1 The major growth factor families involved in wound healing

EGF family	EGF TGF-α Amphiregulin Heparin-binding EGF Pox virus growth factors Cripto
Platelet derived growth factor family	PDGF VEGF
Insulin-like growth factors	Insulin IGF-I IGF-II NGF
TGF-β family	TGF-β1–TGF-β5 Inhibins Activins BMP-1–BMP-7
Fibroblast growth factor family	FGF-1–FGF-7
Hepatocyte Growth Factor	HGF-SF
Trefoil growth factor family	pS2, SP, ITF
Haematopoietic growth factors	Erythropoietin G-CSF, GM-CSF Stem cell factor (c *kit* ligand) IL-1–IL-12

beyond that from which its name derives. It is now known to be a major mitogen for many cell lineages and even has non-related actions such as inhibiting gastric acid secretion. Mouse EGF is highly homologous with the human polypeptide β-urogastrone, originally isolated from the urine of pregnant women and now regarded as the human homologue of rodent EGF (Gregory, 1975); 37 of the 53 amino acids are common to both mouse EGF and URO-EGF, while the six cysteine residues occupy the same relative positions.

All members of the EGF family are synthesized as much larger, membrane-bound, glycosylated precursors, and despite only limited sequence homology, the secreted molecules have six conserved cysteine residues forming three disulfide bonds (Prigent and Lemoine, 1992; Figure 9.2). All these molecules bind to the same receptor, EGFR, sometimes called *c-erb B*-1, a member of the type I family of receptor tyrosine kinases which includes two more related molecules *c-erb B*-2 and *c-erb B*-3. TGF-α, despite only 35% sequence

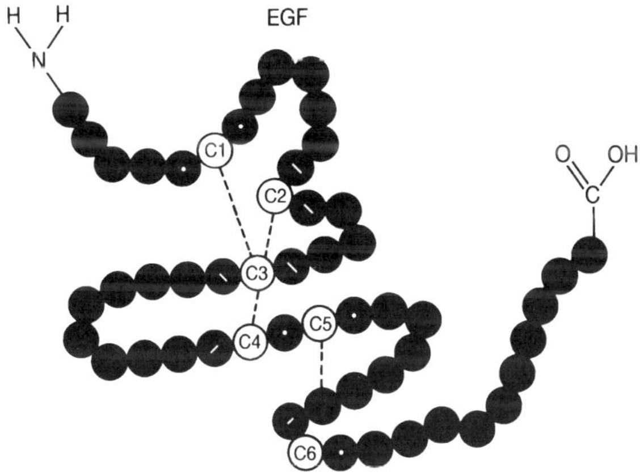

Figure 9.2. Schematic representation of the EGF molecule; there are three disulfide bonds between the cysteine (c) residues in the 53 amino acid peptide.

homology with EGF, has biological activity similar to EGF and binds to the same receptor. As well as being abundant in many tumour cells, TGF-α is also found in many normal cells (Nasim et al., 1992, 1993; Thomas et al., 1992; Alison et al., 1993a). Amphiregulin was isolated from conditioned medium of MCF-7 breast carcinoma cells treated with phorbol ester and can be both stimulatory and inhibitory to cell growth.

There has been considerable interest in the use of EGF and related growth factors for promoting healing in the gastrointestinal tract (Alison and Sarraf, 1994b). It is generally agreed that the effects of any putative growth factor for the gut be best judged when the gut is in a hypoplastic state. This can be achieved by maintenance on isocaloric total parenteral nutrition (TPN), which produces a steady state, basal level of proliferation in the gut, with the direct and indirect effects of food (luminal nutrition) being abolished. Using this approach Goodlad and colleagues (1987a, 1987b, 1992) have monitored the effects of recombinant URO-EGF on rats maintained on TPN. Not surprisingly, there was marked hypoplasia and atrophy of the bowel of intravenously fed (TPN) rats. Recombinant URO-EGF was able to reverse these changes in a dose-dependent manner, restoring levels of proliferation to those seen in orally fed rats. However, these trophic effects of URO-EGF were only seen when the growth factor was administered intravenously, and not when it was administered luminally *via* intragastric cannulae.

The failure of luminal EGF to have a trophic effect may simply

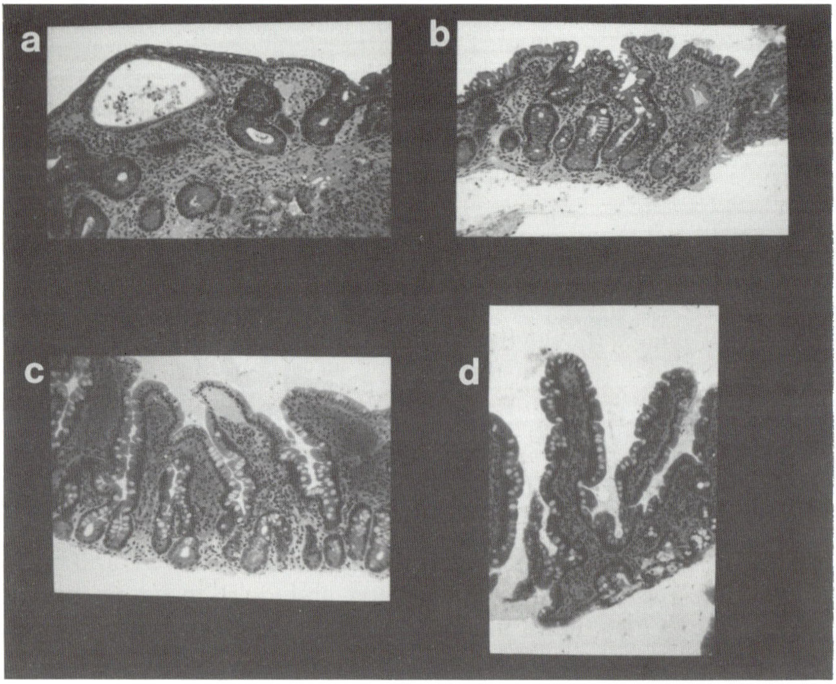

Figure 9.3. Changes in small intestinal histology in an 8-month-old infant suffering from necrotizing enteritis treated with rhEGF (100 ng/kg/h) for a period of 6 days. The mucosa was essentially 'flat' before treatment (a) but showed gradual improvement after 2 (b) and 4 (c) days treatment to be of normal appearance after 7 days (d). (Courtesy of Professor Nick Wright.)

reflect the lack of EGFR on the apical cell membranes, in the small intestine at least, EGF binds to the laterobasal cell membranes but not to the brush border surface (Scheving et al., 1989). If the action of EGF is indeed not luminal, it is possible that the role of EGF may be a paracrine one, as ulceration can induce the growth of a novel cell lineage from the crypt base (Wright et al., 1990a) which secretes EGF via ducts in the lamina propria to pores opening onto the villus surface.

It still remains to be seen whether the systemic proliferative effects of URO-EGF are physiological or pharmacological, but already recombinant EGF has found its way into the clinic where it has proved to be a very potent stimulator of epithelial cell production in the human intestine (Walker-Smith et al., 1985; Sullivan et al., 1991). An 8-month-old girl requiring intensive care, suffering from necrotizing enteritis, was given a continuous intravenous infusion (100 ng/kg/h) of recombinant human EGF (rhEGF) for 6 days. Figure 9.3 illustrates the impressive histological response observed during the first week which eventually led to a complete recovery, and it is highly likely that EGF prevented a fatal outcome in this child. rhEGF has been also used to treat a child with congenital microvillous atrophy, a disorder within the intractable diarrhoea syndrome of infancy. In this condition, there is a failure to elaborate a microvillous border on the lumenal aspect of small intestinal villous cells (Figure 9.4), necessitating some intravenous feeding. rhEGF was able to stimulate crypt cell proliferation in this patient, and though not representing a complete treatment for microvillous atrophy, the results suggest that EGF could be used to treat other conditions requiring an increase to the intestinal mucosal mass, e.g. Crohn's disease, ulcerative colitis, non-responsive coeliac disease, peptic ulceration, mucositis and post-TPN syndrome.

In view of the ability of various members of the EGF family of growth factors to bind to the EGFR, it is not possible to predict the physiological ligand acting on EGFR at a given site. This is especially relevant in the gut where EGFR is detected widely, while EGF has only a limited distribution (Thomas et al., 1992). Accordingly in the gut, TGF-α may be the most important ligand for EGFR. In the human fetal gut, TGF-α is more widely distributed than EGF (Miettinen et al., 1989), and likewise TGF-α is found throughout the human and rodent gastrointestinal tract (Thomas et al., 1992). TGF-α is an acid- and heat-stable polypeptide of 50 amino acids, produced initially as a transmembrane precursor of 160 amino acids from which the active 50 amino acid form is released by proteolytic cleavage (Derynck et al., 1984). Since both EGF and TGF-α promote cell proliferation, stimulate cell migration (Barrandon and Green, 1987) and inhibit gastric acid secretion (Konturek et al., 1984), it is likely that both growth factors play a pivotal role in ulcer healing. Indeed, there is increased expression of TGF-α mRNA and protein in the gastric mucosa shortly after gastric injury to rats (Polk et al., 1992), while bilateral extirpation of the submaxillary/sublingual gland complexes (a rich source of EGF) delays the healing of acetic acid-induced gastric and duodenal ulcers (Konturek et al., 1988). Administration of EGF could accelerate the healing of these gastro-duodenal ulcers in rats, and completely reverse the delay in ulcer healing in the sialoadenectomized animals. EGF has also been implicated in the migration and proliferation of regenerative epithelia in the healing of ileal mucosal defects (Saxena et al., 1992).

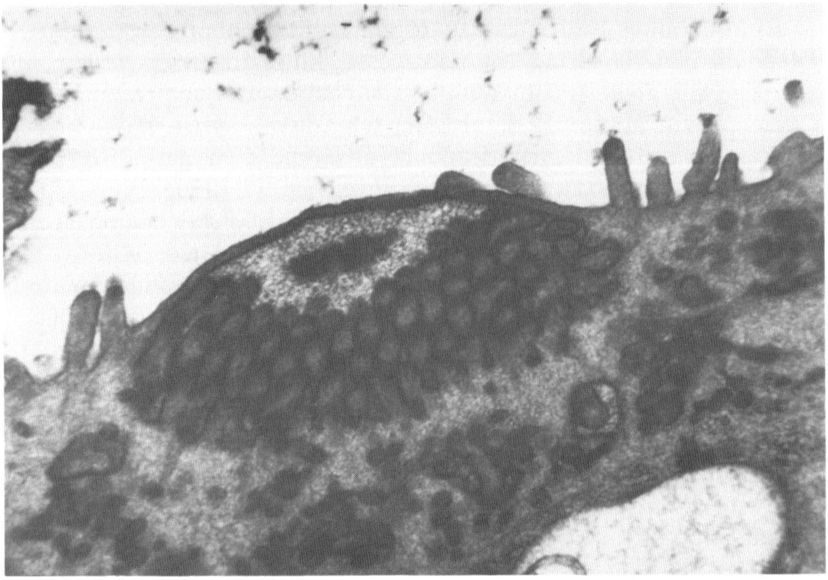

Figure 9.4. Photomicrograph of a small intestinal villous cell from a child suffering from microvillous atrophy; rhEGF was able to increase the crypt cell production rate. (Courtesy of Mr A.D. Phillips, Queen Elizabeth Hospital for Children, Hackney.)

EGF and TGF-α have been also used to promote the healing of cutaneous, corneal and liver injuries, but perhaps their other major clinical application besides that in the gut is in lung maturation and healing. Ryan et al (1994) have shown that both growth factors stimulate type 2 pneumocyte proliferation, the cells which play a critical role in the replenishment of the damaged alveolar epithelium, while EGF may soon be used as a postnatal treatment to promote surfactant development for the premature infant with respiratory distress (Price et al., 1993).

The PDGF family

As a major mitogen for connective tissue cells, platelet-derived growth factor (PDGF) is probably very important in wound healing (Raines et al., 1990). PDGF is a cationic, disulfide-linked dimeric protein with a molecular weight of ~30 kDa; the PDGF family also includes vascular endothelial growth factor (VEGF). The subunits of the PDGF dimer are polypeptides designated A or B chains, and PDGF family can be either homodimeric (AA or BB) or heterodimeric (AB). The B chain is 96% homologous with part of the transforming protein product ($p28^{sis}$) of the simian sarcoma virus which causes sarcomas in baboons. Two distinct PDGF receptor subunits, designated α and β, have been identified (Seifert et al., 1989). High affinity binding of PDGF involves dimers of the receptor (either αα, ββ, or αβ), and results in activation of the tyrosine kinase in the intracellular domain, leading to autophosphorylation of the cytoplasmic domain of the receptor as well as phosphorylation of other intracellular substrates (see below). Fibroblasts, endothelial cells, monocytes and certain tumour cells (along with platelets), are sources of PDGF or PDGF-like molecules, and PDGF functions as a mitogen for mesenchymal cells as well as being a powerful chemoattractant for inflammatory cells (Ross et al., 1986). A recent report (Sundberg et al., 1993) suggests that pericytes (pluripotential stem cells) found in association with the microvasculature in human wound healing situations strongly express the PDGF-β receptor, indicating a role in angiogenesis.

Insulin-like growth factors

Insulin and the insulin-like growth factors (IGFs) have similar structures and biological activities, generally stimulating growth and cellular metabolism. Insulin often acts synergistically with other growth factors while IGF-II has been particularly implicated in fetal development and embryonal neoplasms. IGF-I (formerly called somatomedin C) and IGF-II (formerly called Multiplication Stimulating Activity-MSA) are single chain peptides of 70 and 67 amino acid residues respectively which are highly conserved in different species (Rechler and Nissley, 1990). Growth hormone stimulates the production of IGF-I, primarily in the liver, though IGF-I mRNA can be found in most tissues. IGF-I may have an important role in peripheral nerve regeneration (Kanje et al., 1989).

The transforming growth factor-βs

The TGF-βs form a large family of multifunctional peptide growth factors (Roberts and Sporn, 1990; Sporn and Roberts, 1992). They are active in the form of disulfide-linked dimers, and both homodimers and heterodimers exist. The originally described form of TGF-β is now designated TGF-β1, and there are a number of closely related

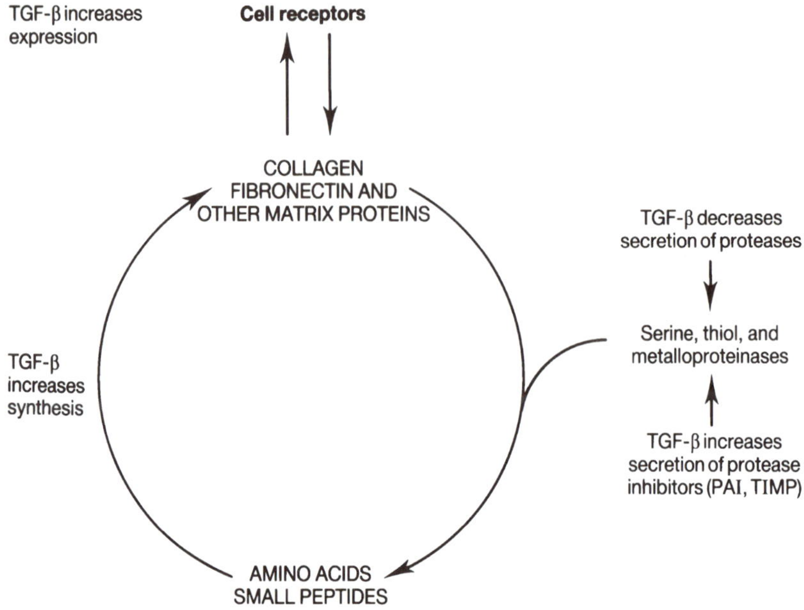

Figure 9.5. Summary of the mechanisms through which TGF-β increases the accumulation of extracellular matrix and the response of the cells to matrix.

peptides (TGF-β2, TGF-β3, TGF-β4, TGF-β5), as well as the more distantly related activins, inhibins and bone morphogenetic proteins (BMPs). The TGF-βs are synthesized as large precursor molecules with the mature form of TGF-β at the C-terminus; this is proteolytically cleaved prior to secretion, but both portions remain together upon secretion as a non-covalent complex of the dimeric latency associated protein (LAP) and the processed dimeric 25 kDa TGF-β. This complex is biologically inactive, and release of TGF-β may be facilitated by action of macrophage-secreted proteases on the LAP. TGF-β is generally held to be stimulatory for the growth of cells of mesenchymal origin and inhibitory for epithelial cells, and may influence wound healing more indirectly through regulating the formation and conservation of extracellular matrix molecules (Figure 9.5). Many members of the TGF-β superfamily show potential in the field of wound healing; exogenously administered recombinant human TGF-β1 (rhTGF-β1) can increase the breaking strength of incisional wounds in rats (Beck et al., 1993) and can also promote osteoblastic activity in rabbits, apparently binding to the periosteum at sites of bone injury (Richardson et al., 1993). Endochondral ossification can be stimulated by osteogenetic protein-1, also called BMP-7 (Asahina et al., 1993).

Fibroblast growth factors

The FGF family currently consists of seven structurally related peptide growth factors, designated FGF-1 to FGF-7 (Hughes and Hall, 1993). Acidic and basic fibroblast growth factors (FGF-1 and FGF-2) are the prototypic members of this family, both characterized by a high affinity for heparin, and synthesized by a wide variety of normal and malignant cells (Gospodarowicz et al., 1987). FGFs are potent stimulators of endothelial proliferation and therefore probably crucial in tumour angiogenesis as well as during wound healing. Basic FGF has shown promise in the healing of ulcers and the growth of skin grafts (Fiddes et al., 1991), and keratinocyte growth factor (KGF; FGF-7) produced by mesenchymal cells, may be the mediator of hypothesized mesenchymal–epithelial interactions since the receptor is found mainly on epidermal keratinocytes, and after wounding, massive increases in KGF mRNA in the underlying dermis precede epidermal proliferation (Werner et al., 1992).

Hepatocyte growth factor

Over the last 2 or 3 years the search for a humoral regulator of liver growth has increasingly concentrated on the role of hepatocyte growth factor, also called scatter factor (HGF-SF). HGF is synthesized from a single precursor molecule of 728 amino acids, which is proteolytically processed to form the mature HGF, a heterodimeric molecule composed of a 69 kDa α chain and a 34 kDa β chain. The α chain contains four kringle domains (double loop structures held together with disulfide bonds) reminiscent of various proteases involved in coagulation and fibrinolysis. The β chain has a 37% homology with the β chain of plasmin. HGF is currently considered to be a pleiotropic factor, produced by mesenchymal cells, influencing epithelial cell growth, motility and morphogenesis. HGF was originally termed 'scatter factor' (Stoker and Perryman, 1985), because the protein from the conditioned medium of human embryonic fibroblasts was able to enhance the local motility (scatter) of a variety of epithelial cells *in vitro*. HGF and scatter factor are identical. The usual target cells for a bioassay of HGF scattering activity are Madin–Darby canine kidney (MDCK) cells, and when

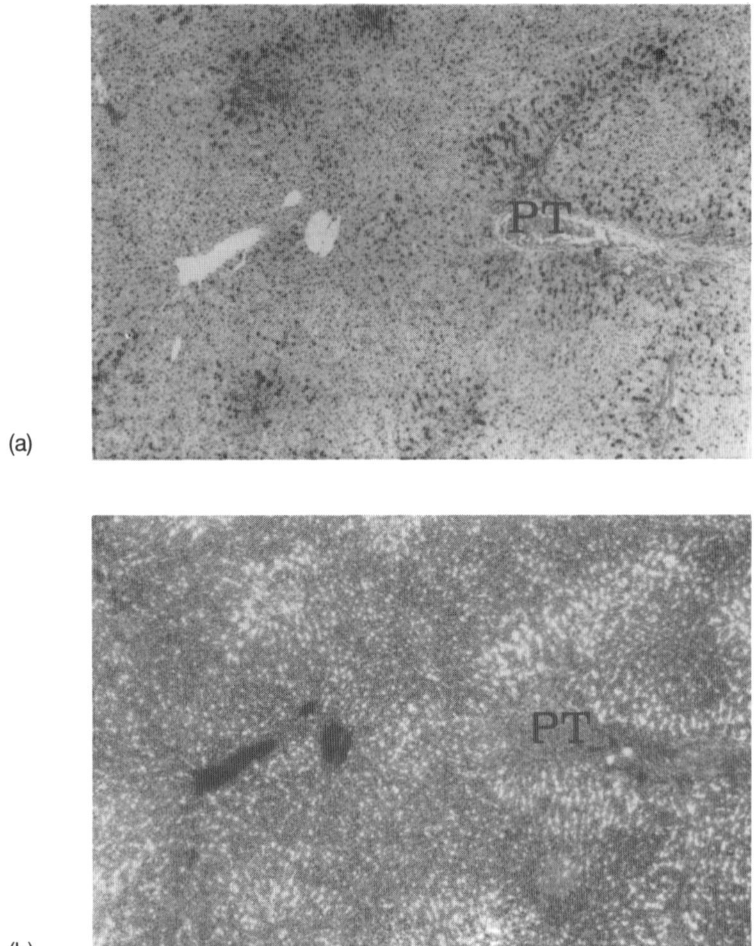

Figure 9.6. HGF expression in the liver after partial hepatectomy as detected by *in situ* hybridization using a ^{35}S antisense riboprobe to HGF mRNA, viewed by bright field (a) and dark field reflected light (b) illumination. HGF expression is confined to sinusoid-lining cells, and here most are close to the portal tracts (PT).

these cells are grown in collagen gels, HGF can also act as a morphogen promoting nephrogenesis (Montesanto et al., 1991).

In the liver, HGF is not produced by hepatocytes, but by non-parenchymal sinusoid-lining cells, principally Ito cells (Figure 9.6). The body of evidence linking enhanced production of HGF with increased hepatocyte proliferation is considerable: serum levels of HGF rise after liver resection in both rat (Kinoshinta et al., 1991) and humans (Tomiya et al., 1992). HGF synthesis in the liver increases after CCl_4 injury (Noji et al., 1990) and partial resection (Zarnegar et al., 1991), high levels of HGF are found in patients with fulminant hepatic failure (Tsubouchi et al., 1989) and HGF is the most potent mitogen for rat hepatocytes *in vitro* (Strain et al., 1991). When hepatocyte regeneration is impaired, relatively undifferentiated cells emerge from the portal space and take over the burden of regenerative growth. These facultative or potential stem cells are called oval cells (Sell, 1990) and in humans they are seen in chronically damaged liver (De Vos and Desmet, 1992). When hepatocyte regeneration is prevented by the presence of cytotoxic carcinogens such as 2-acetylaminofluorene in the partially hepatectomized rat, oval cell proliferation results, and here also, HGF production by sinusoid-lining cells seems important in governing their behaviour (Alison et al., 1993b). A model of HGF activation on target cells such as hepatocytes and oval cells can be proposed (Figure 9.7), and since HGF is distributed throughout the body it is likely that the mitotically active two-chain HGF is produced locally by the action of

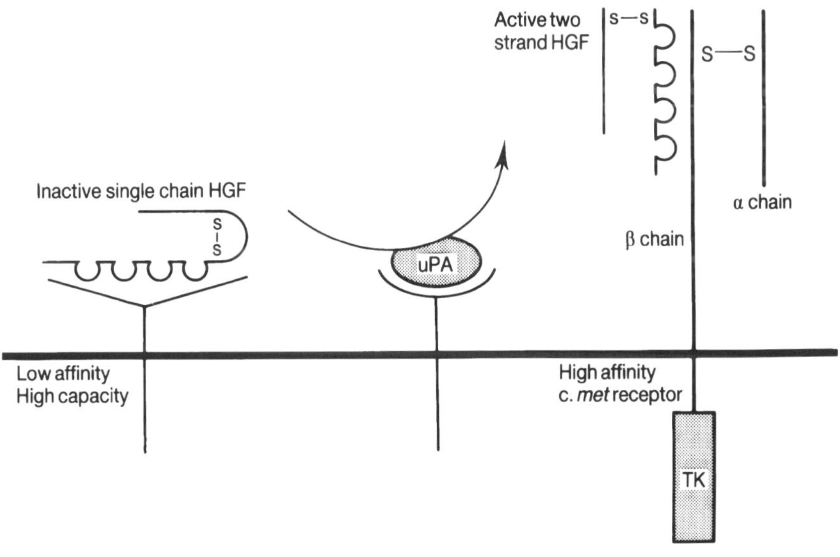

Figure 9.7. Schematic diagram illustrating the way HGF may be activated at the target site and subsequently interacts with the c.*met* receptor, a member of the receptor protein tyrosine kinase family.

plasminogen activators on the inactive single chain molecule (Mars et al., 1993). Of course, you can have too much of a good thing, and high levels of HGF in fulminant hepatic failure do not guarantee survival (Tsubouchi et al., 1992), so perhaps a more effective therapy would be to boost the Ito cell numbers in such extreme cases? These cells are a rich source of growth factors for neighbouring oval cells and hepatocytes.

The trefoil peptides

A new group of peptides has recently gained prominence, particularly in the field of gastroenterology: the trefoil peptides are a highly conserved group of molecules that, in humans at least, have a distinctive pattern of distribution in the gut (Wright et al., 1990b; Hanby et al., 1993). The group takes its title from the characteristic trefoil motif, a three loop ('three leafed') structure secured by disulfide bonds based on cysteine residues (Thim, 1989, 1993). The trefoil peptides known to date have either one, two or four trefoil domains (Poulsom and Wright, 1993).

The first molecule characterized was pS2, a single trefoil, an oestrogen-inducible peptide discovered in the MCF-7 human breast cancer cell line (Masiakowski et al., 1982). Despite its heritage as a tumour-associated peptide, pS2 mRNA and protein is expressed by the foveolar epithelium throughout the length of the normal human stomach (Hanby et al., 1993), though its function remains illusive. pS2 is, however, highly homologous with pancreatic spasmolytic polypeptide (PSP), a larger molecule of 108 amino acids, which has two cysteine-rich trefoil domains (Thim, 1993). This peptide was originally found as a side fraction in the commercial purification of insulin from pig pancreas (Jorgensen et al., 1982a) and has defined physiological effects on the gut, inhibiting gastric acid secretion and intestinal motility as well as stimulating growth (Jorgensen et al., 1982b; Hoosein et al., 1989) – highly desirable qualities for a putative gut growth factor. Homologues of PSP have been identified in many species including humans (Tomasetto et al., 1990) and various rodents, though the 'pancreatic' component of the name was discarded as evidence for expression in human pancreas was not available. Human spasmolytic polypeptide (hSP) is widely expressed by foveolar epithelial cells throughout the human gastric mucosa, but unlike pS2, hSP mRNA expression is also seen at the bottom of gastric antral glands (Hanby et al., 1993) – a region particularly susceptible to ulceration. In the rat stomach rat spasmolytic polypeptide (rSP) is expressed by mucous neck cells just beneath the foveolae. Rat intestinal trefoil factor (rITF), found in the rat small intestine and colon, is a recently described single trefoil peptide (Suemori et al., 1991), the synthesis of which is largely confined to goblet cells (Chinery et al., 1992). In humans too, human intestinal trefoil factor (hITF) is also synthesized by small intestinal and colonic goblet cells (Podolsky et al., 1993).

It has recently been demonstrated that gastric ulceration perturbs the pattern of trefoil peptide expression in humans (Levi et al., 1993), and the tongue of epithelium that grows out to cover the ulcer floor and the regenerative mucosal glands themselves, express trefoil peptide nRNAs at high levels. In rats too, gastric ulcers cause massive increases in rSP and rITF mRNA expression in the regenerative glands (Chinery et al., 1994), strongly suggesting that trefoil peptides are important to the healing process. This notion is supported by the fact that pS2 and hSP are widely expressed in chronic ulcerative conditions such as Crohn's disease. What used to be regarded as pyloric or gastric metaplasia in chronically damaged intestine, is in fact a differentiating cell lineage that initially buds from the bases of intestinal crypts adjacent to the ulcer (Wright et al., 1990a, 1990b). These buds form a ramifying network of tubules in the lamina propria, before forming a duct through the core of an adjacent villus and opening on to the mucosal surface through a pore. This structure has a novel phenotype and it has become known as the Ulcer Associated Cell Lineage (UACL). The UACL synthesizes the trefoil peptides, pS2 and hSP. As the cells migrate through the UACL they sequentially change the pattern of peptide expression: EGF in the basal tubules, hSP in the basal tubules and lower portions of the duct, and pS2 in the upper ductular cells and the surface cells of the lineage on the villi (Wright et al., 1990b). Thus, the UACL seems uniquely capable of mediating, through a paracrine mechanism, the healing of gastrointestinal mucosal injury by the remarkable co-expression of multiple peptide growth factors. Trefoil peptides will undoubtedly find their way into the clinic within a few years – watch this shape!

The haematopoietic growth factors

A number of regulatory molecules have been identified that influence haematopoiesis; many were called colony stimulating factors (CSFs) because of their ability to stimulate *in vitro* colony formation by progenitor cells in semi-solid media, some have now been assigned appropriate names, e.g. erythropoietin, others have retained their

CSF designation, while others have been given an interleukin number.

Almost all patients in the later stages of renal failure were anaemic until recombinant human erythropoietin (rhEPO) became available for therapy. EPO is a 165 amino acid residue glycoprotein (Jelkmann, 1992), and the major stimulus for EPO gene transcription is tissue hypoxia. Most EPO is produced by the kidney, and it is likely that the renal source of EPO is a fibroblast-like population of interstitial cells (Ratcliffe, 1993). EPO acts in concert with other growth factors to stimulate the proliferation and maturation of bone marrow erythroid precursor cells, and rhEPO raises the haematocrit and blood haemoglobin concentration in a dose-dependent way (Faller et al., 1993). The availability of rhEPO was a major advance in clinical medicine, and it abolishes the need for blood transfusions to correct the anaemia associated with chronic renal failure; it also appears useful in alleviating the anaemia of chronic inflammatory and malignant diseases.

At present the two clinically most important CSFs are granulocyte colony stimulating factor (G-CSF) and granulocyte-macrophage CSF (GM-CSF). Both are glycoproteins, produced by a variety of cell types including macrophages, fibroblasts and endothelial cells, particularly in response to cytokines (TNF-α and IFN-γ) and inflammatory stimuli (endotoxin and LPS). GM-CSF stimulates the proliferation of granulocyte and macrophage progenitors, and enhances the function of the differentiated cells, though many other functions have been attributed to the molecule (Burgess, 1990). Likewise, G-CSF is best known for its stimulatory effects on granulocyte precursor proliferation and survival and function of the terminally differentiated cells. Both CSFs are now widely used in the clinic, particularly for the recovery of haematopoiesis after chemotherapy-induced neutropenias and/or pancytopenias (for review see Focus on Growth Factors, 1993, Costello, 1993). Neutropenia is a significant dose-limiting toxicity of many chemotherapeutic regimens, therefore CSFs can reduce the risk of infections, reduce the days of hospitalization and decrease the use of antibiotics. Chemotherapy is often accompanied by autologous marrow infusion, and as might be predicted, the clinical benefits of CSFs are less if the bone marrow has been collected after extensive prior chemotherapy, consistent with the hypothesis that a sufficient number of myeloid precursor target cells need to be available for a significant effect.

Stem cell regulation in the bone marrow is a complex process in which there are both positive and negative influences (Moore, 1991; McCulloch, 1993), and it is quite clear that many of the growth factors can act synergistically. For example, some of the interleukins (e.g. IL-1 and IL-3) act on early progenitor cells which primes them to respond more effectively to other more lineage-restricted haematopoietic growth factors, and so combinations such as IL-3 and GM-CSF are proving very effective in alleviating myelosuppression after chemotherapy for cancer. Stem cell factor (SCF or c.*kit* ligand) is another early acting growth factor, which alone, is predominantly a survival factor (Johnson, 1993), but it synergizes strongly with other growth factors, and now recombinant human SCF is finding clinical use in combination with GM-CSF, G-CSF and EPO in promoting the growth of myeloid and erythroid progenitors.

GROWTH FACTOR SIGNAL TRANSDUCTION: A BRIEF OVERVIEW

Cell surface-associated receptors have a similar overall design being composed of an *extracellular domain* responsible for binding the growth factor, a short hydrophobic *transmembrane domain*, and an *intracellular domain* responsible for initiating the intracellular signal in response to ligand binding. Many of the growth factors considered in this chapter (EGF family, PDGF, FGFs, IGFs, HGF, SCF) bind to transmembrane receptors belonging to a large family of *protein tyrosine kinases* (PTKs), essentially enzymatic proteins with the ability to catalyse the phosphorylation of the amino acid tyrosine in proteins – the phosphorylated forms of many proteins (enzymes) are more active than the non-phosphorylated forms. As a general rule, ligand binding results in receptor dimerization, and leads to receptor autophosphorylation and tyrosine phosphorylation of specific proteins. Further transmission of the ligand-induced signal involves recognition of the phosphorylated tyrosines on the non-catalytic regions of the receptors by cytoplasmic proteins which contain Src homology 2 (SH2) domain sequences. The SH2 region is so called, of course, because of its homology with a conserved domain (SH2) in the Src family of non-receptor protein kinases. The model for this family is $pp60^{c\text{-}src}$ a protein generally associated with the inner surface of the plasma membrane, while the gene responsible for the transforming activity of Rous sarcoma virus was, in fact, derived from the normal cellular gene, c-src.

Examples of proteins that have SH2 domains that can bind to phosphotyrosine sites on growth factor receptors include phospholipase Cγ (PLCγ), the p85 subunit of phosphatidyl inositol (PI) 3-kinase,

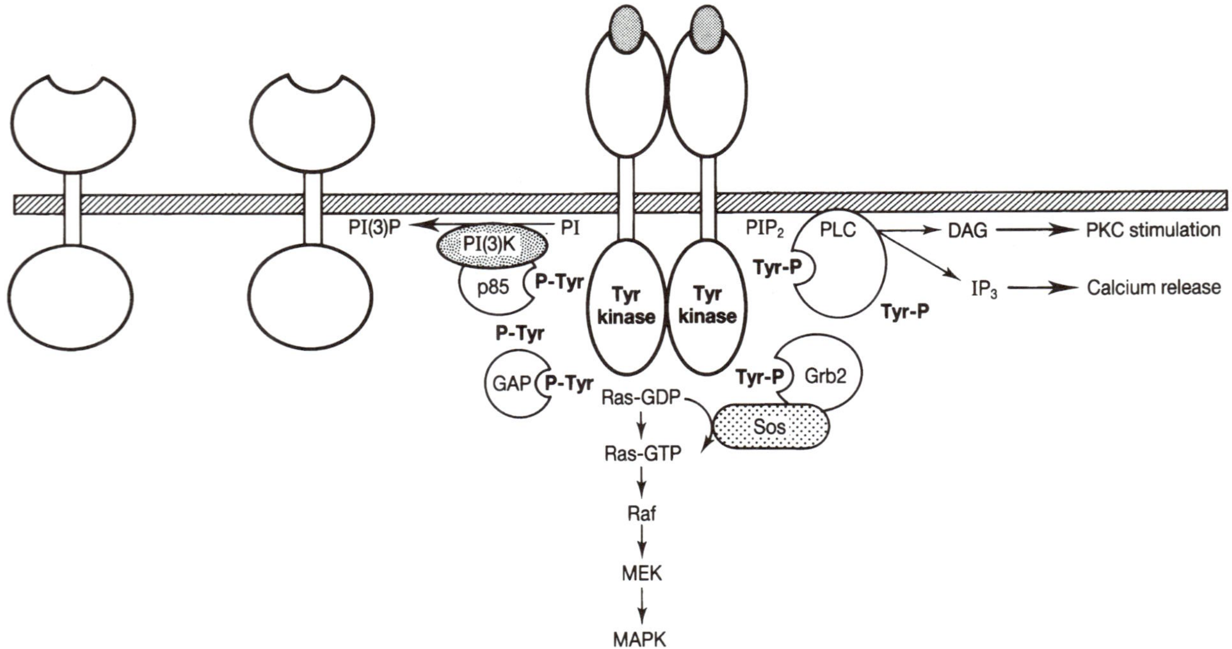

Figure 9.8. Schematic diagram of the recruitment of signal transduction molecules in response to activation of a receptor protein tyrosine kinase (TK) through ligand binding and subsequent TK stimulation and autophosphorylation (See text for further details).

GTPase-activating protein (GAP) and Grb-2 (growth factor receptor bound protein 2). Thus, the tyrosine-phosphorylated receptors are acting as a 'magnet' for enzymes whose substrates are plasma membrane-associated (Figure 9.8), and the enzymes in turn are generating more 'downstream' signalling molecules. The enzyme PI 3-kinase phosphorylates inositol lipids at the 3 position, PLCγ generates inositol trisphosphates which are signals for intracellular calcium release and diacylglycerol which is an activator of protein kinase C, GAP stimulates the GTPase activity of Ras, while Grb2 is an adaptor protein which binds to the Ras guanine-nucleotide exchange factor, Sos, which interacts with the Ras–GDP complex causing the dissociation of GDP from Ras and allowing the formation of the activated Ras–GTP complex (Panaretto, 1994; Johnson and Vaillancourt, 1994). In turn, the serine–threonine protein kinase Raf is activated by Ras–GTP, which subsequently phosphorylates and activates MEK (a threonine/tyrosine kinase), which then phosphorylates and activates another serine–threonine protein kinase termed MAPK or ERK1 (Mitogen Activated Protein Kinase or Extracellular signal Regulated Kinase).

Further cellular targets of MAPK are being established and, of course, in time, manipulation of these pathways for therapeutic benefit will occur in much the same way as the sequencing and cloning and production of recombinant growth factors for clinical use has gathered momentum.

REFERENCES

Alison, M.R. (1986) Regulation of hepatic growth. *Physiological Reviews* **66**: 499–541.

Alison, M.R. (1992) Repair and regenerative responses. In McGee, J.O.D., Isaacson, P.G., Wright, N.A. (eds) *Oxford Textbook of Pathology*, Vol. 1, pp. 365–389. Oxford: Oxford University Press.

Alison, M.R., Sarraf, C.E. (1994a) Liver cell death: patterns and mechanisms. *Gut* **35**: 577–581.

Alison, M.R., Sarraf, C.E. (1994b) The role of growth factors in gastro-intestinal cell proliferation. *Cell Biology International* **18**: 1–10.

Alison, M.R., Wright, N.A. (1979) Testosterone induced cell proliferation in the accessory sex glands of mice at various times after castration. *Cell and Tissue Kinetics* **12**: 461–475.

Alison, M.R., Wright, N.A. (1993) Growth factors and growth factor receptors. *British Journal of Hospital Medicine* **49**: 774–790.

Alison, M.R., Nasim, M.M., Anilkumar, T.V., Sarraf, C.E. (1993a) The expression of transforming growth factor α in a variety of epithelial tissues. *Cell Proliferation* **26**: 449–460.

Alison, M.R., Poulsom, R., Jeffery, R. et al. (1993b) Expression of hepatocyte growth factor mRNA during oval cell activation in the rat liver. *Journal of Pathology* **171**: 291–299.

Asahina, I., Sampath, T.K., Nishimura, I. et al. (1993) Human osteogenic protein-1 induces both chondroblastic and osteoblastic differentiation of osteoprogenitor cells derived from newborn rat calvaria. *Journal of Cell Biology* **123**: 921–933.

Barrandon, Y., Green, H. (1987) Cell migration is essential for sustained growth of keratinocyte colonies: the roles of transforming growth factor α and epidermal growth factor. *Cell* **50**: 1131–1137.

Beck, L.S., DeGuzman, L., Lee, W.P. et al. (1993) One systemic administration of transforming growth factor-β1 reverses age- or glucocorticoid-impaired wound healing. *Journal of Clinical Investigation* **92**: 2841–2849.

Burgess, A.W. (1990) Granulocyte-macrophage colony-stimulating factor. In Sporn, M.B., Roberts, A.B. (eds) *Peptide Growth Factors and Their Receptors I*, pp. 723–745. Berlin: Springer-Verlag.

Chinery, R., Poulsom, R., Rogers, L.A. et al. (1992) Localization of intestinal trefoil-factor mRNA in rat stomach and intestine by hybridization in situ. *Biochemical Journal* **285**: 5–8.

Chinery, R., Ashwood, P., Alison, M.R. et al. (1994) Healing of cryoprobe-induced ulcers in rats occurs with sequential expression of spasmolytic polypeptide (SP), intestinal trefoil factor (ITF), EGF, and TGFa mRNAs. *Journal of Pathology* **172** (suppl.): 95A.

Cohen, S. (1962) Isolation of a mouse submaxillary gland protein accelerating incisor eruption and eyelid opening in the new-born animal. *Journal of Biological Chemistry* **237**: 1555–1562.

Costello, R.T. (1993) Therapeutic use of granulocyte-macrophage colony-stimulating factor (GM-CSF). *Acta Oncologica* **32**: 403–408.

Dallman, M.F. (1985) Control of adrenocortical growth in vivo. *Endocrine Research* **10**: 213–242.

Derynck, R., Roberts, A.B., Winkler, et al. (1984) Human transforming growth factor-α: precursor structure and expression in *E. coli*. *Cell* **38**: 287–297.

De Vos, R., Desmet, V. (1992). Ultrastructural characteristics of novel epithelial cell types identified in human pathologic liver specimens with chronic ductular reaction. *American Journal of Pathology* **140**: 1441–1450.

DeLarco, J.E., Todaro, G.J. (1978). Growth factors from murine sarcoma virus-transformed cells. *Proceedings of the National Academy of Sciences, USA* **75**: 4001–4005.

Faller, B., Slingeneyer, A., Waller, M. et al. (1993) Daily subcutaneous administration of recombinant erythropoietin (rhEPO) in peritoneal dialysis patients: a european dose–response study. *Clinical Nephrology* **40**: 168–175.

Fiddes, J.C., Hebda, P.A., Hayward, P. et al. (1991) Pre-clinical wound healing studies with recombinant human basic fibroblast growth factor. *Annals of the New York Academy of Sciences* **638**: 316–328.

Focus on Growth Factors (1993) **4(1)**. London: Mediscript.

Goodlad, R.A., Wilson, T.J.G., Lenton, W. et al. (1987a) Proliferative effects of urogastrone-EGF on the intestinal epithelium. *Gut* **28** S: 37–43.

Goodlad, R.A., Wilson, T.J.G., Lenton, W. et al. (1987b). Intravenous but not intragastric urogastrone-EGF is trophic to the intestine of parenterally fed rats. *Gut* **28**: 573–582.

Goodlad, R.A., Lee, C.Y., Wright, N.A. (1992) Cell proliferation in the small intestine and colon of intravenously fed rats: effects of urogastrone-epidermal growth factor. *Cell Proliferation* **25**: 393–404.

Gospodarowicz, D., Neufeld, G., Schweigerer, L. (1987). Fibroblast growth factor: structural and biological properties. *Journal of Cellular Physiology Supplement* **5**: 15–26.

Gregory, H. (1975) Isolation and structure of urogastrone and its relationship to epidermal growth factor. *Nature* **257**: 325–327.

Grondahl-Hansen, J., Lund, L.R., Ralfkiaer, E. et al. (1988) Urokinase and tissue-type plasminogen activators in keratinocytes during wound re-epithelialization *in vivo*. *Journal of Investigative Dermatology* **90**: 790–795.

Hanby, A.M., Poulsom, R., Singh, S. et al. (1993) Spasmolytic polypeptide is a major antral peptide: spasmolytic polypeptide and pS2 in the stomach. *Gastroenterology* **105**: 1110–1116.

Harris, R.C., Meyer, T.W., Brenner, B.M. (1986) Nephron adaptation to renal injury. In Brenner, B.M., Rector, F.C. (eds) *The Kidney*, 3rd edn., pp 1553–1585. Philadelphia: W.B. Saunders.

Herron, G.S., Werb, Z., Dwyer, K., Banda, M.J. (1986a) Secretion of metalloproteinases by stimulated capillary endothelial cells. [1]. Production of procollagenase and prostromelysin exceeds expression of proteolytic activity. *Journal of Biological Chemistry* **261**: 2810–2813.

Herron, G.S., Banda, M.J., Clark, E.J., Gavrilovic, J., Werb, Z. (1986b) Secretion of metalloproteinases by stimulated capillary endothelial cells. [11]. Expression of collagenase and stromelysin activities is regulated by endogenous inhibitors. *Journal of Biological Chemistry* **261**: 2814–2818.

Hoosein, N.M., Thim, L., Jorgensen, K.H. et al. (1989) Growth stimulatory effects of pancreatic spasmolytic polypeptide on cultured colon and breast tumour cells. *FEBS Letters* **247**: 303–306.

Hughes, S.E., Hall, P.A. (1993) The fibroblast growth factor and receptor multigene families. *Journal of Pathology* **170**: 219–221.

Jelkman, W. (1992) Erythropoietin: structure, control of production, and function. *Physiological Reviews* **72**: 449–489.

Johnson, G.L., Vaillancourt, R.R. (1994) Sequential protein kinase reactions controlling cell growth and differentiation. *Current Opinion in Cell Biology* **6**: 230–238.

Johnson, G.R. (1993) Stem cell factor: a growth factor with many identities. *Cancer Topics* **9**: 106–108.

Jorgensen, K.D., Diamant, B., Jorgensen, K.H. et al. (1982a) Pancreatic spasmolytic polypeptide. III. Pharmacology of a new porcine pancreatic polypeptide with spasmolytic and gastric acid secretion inhibitory effects. *Regulatory Peptides* **3**: 231–293.

Jorgensen, K.H., Thim, L., Jacobsen, H.E. (1982b) Pancreatic spasmolytic polypeptide (PSP). I. Preparation, and initial chemical characterisation of a new polypeptide from porcine pancreas. *Regulatory Peptides* **3**: 209–219.

Kanje, M., Skottner, A., Sjoberg, J. et al. (1989) Insulin-like growth factor I (IGF-I) stimulates regeneration of the rat sciatic nerve. *Brain Research* **486**: 396–398.

Kinoshinta, T., Hirao, S., Matsumoto, K. et al. (1991) Possible endocrine control by hepatocyte growth factor of liver regeneration after partial hepatectomy. *Biochemical Biophysical Research Communications* **177**: 330–335.

Konturek, S.J., Cieszkowski, M., Jaworek, J. et al. (1984) Effects of epidermal growth factor on gastrointestinal secretions. *American Journal of Physiology* **246**: G580–G586.

Konturek, S.J., Dembinski, A., Warzecha, Z. et al. (1988) Role of epidermal growth factor in healing of chronic gastroduodenal ulcers in rats. *Gastroenterology* **94**: 1300–1307.

Levi, S., Goodlad, R.A., Lee, C.Y. et al. (1993) Effects of cell proliferation and differentiation on ulcer healing. *European Journal of Gastroenterology and Hepatology* **5** (suppl. 3): S39–S43.

McCulloch, E.A. (1993) Stem cell renewal and determination during clonal expansion in normal leukaemic haemopoiesis. *Cell Proliferation* **26**: 399–425.

Maibach, H.I., Rovee, D.T. (1972) *Epidermal Wound Healing*. Chicago: Year Book Medical Publishers.

Mars, W.M., Zarnegar, R., Michalopoulos, G.K. (1993) Activation of hepatocyte growth factor by the plasminogen activators uPA and tPA. *American Journal of Pathology* **143**: 949–958.

Masiakowski, P., Breathnach, R., Bloch, J. et al. (1982) Cloning of cDNA sequences of hormone-regulated genes from the MCF-7 human breast cancer cell line. *Nucleic Acid Research* **24**: 7895–7903.

Mead, J.E., Fausto, N. (1989) Transforming growth factor α may be a physiological regulator of liver regeneration by means of an autocrine mechanism. *Proceedings of the National Academy of Sciences, USA* **86**: 1558–1562.

Miettinen, P.J., Perheentupa, J., Otonkoski, T. et al. (1989) EGF- and TGF-alpha-like peptides in human foetal gut. *Pediatric Research* **26**: 25–30.

Montesanto, R., Matsumoto, K., Nakamura, T. et al. (1991) Identification of a fibroblast-derived epithelial morphogen as hepatocyte growth factor. *Cell* **67**: 901–908.

Moore, M.A.S. (1991) Clinical implications of positive and negative hematopoietic stem cell regulators. *Blood* **78**: 1–19.

Moscatelli, D., Rifkin, D.B. (1988) Membrane and matrix localization of proteinases: a common theme in tumor cell invasion and angiogenesis. *Biochimica et Biophysica Acta* **948**: 67–85.

Nasim, M.M., Thomas, D.M., Alison, M.R., Filipe, M.I. (1992) Transforming growth factor-alpha expression in normal gastric mucosa, intestinal metaplasia, dysplasia and gastric carcinoma – an immunohistochemical study. *Histopathology* **20**: 339–343.

Nasim, M.M., Ahnen, D., Thomas, D.M. et al. (1993) Expression of transforming growth factor α, epidermal growth factor receptor and proliferating cell nuclear antigen in gastric carcinoma: an immuno-histochemical study. *International Journal of Oncology* **2**: 191–196.

Noji, S., Tashiro, K. Koyama, E. et al. (1990) Expression of hepatocyte growth factor gene in endothelial and Kupffer cells of damaged rat livers, as revealed by *in situ* hybridisation. *Biochemical Biophysical Research Communications* **173**: 42–47.

Panaretto, B.A. (1994) Aspects of growth factor signal transduction in the cell cytoplasm. *Journal of Cell Science* **107**: 747–752.

Podolsky, D.K., Lynch-Devaney, K., Stows, J.L. et al. (1993) Identification of human intestinal trefoil factor. *Journal of Biological Chemistry* **268**: 6694–6702.

Polk, W.H., Dempsey, P.J., Russell, W.E. et al. (1992) Increased production of transforming growth factor α following acute gastric injury. *Gastroenterology* **102**: 1467–1474.

Potten, C.S., Hendry, J.H., Moore, J.V., Chwalinski, S. (1983) Cytotoxic effects in gastrointestinal epithelium (as exemplified by small intestine). In Potten, C.S., Hendry, J.H. (eds) *Cytotoxic Insult to Tissue*, pp. 105–152. Edinburgh: Churchill Livingstone.

Poulsom, R., Wright, N.A. (1993) Trefoil peptides: a newly recognised family of epithelial mucin-associated molecules. *American Journal of Physiology* **265**: G205–G213.

Price, L.T., Chen, Y., Frank, L. (1993) Epidermal growth factor increases antioxidant enzyme and surfactant system development during hypoxia and protects fetal rat lungs *in vitro* from hyperoxic toxicity. *Pediatrics Research* **34**: 577–585.

Prigent, S.A., Lemoine, N.R. (1992) The type I (EGFR-related) family of growth factor receptors and their ligands. *Progress in Growth Factor Research* **4**: 1–24.

Raines, E.W., Bowen-Pope, D.F., Ross, R. (1990) Platelet-derived growth factor. In Sporn, M.B., Roberts, A.B. (eds) *Peptide Growth Factors and Their Receptors I*, pp 173–262. Berlin: Springer-Verlag.

Ratcliffe, P.J. (1993) Molecular biology of erythropoietin. *Kidney International* **44**: 887–904.

Rechler, M.M., Nissley, S.P. (1990) Insulin-growth factors. In Sporn, M.B., Roberts, A.B. (eds) *Peptide Growth Factors and Their Receptors I*, pp 263–367. Berlin: Springer-Verlag.

Richardson, L., Zioncheck, T.F., Amento, E.P. et al. (1993) Characterization of radioiodinated recombinant human TGF-β_1 binding to bone matrix within rabbit skull defects. *Journal of Bone and Mineral Research* **8**: 1407–1414.

Roberts, A.B., Sporn, M.B. (1990) The transforming growth factor-βs. In Sporn, M.B., Roberts, A.B. (eds) *Peptide Growth Factors and Their Receptors I*, pp 419–472. Berlin: Springer-Verlag.

Ross, R., Raines, E.W., Bowen Pope, D.F. (1986) The biology of platelet-derived growth factor. *Cell* **46**: 155–169.

Ryan, R.M., Mineo-Kuhn, M.M., Kramer, C.M. et al. (1994) Growth factors alter neonatal type II alveolar epithelial cell proliferation. *American Journal of Physiology* **266**: L17–L22.

Saxena, S.K., Thompson, J.S., Sharp, J.G. (1992) Role of epidermal growth factor in intestinal regeneration. *Surgery* **11**: 318–325.

Scheving, L.A., Shiurba, R.A., Nguyen, T.D. et al. (1989) Epidermal growth factor receptor of the intestinal enterocyte. Localization to laterobasal but not brush border membrane. *Journal of Biological Chemistry* **264**: 1735–1741.

Seifert, R.A., Hart, C.E., Phillips, P.E. et al. (1989) Two different subunits associate to create isoform-specific platelet-derived growth factor receptors. *Journal of Biological Chemistry* **264**: 8771–8778.

Sell, S. (1990) Is there a liver stem cell? *Cancer Research* **50**: 3811–3815.

Sporn, M.B., Roberts, A.B. (1985) Autocrine growth factors and cancer. *Nature* **313**: 745–747.

Sporn, M.B., Roberts, A.B. (1992) Transforming growth factor-β: recent progress and new challenges. *Journal of Cell Biology* **119**: 1017–1021.

Stoker, M., Perryman, M. (1985) An epithelial scatter factor released by embryo fibroblasts. *Journal of Cell Science* **77**: 203–209.

Strain, A.J., Ismail, T., Tsubouchi, H. et al. (1991) Native and recombinant human hepatocyte growth factors are highly potent promoters of DNA synthesis in both human and rat hepatocytes. *Journal of Clinical Investigation* **87**: 1853–1857.

Suemori, S., Lynch-Devaney, K., Podolsky, D.K. (1991) Identification and characterisation of rat intestinal trefoil factor: tissue- and cell-specific member of the trefoil protein family. *Proceedings of the National Academy of Sciences, USA* **88**: 11017–11021.

Sullivan, P.B., Brueton, M., Tabara, Z.B. et al. (1991) Epidermal growth factor in necrotising enteritis. *Lancet* **338**: 53–54.

Sundberg, C., Ljungstrom, M., Lindmark, G. et al. (1993) Microvascular pericytes express platelet-derived growth factor-β receptors in human healing wounds and colorectal adenocarcinoma. *American Journal of Pathology* **143** 1377–1388.

Thim, L. (1989) A new family of growth factor-like peptides. 'Trefoil' disulphide loop structures as a common feature in breast cancer associated peptide (pS2), pancreatic spasmolytic polypeptide (PSP), and frog skin peptides (spasmolysins). *FEBS Letters* **250**: 85–90.

Thim, L., Norris, K., Norris, F. et al. (1993) Purification and characterization of the trefoil peptide human spasmolytic polypeptide (hSP) produced in yeast. *FEBS Letters* **318**: 345–352.

Thomas, D.M., Nasim, M.M., Gullick, W.J. et al. (1992) Immunoreactivity of transforming growth factor alpha in the normal adult gastrointestinal tract. *Gut* **33**: 628–631.

Thurlbeck, W.M. (1983) Postpneumonectomy compensatory lung growth. *American Review of Respiratory Diseases* **128**: 965–967.

Tomasetto, C., Rio, M., Gautier, C. et al. (1990) hSP, the domain-duplicated homolog of pS2 protein, is co-expressed with pS2 in stomach but not in breast carcinoma. *EMBO Journal* **9**: 407–414.

Tomiya, T., Tani, M., Yamada, S. et al. (1992) Serum hepatocyte growth factor levels in hepatectomized and nonhepatectomized surgical patients. *Gastroenterology* **103**: 1621–1624.

Tsubouchi, H., Hirono, S., Gohda, E. et al. (1989) Clinical significance of human hepatocyte growth factor in blood from patients with fulminant hepatic failure. *Hepatology* **9**: 875–881.

Tsubouchi, H., Kawakami, S., Hirono, S. et al. (1992) Prediction of outcome in fulminant hepatic failure by serum human hepatocyte growth factor. *Lancet* **340**: 307.

Walker-Smith, J.A., Phillips, A.D., Walford, N. et al. (1985) Intravenous epidermal growth factor/urogastrone increases small intestinal cell proliferation in congenital microvillous atrophy. *Lancet* **11**: 1239–1240.

Weller, R.O., Swash, M., McLellan, D.L. et al. (1983) *Clinical Neuropathology*. Berlin: Springer-Verlag.

Werner, S., Peters, K.G., Longaker, M.T. et al. (1992) Large induction of keratinocyte growth factor expression in the dermis during wound healing. *Proceedings of the National Academy of Sciences, USA* **89**: 6896–6900.

Wright, N.A., Alison, M.R. (1984) *The Biology of Epithelial Cell Populations*, Vols 1 and 2. Oxford: Clarendon Press.

Wright, N.A., Pike, C., Elia, G. (1990a) Induction of a novel epidermal growth factor-secreting cell lineage by mucosal ulceration in human gastrointestinal stem cells. *Nature* **343**: 82–85.

Wright, N.A., Poulsom, R., Stamp, G.W.H. et al. (1990b) Epidermal growth factor (EGF/URO) induces expression of regulatory peptides in damaged human gastrointestinal tissues. *Journal of Pathology* **162**: 279–284.

Wynford-Thomas, D., Stringer, B.M.J., Harach, H.R. et al. (1982) Goitrogen-induced thyroid growth in the rat: a quantitative morphometric study. *Journal of Endocrinology* **94**: 131–140.

Zarnegar, R., DeFrances, M.C., Kost, D.P. et al. (1991) Expression of hepatocyte growth factor mRNA in regenerating rat liver after partial hepatectomy. *Biochemical Biophysical Research Communications* **177**: 559–565.

10

Muscle Dysfunction in Critical Illness

John Coakley, Richard Ross

INTRODUCTION

Weakness during the course, of, or following, critical illness has been attributed principally to muscle wasting, due to the combination of immobility, starvation and the catabolic response to illness or injury (Lee, 1982). It has now been recognized, however, that in many cases loss of muscle mass cannot be prevented by nutritional support alone, and that nitrogen loss may be an inevitable consequence of critical illness (Elwyn, 1987). During the last decade there have been reports of myopathies and peripheral neuropathies in the critically ill and these may also cause severe weakness. The final result of muscle weakness, whatever the cause, is prolonged dependency on ventilatory support and lengthy rehabilitation.

There are many who have attributed the development of these neuromuscular disorders to adverse effects of drug therapy, but this is almost certainly an oversimplification. The more widespread use of neurophysiological studies, recently combined with histological and histochemical examination of muscle biopsy samples, has enabled investigators to characterize these abnormalities more clearly. In this chapter we will discuss the nature, incidence, aetiology, and importance of acquired neuromuscular disorders in the critically ill, and some mechanisms by which they could be ameliorated.

ACQUIRED MUSCLE DISEASE IN CRITICAL ILLNESS

It is difficult to study the isolated effects on muscle of prolonged immobility, since only the critically ill remain recumbent for any length of time. Information has mostly been obtained from other patient populations. In otherwise healthy young adults, immobilization of a fractured limb resulted in a reduction in mean muscle fibre area of approximately 40% after 6 to 7 weeks (Sargeant et al., 1977). Disuse atrophy may persist for many years, although aggressive rehabilitation physiotherapy accelerates recovery (Rutherford et al., 1990). It is not clear how relevant the former observation is to the critically ill, but clearly immobility and disuse may exacerbate any of the neuromuscular disorders acquired during intensive therapy.

Muscle wasting is universal in severe malnutrition, but there are few histological studies of the effect of starvation on muscle. Obese patients treated by starvation (400 kcal/day), were found to have type II muscle fibre atrophy. It is not clear whether the histological abnormalities accounted for the disordered muscle physiology, but it was suggested that deranged internal chemistry of the muscle was the more likely explanation (Russell et al., 1984).

The first reports of weakness complicating critical illness were in patients requiring mechanical ventilation for acute severe asthma who received high-dose intravenous steroid therapy (McFarlane and Rosenthal, 1977; Van Marle and Woods, 1980). One patient required mechanical ventilation for eight days, and received hydrocortisone in addition to muscle relaxants and sedatives. When the muscle relaxants were withdrawn there was profound, distal weakness and only a slow recovery over several months. Neurophysiological studies showed normal nerve conduction velocities, with low amplitude motor potentials suggestive of a myopathy (McFarlane and Rosenthal, 1977). A second patient required similar treatment but also received subcutaneous terbutaline. Although the clinical features were similar to the first case there was no neurophysiological evidence of a myopathy, but muscle biopsy showed a vacuolar myopathy with regenerating fibres (Van Marle and Woods, 1980). While some of these abnormalities may occur in steroid myopathy the associated elevation of creatine kinase (CK) activity was somewhat atypical, and subsequent reports have suggested that subcutaneous terbutaline treatment may lead to elevated plasma CK activities (Sykes et al., 1991). A number of cases of myopathy, perhaps related to steroids and muscle relaxants, complicating severe asthma requiring mechanical ventilation have been reported (Knox et al., 1986; Williams et al., 1988; Douglass et al., 1992; Griffin et al., 1992). Rhabdomyolysis has also been reported in two patients with status asthmaticus who received both steroids and muscle relaxants (Barrett et al. 1993).

There have been few descriptions of the histological muscle abnormalities which accompany critical illness. Three patients with peripheral vascular disease who developed acute renal failure were found to have elevated plasma CK activity. Histological examination of biopsy samples from the anterior tibial muscle revealed varying degrees of damage, and in one patient, myoglobin casts were present in the renal tubules, suggesting that rhabdomyolysis had precipitated the renal failure (Coakley et al., 1990). A further 28 cases were subsequently reported in detail (Helliwell et al., 1991). Twelve patients had atrophy of type I or II fibres in serial muscle biopsies, and more strikingly there was a necrotizing myopathy in 15 of the 31 patients. In only nine patients was muscle histology normal. At post mortem examination the renal tubules contained myoglobin in five of seven patients who died, again suggesting that there was an association between muscle damage and renal failure. This is a well recognized complication of severe muscle breakdown (Bywaters and Beall, 1941) and although usually seen in the context of severe trauma with gross muscle damage, may occur in association with sepsis (El Nahas et al., 1983) and drug overdose (Hojgaard et al., 1988; Rumpf et al., 1984).

Helliwell et al. (1991) demonstrated that severe necrotizing myopathy may be associated with sepsis, acute renal failure and a poor prognosis (mortality was about 70% in those with necrotizing myopathy) in a proportion of critically ill patients. It also highlighted the importance of histological examination of muscle biopsy specimens before drawing conclusions about biochemical abnormalities of muscle, the interpretation of which might be rendered difficult in the presence of muscle necrosis.

Recently we obtained muscle biopsies from 23 critically ill patients for histological examination. Patients were recruited prospectively on the basis of an anticipated intensive care unit stay of more than 7 days and were representative of our ITU patient population in terms of APACHE II scores and overall mortality (Coakley et al., 1993). Abnormal muscle histological features (diffuse atrophy of both muscle fibre types, type 2 fibre type atrophy, myopathy and neurogenic atrophy) were seen in all but one of the patients. In a few patients there was muscle necrosis, although in none was this as severe as that reported previously (Helliwell et al., 1991). Electron microscopy suggested that there was myofibrillar disruption and abnormalities of mitochondrial structure. Since then we have examined serial muscle biopsies and have documented progressive histological changes, consistent with a worsening myopathy (Yarwood et al., 1994).

Previously undiagnosed muscle disease may also be seen in the critical care setting, and may mimic the neuromuscular complications of severe illness leading to confusion about the cause of the weakness (Borgeat et al., 1992). There are of course other causes of acute muscle damage in the critically ill, one of the most obvious being that related to ischaemia and reperfusion injury (Adiseshiah, et al., 1992). In severe cases this may be of sufficient severity to lead to acute renal failure, and in renal failure of uncertain aetiology we recommend a search for occult rhabdomyolysis (Coakley et al., 1990).

ACQUIRED PERIPHERAL NERVOUS DISEASES IN CRITICAL ILLNESS

Four patients developed profound weakness following intensive care for sepsis and respiratory failure (Roelofs et al., 1983). The weakness was worse proximally, reflexes were decreased or absent, but there was no sensory or cranial nerve deficit. Electromyogram findings suggested denervation but motor nerve conduction velocities were essentially normal, suggesting an acute axonal neuropathy. Muscle biopsy findings included type 2 fibre atrophy and mild fibre type grouping in one biopsy. A further four patients were found to have severe generalized weakness, but no sensory loss, following episodes of severe hypotension (Rivner et al., 1983). Neurophysiological examinations suggested major neuropathic damage. At follow up 2–4 months later the clinical and neurophysiological abnormalities had improved, with complete resolution in two cases. These two papers were probably the first to describe the condition now known as critical illness neuropathy.

The majority of the work relating to this disorder has been from the University of Western Ontario (Bolton et al., 1984, 1986; Zochodne et al., 1987; Witt et al., 1991). Five patients had severe generalized flaccid weakness following a prolonged period of intensive care and were consequently difficult to wean from mechanical ventilatory support (Bolton et al., 1984). Limb reflexes were sometimes diminished. Neurophysiological study revealed a peripheral motor and sensory polyneuropathy of variable severity, characterized by normal nerve conduction velocities, with reduced compound muscle action potentials, and a variable reduction in sensory action potentials. There was spontaneous activity on needle electrode examination of the muscles. 'Critical illness neuropathy' can be differentiated from Guillain–Barre syndrome since cerebrospinal fluid protein is normal and there is no other evidence of demyelination (Bolton et al., 1986).

A patient with pancreatitis and septicaemia with an axonal neuropathy was the first case from the UK of critical illness neuropathy, in which it was suggested that the condition might be underdiagnosed (Williams et al., 1986). A summary paper from the Canadian group described a total of 19 intensive care patients who had developed weakness (Zochodne et al., 1987), 17 of whom had neurophysiological evidence of an axonal neuropathy. This was confirmed in nine cases on post mortem examination. Extensive denervation atrophy was found in all muscle groups examined.

We reported a variant of critical illness neuropathy with a predominantly motor syndrome in patients receiving mechanical ventilation for obstructive airways disease who presented with clinical features very similar to those of the critical illness neuropathy (Coakley et al., 1991). Although one of the three patients might have been suffering from critical illness neuropathy in the other cases the compound muscle action potentials were markedly reduced but with preservation of sensory action potentials. There was diffuse fibrillation in all muscles examined, suggesting neuropathic damage; the lesion appeared to be either in the distal portion of the motor neurone or at the neuromuscular junction. Nerve condition velocities were within the normal range. Muscles supplied by the cranial nerves were less affected and on repetitive stimulation in one patient there was no evidence of prolonged neuromuscular blockade. In another, administration of an anti-cholinesterase failed to improve muscle strength. The clinical and neurophysiological features eventually resolved in all patients over a period of months. More recently a series of neurophysiologically similar cases have been reported in patients with acute respiratory failure from a variety of causes (Gorson and Roper, 1993).

There have only been two prospective studies of the neuromuscular complications of intensive care in recent years. The first examined 43 patients out of a total of 1167 consecutive admissions to an intensive care unit over a 14-month period (Witt et al., 1991). Patients were recruited on the basis of proven sepsis and multiple organ failure. On clinical neurological examination 15 had signs of polyneuropathy. More detailed examination by neurophysiological studies demonstrated an axonal neuropathy in 30 (70%) of the 43 patients. In this group of patients with multiple organ dysfunction, abnormalities of the peripheral nervous system represented the fourth most common organ system failure. As would be expected in such a group of patients mortality was high with 20 of the 43 patients dying. For those who did survive, however, the prognosis for significant improvement of the neuropathy was good.

In our prospective study of patients remaining in intensive care for more than 7 days (Coakley et al., 1993) the incidence of neurophysiological abnormalities was 80%. On careful examination after discharge from intensive care surviving patients were all weak; in some weakness was extreme. In the most severe cases weaning from ventilatory support was prolonged and hospital discharge delayed by the need for rehabilitation. We have performed electrophysiological studies in 33 patients requiring intensive care for more than 7 days (Hinds et al., 1994). We found the majority of patients to have findings similar to those previously described in critical illness, that is of a predominantly axonal mixed sensory and motor neuropathy.

There was a challenging group in which compound muscle action potentials were greatly reduced, but sensory action potentials preserved. We do not believe that this group of patients, which includes those patients previously reported as having neurogenic weakness (Coakley et al., 1992) can be classified as having a conventional neuropathy since there was no evidence of sensory involvement. We would prefer to describe this syndrome as the *Critical Illness Neurological Syndrome*. Patients reported by Gorson and colleagues probably had the same syndrome. Similar neurophysiological findings have recently been described in seven patients with necrotizing myopathy who had received neuromuscular blocking drugs, although only three had evidence of prolonged neuromuscular blockade (Zochodne et al., 1994).

NEUROMUSCULAR DISORDERS

Relationship between Neurological and Muscular Abnormalities

Thus far we have been unable to find an obvious relationship between the neurophysiological abnormalities and the histological findings, although profound reductions in compound muscle action potential may be associated with histological features of denervation. This suggests that both muscle histological and neurophysiological investigations are required to define the precise nature of neuromuscular disorders in any individual patient.

Aetiology of Neuromuscular Disorders

The aetiology of these disorders remains elusive. It is tempting to ascribe some, or all, of these acquired neuromuscular abnormalities to the administration of drugs, and the frequent use of muscle relaxants has led many to incriminate the persisting effects of these agents. The first report to link muscle relaxants with weakness (Op de Coul et al., 1985) was of 12 patients who presented with weakness following mechanical ventilation facilitated by intermittent pancuronium. The clinical features were indistinguishable from the subsequent reports of critical illness neuropathy. Neurophysiological studies revealed normal nerve conduction velocities with muscle denervation and in some cases re-inervation. Muscle biopsy showed features of neurogenic atrophy, although in some there was muscle fibre necrosis. Histological examination of nerves suggested axonal involvement. Overall the clinical and laboratory features were highly suggestive of critical illness neuropathy. At the time this paper was accepted for publication this condition had not been adequately defined and the authors therefore ascribed the weakness to the use of pancuronium, perhaps exacerbated by the concomitant administration of drugs known to affect neuromuscular transmission such as the aminoglycosides or conditions which hinder pancuronium excretion such as hepatic or renal failure.

In their early reports of critical illness neuropathy Bolton's group did not describe the sedative and muscle relaxant regimens used to facilitate mechanical ventilation and in a later prospective study (Witt et al., 1991) said that there was no relationship between neuropathy and drug administration, but provided no clear details of drug administration. In other reports of critical illness neuropathy (Rivner et al., 1983; Roelofs et al., 1983; Williams et al., 1986) there was no mention of the use of neuromuscular blocking agents. However, in a study of 15 patients who developed critical illness neuropathy (Coronel et al., 1990) only six patients had received muscle relaxants. Moreover in our study (Hinds et al., 1994) one patient developed critical illness neuropathy without having received any muscle relaxants. It also seems unlikely that muscle relaxants could account for the sensory abnormalities in critical illness neuropathy or that they could precipitate axonal damage. They might, however, be implicated in the development of disuse atrophy.

Although, conventionally, critical illness neuropathy is said to be associated with sepsis and multiple organ failure this is not invariably the case. In our series both critical illness neuropathy (Coakley et al., 1993; Hinds et al., 1994) and abnormal muscle histology (Coakley et al., 1993; Yarwood et al., 1994) have been observed in the absence of sepsis and in those with only one organ failure. In their prospective study Witt et al. (1991) examined a variety of abnormalities possibly associated with the development of a neuropathy but found positive associations only with factors reflecting the severity of the illness. There was no evidence implicating muscle relaxants or steroids.

It might be argued that the purely motor lesion which we originally described as 'neurogenic weakness' in patients mechanically ventilated for obstructive airways disease could be related to the administration of muscle relaxants. In our original publication (Coakley et al., 1992) we suggested that this was unlikely since weakness and neurophysiological abnormalities persisted for many weeks, or even months, after muscle relaxants had been discontinued. In other studies (Coronel et al., 1990) neurophysiological investigations were performed at the earliest 20 days and in one case 85 days after cessation of muscle relaxants. Neurophysiologically-similar cases have been reported and importantly one of these patients had not received any muscle relaxants (Gorson and Roper, 1993). We can not, however, exclude some form of reversible damage to the motor end plate induced by prolonged neuromuscular blockade. Interestingly, pathological alterations in motor end plates at both the light microscopical and ultrastructural level in two critically ill patients have been described (Wokke and Jennekens, 1988). The authors suggested that pharmacological denervation might explain the histological abnormalities they observed. It has been suggested (Segredo et al., 1992) that prolonged, but reversible, neuromuscular blockade after long-term administration of vecuronium may be responsible for persistent paralysis in some cases. This syndrome only occurred in those with renal failure and was related to the accumulation of an active metabolite, 3-desacetylvecuronium. Although some of our patients received long-term vecuronium infusions, only one of these had renal impairment. Most of our patients with critical illness neuropathy requiring muscle relaxants had been given atracurium which has not yet been implicated in the syndrome. Moreover all the patients in our first report of neurogenic weakness were receiving β_2-agonists and it is known that intravenous salbutamol may potentiate the effect of muscle relaxants (Salib and Donati, 1993) (although the importance of this in the critically ill is unclear). Finally, the possibility that prolonged immobility, perhaps exacerbated by muscle relaxants, adversely effects the neuromuscular junction should not be discounted.

Steroid therapy can undoubtedly precipitate a myopathy characterized by proximal weakness, together with wasting, and moderately diminished reflexes. This may occur acutely, following short-term use in severe asthmatics (Knox et al., 1986) or following chronic therapy as in patients with connective tissue diseases (Askari et al., 1976). The administration of very high doses of steroids may therefore be responsible for weakness and difficulty weaning from mechanical ventilation in a few patients with obstructive airways disease. In our prospective study we could not, however, discern any relationship between steroid therapy and acquired neuromuscular disorders (Coakley et al., 1993). Some authors have suggested a link with the combined use of corticosteroids and muscle relaxants (Kupfer et al., 1987; Griffin et al., 1992; Barrett et al., 1993) although others feel that steroids alone are the likely culprit (Douglass et al., 1992). In one report (Williams et al., 1988), however, no neuromuscular blocking agents were used but there was evidence of rhabdomyolysis. The pattern of the rise and fall in plasma creatine kinase in these patients strongly suggested muscle damage occurring as early as 24 h after admission.

Importance of Neuromuscular Disorders

Acquired neuromuscular disorders are extremely common in long-stay intensive care patients and weakness can be extreme. When there is respiratory muscle involvement there will inevitably be prolonged dependence on respiratory support. This latter problem may have been underestimated in the past, and has been dismissed as unlikely to cause major difficulties in weaning from mechanical ventilation (Branthwaite, 1988). Our own experience, and that of others (Bolton et al., 1986; Witt et al., 1991) leads us to refute this suggestion. In some cases the weakness may be relatively mild, and may escape detection unless specifically looked for. Even when the weakness is noted it is often attributed to immobility and malnutrition alone. It cannot be emphasized too strongly that affected patients will recover normal neuromuscular function provided they survive the underlying illness, although both intensive care and hospital stay may be prolonged, initially due to difficulty in weaning from ventilatory support and subsequently due to immobility.

Prevention of these disorders would, therefore, shorten hospital stay and facilitate rehabilitation as well as, perhaps, reducing morbidity and mortality. This is not likely to be simple since the aetiology remains obscure and is probably multifactorial. Obviously in some cases there will be simple explanations such as prolonged immobility associated with disuse atrophy or malnutrition leading to negative nitrogen balance. There is no evidence to date that any specific group of drugs should be avoided and in particular corticosteroids, except in very high doses, appear to have no definite role in the development of neuromuscular abnormalities. Although it is understandable that many have blamed muscle relaxants it would seem that in most cases acquired neuromuscular disorders are unrelated to the use of these agents. Nevertheless we would recommend avoiding the use of muscle relaxants when possible and would suggest that in most instances atracurium is least likely to lead to difficulties. The position with prolonged infusions of vecuronium is less certain and this drug should certainly be avoided in those with renal failure in whom atracurium is the obvious choice.

The expected abnormalities of neuromuscular investigations in the various conditions which may complicate critical illness are shown in Table 10.1.

AMELIORATION OF MUSCLE WASTING

The hormonal responses (Chernow and Anderson, 1985) to critical illness probably play a role in catabolism. This has led to increasing interest in hormonal manipulation, particularly of growth hormone (GH) and insulin-like growth factor-I (IGF-I), as a means of overcoming catabolism.

Growth Hormone

Growth hormone has direct effects, such as lipolysis and insulin antagonism (Davidson, 1987), and indirect anabolic actions which are mediated by IGF-I (Isaksson et al., 1987). The availability of biosynthetic GH has stimulated interest in treatment of critically ill patients to overcome muscle wasting. Some studies have shown that supraphysiological doses of GH can promote positive nitrogen balance in certain patient groups: post-operative patients (Ward et al., 1987); those receiving parenteral nutrition (Ponting et al., 1988); patients with chronic lung disease (Suchner et al., 1990); victims of burns (Herndon et al., 1990). In patients undergoing cholecystectomy, the fall in muscle glutamine and polyribosome index and the increase in whole body nitrogen loss were all diminished by treatment with GH (Hammarquist et al., 1992). Few studies have looked at outcome measures, although a recent study in 180 patients undergoing cholecystectomy demonstrated that GH treatment reduced the infection rate and length of hospital stay (Vara-Thorbeck et al., 1993).

Critically ill septic patients appear to be more resistant to GH, either showing no response or a poor response (Dahn et al., 1988; Douglas et al., 1990; Gottardis et al., 1991; Gatzen et al., 1992;

Table 10.1 Abnormalities found in various syndromes causing weakness in critical illness

	Necrotizing myopathy	Other myopathy	CIN	CINS	GBS
Nerve conduction velocity	Normal	Normal	Normal	Normal	Reduced
CMAP	Normal	Normal	Reduced	Reduced	
SAP	Normal	Normal	Reduced	Normal	
CSF protein	Normal	Normal	Normal	Normal	Raised
Creatine kinase	Raised	Normal	Normal	Normal	Normal or raised
Reflexes	May be reduced	Normal or raised	Reduced	Reduced	Absent
Muscle biopsy	Necrosis	Variable	Variable	Atrophy	Atrophy or Necrosis
EMG	Myopathic	Myopathic	Denervation	Denervation	Denervation

CIN, critical illness; CINS, critical illness neurological syndrome; GBS, Gullain–Barre syndrome; CMAP, compound muscle action potential; SAP, sensory action potential; CSF, cerebrospinal fluid.

Voerman et al., 1992). Critically ill patients have high basal growth hormone levels with low IGF-I levels (Ross et al., 1991). It may be that there is an adaptive change in critically ill patients, with a reduction in the indirect anabolic of GH (mediated through IGF-I) and an increased direct effect leading to lipolysis and insulin antagonism. This would increase the availability of energy substrates.

Insulin-like Growth Factor-I

IGF-I is a small protein of 70 amino acids. It is structurally similar to insulin, and exhibits insulin-like effects on classical insulin target tissues. However, it also has major promoting effects on the proliferation and differentiation of cells. Growth promoting activity has been shown *in vivo* in both animals and humans (Zap and Froesch, 1986). Its metabolic effects differ from insulin, although controversy remains over which actions are mediated by the insulin or IGF-I receptor; IGF-I enhances uptake of glucose by muscle (which has abundant IGF-I receptors) but has little effect on hepatic production of glucose as the liver has few IGF-I receptors (Jacob et al., 1989).

IGF-I acts as both an endocrine and a paracrine/autocrine hormone. It is synthesized in most body tissues, including muscle. Circulating IGF-I is principally synthesized in the liver and thereafter its activity is modified by binding proteins. Six binding proteins have so far been identified, but their biological roles have not yet been clearly defined. Two important circulating binding proteins are IGFBP-3 – a large molecular weight complex that acts primarily as a carrier protein, and like IGF-I is synthesized in the liver and is GH dependent; and the smaller IGFBP-1 – apparently regulated by insulin and glucose levels. The majority of circulating IGF-I is normally protein-bound (Hardouin et al., 1989).

Like GH, IGF-I has now also been synthesized by recombinant techniques, and is thus available as a potential treatment for protein catabolism in critical illness. A number of authors have shown low circulating levels of IGF-I in critical illness (Hawker et al., 1987; Ross et al., 1991), and IGF-I production has been shown to be inhibited in sepsis (Dahn et al., 1988). IGF-I should reduce net protein breakdown and enhance hepatic muscle uptake of exogenous amino acids and glucose, thus promoting repletion of protein and glycogen. IGF-I appears to affect protein kinetics primarily by decreasing breakdown (Jacob et al., 1989) in the same way as insulin (Gelfand and Barrett, 1987). This is especially relevant, as it appears that increased whole body protein breakdown is the major cause of catabolism in patients with multiple organ failure (Arnold et al., 1993).

Intravenous administration of IGF-I briefly causes a rise in the free hormone concentration sufficient to cause hypoglycaemia through its action at the insulin receptors, but subcutaneous injection appears to minimize this problem (Froesch et al., 1990). Subcutaneous IGF-I has been given safely to patients following major gastrointestinal surgery (Miell et al., 1992). Combination therapy with GH and IGF-I has shown a potent anabolic effect in fasted man (Kupfer et al., 1993). Combination therapy has a number of theoretical advantages, maximizing the effects of GH and IGF-I on muscle and producing balanced glycaemia (Clemmons et al., 1992).

Whether the use of IGF-I becomes more widespread in the treatment of catabolism depends upon its efficacy in reducing nitrogen loss, and whether the catabolism *per se* determines length of stay or whether it is more dependent upon the neuromuscular complications independent of catabolism.

CONCLUSION

Catabolism, together with the neuromuscular complications of critical illness which occur despite optimal nutritional support, inevitably leads to prolonged intensive care and hospital stay, and thus increased morbidity and mortality. Any therapies that reverse this will benefit patients. Intensive care is expensive, and thus any treatment which may reduce the length of stay and of subsequent rehabilitation may well prove cost-effective.

ACKNOWLEDGEMENTS

We would like to thank the Joint Research Board of St Bartholomew's Hospital, the Locally Organised Research Scheme of the North East Thames Regional Health Authority, the Intensive Care Society and the Frances and Augustus Newman Foundation for funding much of our research. We also thank our colleagues on the Intensive Care Unit of St Bartholomew's Hospital at Smithfield and Homerton and collaborators in the Departments of Neurophysiology and Histopathology. We are grateful to Pharmacia for financial support of our studies.

REFERENCES

Adiseshiah, M., Round, J.M., Jones, D.A. (1992) Reperfusion injury in skeletal muscle: a prospective study in patients with acute limb ischaemia and claudicants treated by revascularization. *British Journal of Surgery* **79**: 1026–1029.

Arnold, J., Campbell, I.T., Samuels, T.A. et al. (1993) Increased whole body protein breakdown predominates over increased whole body protein synthesis in multiple organ failure. *Clinical Science* **84**: 655–661.

Askari, A.L.I., Vignos, P.J., Moskowitz, R.W. (1976) Steroid myopathy in connective tissue disease. *American Journal of Medicine* **61**: 485–492.

Barrett, S.A., Mourani, S., Villareal, C.A., Gonzales, J.M., Zimmerman, J.I. (1993) Rhabdomyolysis associated with status asthmaticus. *Critical Care Medicine* **21**: 151–153.

Bolton, C.F., Gilbert, J.J., Hahn, A.F. et al. (1984) Polyneuropathy in critically ill patients. *Journal of Neurology, Neurosurgery and Psychiatry* **47**: 1223–1231.

Bolton, C.F., Laverty, D.A., Brown, J.D. et al. (1986) Critically ill polyneuropathy: electrophysiological studies and differentiation from Guillan–Barre syndrome. *Journal of Neurology, Neurosurgery and Psychiatry* **49**: 563–573.

Borgeat, A., Pizzolato, G., Cox, J.N., Suter, P.M. (1992) Latent dystrophic myopathy revealed by unsuccessful weaning from mechanical ventilation. *Intensive Care Medicine* **18**: 427–429.

Branthwaite, M.A. (1988) Getting a patient off a ventilator. *British Journal of Diseases of the Chest* **82**: 16–22.

Bywaters, E.G.L., Beall, D., (1941) Crush injuries and renal function. *British Medical Journal* **i**: 427–432.

Chernow, B., Anderson, D.M. (1985) Endocrine responses to critical illness. *Seminars in Respiratory Medicine* **7**: 1.

Clemmons, D.R., Smith-Banks, A., Underwood, L.E. (1992) Reversal of diet-induced catabolism by infusion of recombinant insulin-like growth factor-1 on postburn hypermetabolism. *Surgery* **108**: 161–164.

Coakley, J.H., Edwards, R.H.T., McClelland, P., Bone, J.M., Helliwell, T.R. (1990) Occult skeletal muscle necrosis associated with renal failure. *British Medical Journal* **301**: 370.

Coakley, J.H., Nagendran, K., Ormerod, I.E.D., Ferguson, C.N., Hinds, C.J. (1992) Prolonged neurogenic weakness in patients receiving mechanical ventilation for acute airflow limitation. *Chest* **101**: 1413–1416.

Coakley, J.H., Nagendran, K., Honavar, M., Hinds, C.J. (1993) Preliminary observations on the neuromuscular abnormalities in patients with organ failure and sepsis. *Intensive Care Medicine* **19**: 323–328.

Coronel, B., Mercatello, A., Couturier, J.C. et al. (1990) Polyneuropathy: potential cause of difficult weaning. *Critical Care Medicine* **18**: 486–489.

Dahn, M.S., Lange, M.P., Jacobs, L.A. (1988) Insulin-like growth factor-I production is inhibited in human sepsis. *Archives of Surgery* **123**: 1409–1414.

Davidson, M.B. (1987) Effect of growth hormone on carbohydrate and lipid metabolism. *Endocrine Review* **8**: 115–130.

Douglas, R.G., Humberstone, D.A., Haystead, A., Shaw, J.H.F. (1990) Metabolic effects of recombinant human growth hormone: Isotopic studies in the postabsorptive state and during total parenteral nutrition. *British Journal of Surgery* **77**: 785–790.

Douglass, J.A., Tuxen, D.V., Horne, M. et al. (1992) Myopathy in severe asthma. *American Review of Respiratory Disorders* **146**: 517–519.

El Nahas, A.M., Farrington, K., Quyyumi, S., Sweny, P. (1983) Rhabdomyolysis and systemic infection. *British Medical Journal* **286**: 349–350.

Elwyn, D.H. (1987) Protein metabolism and requirements in critically ill patients. *Critical Care Clinics* **3**: 57–69.

Froesch, E.R., Guler, H., Schmid, C. et al. (1990) Therapeutic potential of insulin-like growth factor-I. *Trends in Endocrinology and Metabolism* **1**: 254–260.

Gatzen, C., Scheltinga, M.R., Kimbrough, T.D. et al. (1992) Growth hormone attenuates the abnormal distribution of body water in critically ill surgical patients. *Surgery* **112**: 181–187.

Gelfand, R., Barrett, E.J. (1987) Effect of physiologic hyperinsulinaemia on skeletal muscle protein synthesis and breakdown in man. *Journal of Clinical Investigation* **80**: 1–6.

Gorson, K.C., Roper, A.H. (1993) Acute respiratory failure neuropathy: A variant of critical illness polyneuropathy. *Critical Care Medicine* **21**: 267–271.

Gottardis, M., Benzer, A., Koller, W. et al. (1991) Improvement of septic syndrome after administration of recombinant human growth hormone? Journal of Trauma **31**: 81–86.

Griffin, D., Fairman, N., Coursin, D., Rawsthorne, L., Grossman, J.E. (1992) Acute myopathy during treatment of status asthmaticus with corticosteroids and steroidal muscle relaxants. *Chest* **102**: 510–514.

Hammarquist, F., Stromberg, C., Van der Decken, A. et al. (1992) Biosynthetic human growth hormone preserves both muscle protein synthesis and the decrease in muscle free glutamine, and improves whole body nitrogen economy after operation. *Annals of Surgery* **216**: 184–191.

Hardouin, S., Gourmelen, M., Noguiez, P. et al. (1989) Molecular forms of serum insulin-like growth factor (IGF) binding proteins in man: relationships with growth hormone and IGFs and physiological significance. *Journal of Clinical Endocrinology and Metabolism* **69**: 1291–1301.

Hawker, F.H., Stewart, P.M., Baxter, R.C. (1987) Relationship of somatomedin/insulin-like growth factor-I levels to conventional nutritional indices in critically ill patients. *Critical Care Medicine* **15**: 732–736.

Helliwell, T.R., Coakley, J.H., Wagenmakers, A.J. et al. (1991) Necrotising myopathy in critically ill patients. *Journal of Pathology* **164**: 307–314.

Herndon, D.N., Barrow, R.E., Kankel, K.R. et al. (1990) Effects of recombinant human growth hormone on donor site healing in severely burnt children. *Annals of Surgery* **212**: 424–429.

Hinds, C.J., Yarwood, G.D., Coakley, J.H. (1994) Acquired neuromuscular abnormalities in intensive care patients. In Vincent, J.L. (ed.) *Yearbook of Intensive Care and Emergency Medicine*, pp. 655–667. Berlin: Springer Verlag.

Hojgaard, A.D., Anderson, P.T., Moller-Petersen, J. (1988) Rhabdomyolysis and acute renal failure following an overdose of doxepin and nitrazepam. *Acta Medica Scandinavica* **223**: 79–82.

Isaksson, O.G.P., Lindahl, A., Nilssen, A. et al. (1987) Mechanism of the stimulating effect of growth hormone on longitudinal bone growth. *Endocrine Reviews* **8**: 426–438.

Jacob, R., Barrett, E., Plewe, G. et al. (1989) Acute effects of insulin-like growth factor-I on glucose and amino acid metabolism in the awake fasted rat. *Journal of Clinical Investigation* **83**: 1717–1723.

Knox, A.J., Mascie-Taylor, B.H., Muers, M.F. (1986) Acute hydrocortisone myopathy in acute severe asthma. *Thorax* **41**: 411–412.

Kupfer, Y., Okrent, D.G., Twersky, R.A., Tessler, S. (1987) Disuse atrophy in a ventilated patient with status asthmaticus receiving neuromuscular blockade. *Critical Care Medicine* **15**: 795–796.

Kupfer, S.R., Underwood, L.E., Baxter, R.C., Clemmons, D.R. (1993) Enhancement of the anagolic effects of growth hormone and insulin-like growth factor I by use of both agents simultaneously. *Journal of Clinical Investigation* **91**: 391–396.

Lee, H.A. (1982) Intravenous feeding. In Sherwood Jones, E. (ed.) *Intensive Care*, pp 1–30. Lancaster: MTP Press.

McFarlane, I.A., Rosenthal, F.D. (1977) Severe myopathy after status asthmaticus. *Lancet* **ii**: 615.

Miell, J.P., Taylor, A.M., Jones, J. et al. (1992) Administration of human recombinant insulin-like growth factor-I to patients following major gastro-intestinal surgery. *Clinical Endocrinology* **37**: 542–551.

Op de Coul, A.A.W., Lambregts, P.C.L.A., Koeman, J. et al. (1985) Neuromuscular complications in patients given Pavulon (pancuronium bromide) during artificial ventilation. *Clinical Neurology and Neurosurgery* **87**: 17–22.

Ponting, G.A., Halliday, D., Teale, J.D. et al. (1988) Post-operative positive nitrogen balance with intravenous hyponutrition and growth hormone. *Lancet* **i**: 438–440.

Rivner, M.H., Kim, S., Grenberg, M., Swift, T.R., Swift, T.R. (1983) Reversible generalised paresis following hypotension: a new neurological entity. *Neurology* **33** (suppl. 2): 164.

Roelofs, R.I., Cerra, F., Beilka, N. et al. (1983) Prolonged respiratory insufficiency due to acute motor neuropathy; a new syndrome? *Neurology* **33** (suppl. 2): 240.

Ross, R.J.M., Miell, J., Freeman, E. et al. (1991) Critically ill patients have high basal growth hormone levels with attenuated oscillatory activity associated with low levels of insulin-like growth factor-I. *Clinical Endocrinology* **35**: 47–54.

Rumpf, K.W., Wagner, H., Criee, C.-P. et al. (1984) Rhabdomyoloysis after theophylline overdose. *Lancet* **i**: 1451–1452.

Russell, D.McR., Walker, P.M., Leiter, L.A. et al. (1984) Metabolic and structural changes in skeletal muscle during hypocaloric dieting. *American Journal of Clinical Nutrition* **39**: 503–513.

Rutherford, O.M., Jones, D.A., Round, J.M. (1990) Long-lasting unilateral muscle wasting and weakness following injury and immobilisation. *Scandinavian Journal of Rehabilitation Medicine* **22**: 33–37.

Salib, Y., Donati, F. (1993) Potentiation of pancuronium and vecuronium neuromuscular blockade by intravenous salbutamol. *Canadian Journal of Anaesthesia* **30**: 50–53.

Sargeant, A.J., Davies, C.T.M., Edwards, R.H.T., Maunder, C., Young, A. (1977) Functional and structural changes after disuse. *Clinical Science and Molecular Medicine* **52**: 337–342.

Segredo, V., Caldwell, J.E., Matthay (1992) Persistent paralysis in critically ill patients after long term administration of vecuronium. *New England Journal of Medicine* **327**: 524–528.

Suchner, U., Roehkopf, M.M., Kankel, K.R. et al. (1990) Growth hormone and pulmonary disease. *Archives of Internal Medicine* **150**: 1225–1230.

Sykes, A.P., Lawson, N., Finnegan, J.A., Ayres, J.G. (1991) Creatine kinase activity in patients with brittle asthma treated with long term subcutaneous terbutaline. *Thorax* **46**: 580–583.

Van Marle, W., Woods, K.L. (1980) Acute hydrocortisone myopathy. *British Medical Journal* **281**: 271.

Vara-Thorbeck, R., Guerrero, J.A., Rosell, J., Ruiz-Requena, R., Capitán, J.M. (1993) Exogenous growth hormone: Effects on the catabolic response to surgically produced acute stress and on postoperative immune function. *World Journal of Surgery* **17**: 530–538.

Voerman, J.H., Strack van Schindel, R.J.M., Groenveld, A.B.J. et al. (1992) Effects of recombinant human growth hormone in patients with severe sepsis. *Annals of Surgery* **21**: 648–655.

Ward, H.C., Halliday, D., Sim, J.W. (1987) Protein and energy metabolism with biosynthetic human growth hormone after gastrointestinal surgery. *Annals of Surgery* **206**: 56–61.

Williams, A.C., Sturman, S., Kelsey, S., Curran, F.T., Finnegan, J.A. (1986) The neuropathy of the critically ill. *British Medical Journal* **293**: 790–791.

Williams, T.J., O'Hehir, R.E., Czarny, D., Horne, M., Bowes, G. (1988) Acute myopathy in severe acute asthma treated with intravenously administered corticosteroids. *American Review of Respiratory Disorders* **137**: 460–463.

Witt, N.J., Zochodne, D.W., Bolton, C.F. (1991) Peripheral nerve function in sepsis and multiple organ failure. *Chest* **99**: 176–184.

Wokke, J.H.J., Jennekens, G.F.I. (1988) Histological investigations of muscle atrophy and end plates in two critically ill patients with generalised weakness. *Journal of Neurological Sciences* **88**: 95–106.

Yarwood, G., Honavar, M., Hinds, C.J., Coakley, J.H. (1994) Prospective study of sequential change in muscle histology in the critically ill. *Clinical Intensive Care* **3**: 156.

Zap, F.J., Froesch, E.R. (1986) Insulin-like growth factors/somatomedins: Structure, secretion, biological actions and physiological role. *Hormonal Regulation* **24**: 121.

Zochodne, D.W., Bolton, C.F., Wells, G.A. et al. (1987) Critical illness polyneuropathy: A complication of sepsis and multiple organ failure. *Brain* **110**: 819–842.

Zochodne, D.W., Ramsay, D.A., Saly, V., Shelley, S., Moffatt, S. (1994) Acute necrotising myopathy of intensive care: Electrophysiological studies. *Muscle and Nerve* **17**: 285–292.

11

Surfactant Physiology and Therapy in Acute Lung Injury

Peter D. Macnaughton, Timothy W. Evans

INTRODUCTION

The administration of exogenous surfactant to premature infants with respiratory distress syndrome (RDS) secondary to inadequate endogenous surfactant stores is now an established therapy (Avery and Merrit, 1991). A number of prospective, randomized, controlled trials have confirmed that the tracheal instillation of a range of different surfactant preparations reduces the incidence of complications such as pneumothorax and bronchopulmonary dysplasia and mortality by around 30% (Hennes et al., 1991). Although abnormalities of surfactant function have been described in the acute respiratory distress syndrome (ARDS) in adults, their precise role in the pathophysiology of the condition is unclear. A number of case reports have suggested that surfactant therapy may be beneficial in ARDS and multicentre trials are ongoing.

HISTORY

The influence of surface tension forces on the mechanical properties of the lung was first elucidated by Von Neergaard, who demonstrated that the pressure required to inflate an excised lung was considerably less when it was filled with saline than with air (Von Neergaard, 1929). The presence of a surface tension-reducing agent maintaining alveolar patency was first suggested following the observation of the great stability of the bubbles within the fluid expressed from lungs (Pattle, 1955). The potent properties of saturated phosphatidylcholine (DPPC), which was the main component of the lipoprotein mixture obtained from lung washings was identified subsequently (Clements, 1957). When it was demonstrated that the lungs of neonates dying from RDS were deficient in surfactant, the potential for replacement therapy was envisioned (Avery and Mead, 1959). However, the failure of treatment with pure DPPC to alter outcome in RDS highlighted the important functions of the other phospholipids and proteins within the surfactant system. The subsequent development of preparations whose composition more closely reflected endogenous surfactant allowed the efficacy of this therapy in RDS to be demonstrated.

SURFACTANT STRUCTURE AND PHYSIOLOGY

Pulmonary surfactant is a complex mixture of phospholipids (85%), neutral lipids (5%) and proteins (10%) produced by the type II alveolar cells (Notter, 1989). The largest single component is DPPC which has the most potent surface tension-reducing properties. Also present is phosphatidylglycerol (DPPG) which is thought to have an important role in the formation of the DPPC monolayer at the alveolar air–water interface. There are at least three different surfactant specific proteins; SP-A, SP-B and SP-C (Weaver and Whitsett, 1988). SP-A is the most important functionally and is secreted into the alveolar space as a complex, hydrophilic, glycosylated protein of 650 kDa. It binds to DPPC promoting the formation of tubular myelin which appears to be an essential intermediate step in the construction of the DPPC monolayer. SP-A also regulates the metabolic pathways secreting surfactant into the alveolar space and its subsequent re-uptake into the type II cell. All the surfactant-specific proteins are thought to promote the adsorption and spreading of DPPC at the air–liquid interface.

DPPC is synthesized in the endoplasmic reticulum and packaged into lamellar bodies which are then exocytosed into the alveolar lumen where they unravel to form tubular myelin and loose membranous structures (Wright and Clements, 1987). These particular forms promote rapid surface adsorption of the surfactant. Once formed, the surface film becomes almost pure DPPC by preferentially extruding the other protein and lipid constituents. The formation of the surface film is thought to be a dynamic process (Figure 11.1) with continual secretion of newly synthesized surfactant which is incorporated into the monolayer with release of small vesicular structures which are then taken back into the type II cells. The validity of this model is supported by the identification of two distinct aggregate forms of alveolar surfactant (Yamada et al., 1990). Large aggregates contain tubular myelin and have good adsorption characteristics with a low

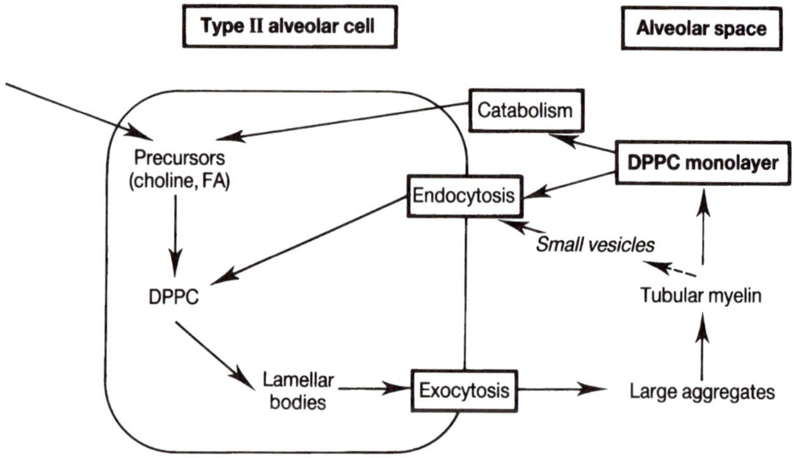

Figure 11.1. Surfactant metabolic pathways (simplified).

surface tension. The smaller vesicular structures do not adsorb well and have no surface tension-reducing properties.

At birth the air–water interface rapidly expands from an area of approximately 2 cm^2 in the pharynx to 3 m^2 within the lungs. Surfactant lines this interface and its ability to spread rapidly and reduce surface tension minimizes the forces required to inflate the lungs in these first few vital breaths. In addition, surfactant is thought to be essential in maintaining alveolar patency throughout life. The classic and most commonly accepted alveolar model dictates that surfactant maintains alveolar stability by its surface tension reducing properties. However, Laplaces law:

$$\delta P = \frac{2\sigma}{R}$$

predicts that surface tension (σ) must be lowered to negligible values due to the small alveoli radii (R) during expiration. This model has been challenged as it implies an unrealistic value of surface free energy (Bangham, 1991) and an alternative hypothesis is that the stability of the alveolus during expiration is due to the DPPC monolayer becoming a highly rigid and solid structure capable of sustaining a very high surface pressure. In a model which also plays down the surface tension-reducing properties of surfactant, the idea of a continuous air–water interface has been rejected and a 'discontinuous theory' put forward, whereby the hydrophobic surfactant pushes water to the corners of the alveoli. Surface tension forces then act to drive water out of the alveolar space, maintaining a dry airspace (Hills, 1987). Whatever the correct model, the formation of a surfactant monolayer over the alveolar surface appears to be central to its ability to prevent alveolar collapse.

Importantly, surfactant has recently been recognized as significant in host defence and immune interactions, promoting alveolar macrophage phagocytosis and bacterial killing. The surfactant protein SP-A may be the most important component interacting with macrophages. A recent study has demonstrated that SP-A binds to specific sites on *Pneumocystis carinii* (Zimmermann et al., 1992) and the observation that the synthetic non-protein containing surfactant, Exosurf, inhibits endotoxin stimulated cytokine release from human alveolar macrophages implies an anti-inflammatory function for the phospholipids (Thomassen et al., 1992). The clinical significance of these observations is presently unclear.

SURFACTANT ABNORMALITY IN ACUTE LUNG INJURY

In the first description of ARDS, the pathological similarities with the neonatal condition were recognized and it was postulated that the surface-active material lining the lungs was abnormal (Ashbaugh et al., 1967). The presence of hyaline membranes were noted and the surface tension of post mortem lung extracts was seen to be abnormally high. It is now clear that although ARDS may arise from a range of different insults, the final common pathway is an increase in alveolar capillary permeability. A number of processes may be involved in this process, including complement and leukocyte activation within the lungs, resulting in the release of oxygen-derived free radicals and various inflammatory mediators such as the interleukins and tumour necrosis factor. The damage to the alveolar capillary membrane results in high permeability pulmonary oedema. Despite the advance in our understanding of the pathophysiology underlying ARDS, mortality remains approximately 50% and current therapy remains essentially supportive (Macnaughton and Evans, 1992).

A number of studies have confirmed an associated abnormality of the surfactant system in ARDS, demonstrating an abnormal surface activity of the surfactant obtained from post mortem lung washings and possibly resulting in the abnormal pressure–volume relationship measured in intact lungs (Petty et al., 1979). Bronchoalveolar lavage (BAL) has revealed an altered phospholipid profile and a marked reduction in the surface activity in patients with ARDS (Hallman et al., 1982). Most studies have described a reduction in both DPPC and

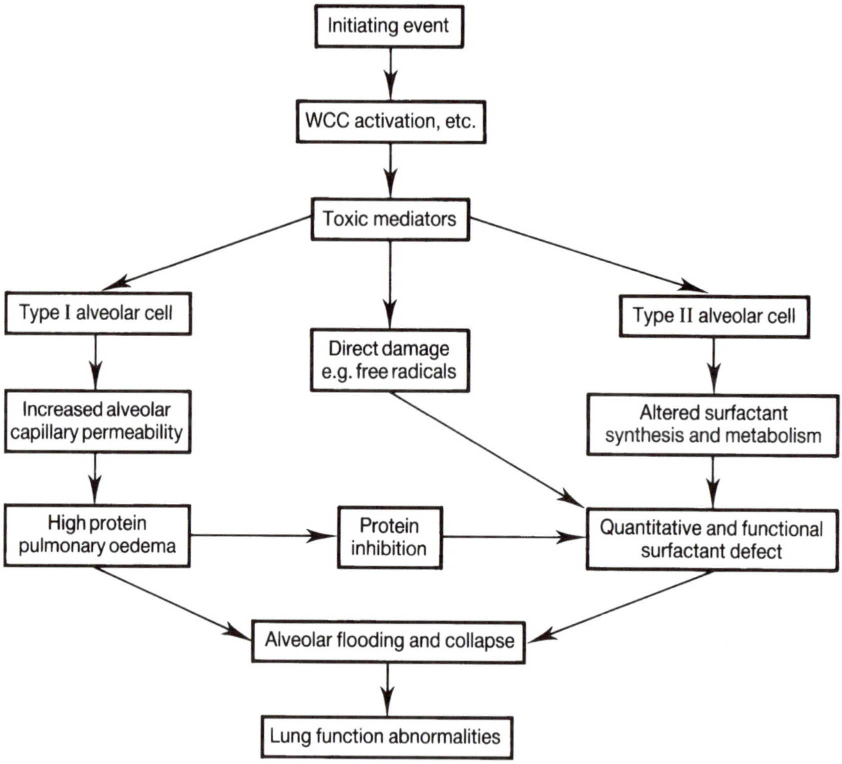

Figure 11.2. Mechanisms of surfactant dysfunction in ARDS.

DPPG associated with an increase in the amounts of non surface-active lipids such as phosphotidylinositol and sphingomyelin. In addition, a reduction in the quantity of surfactant proteins has also been described (Gregory et al., 1991). In a prospective study of patients with multiple trauma who developed ARDS, Pison et al. demonstrated that the reduction in DPPC and loss of surface activity correlated with the degree of respiratory failure (Pison et al., 1989). It is unclear whether the size of the total surfactant pool is affected in ARDS. Animal studies employing extensive lung lavage suggest that the pool size in normal adults is probably 10–15 mg lipid/g and that the effect of lung injury depends upon the response of the type II cells. Thus, exposure to 100% oxygen which is associated with cell damage causes a reduction in surfactant pool size (Holm et al., 1985) while radiation pneumonitis which causes a hyperplastic response results in an increase in pool size (Gross, 1991). Accurate quantification of pool size in patients is not possible, but analysis of BAL samples has not demonstrated a consistent reduction in the total phospholipids recoverable.

A number of mechanisms have been proposed to explain the surfactant abnormalities which have been described in ARDS (Figure 11.2). The processes which destroy the alveolar capillary barrier may also damage the type II pneumocyte and adversely affect surfactant synthesis and metabolism. A reduction in the number of surfactant-containing lamellar bodies within the type II cells has been described in patients with acute lung injury following trauma (Schlag and Redl, 1985). Animal studies also suggest that the conversion of surfactant to its active forms within the alveolar space may also be adversely affected in acute lung injury. Thus, a fivefold increase in the inactive small aggregates has been demonstrated in an animal model of acute lung injury (Lewis et al., 1990). Surfactant may be damaged directly by oxygen derived free radicals (Seeger et al., 1985a) and by phospholipase (Holm et al., 1991). A further mechanism impairing surfactant function is the inhibition exerted by the presence of plasma proteins within the alveolar space. Fibrin degradation products appear to be the most potent inhibitors with albumin having the least effect (Seeger et al., 1985b). However, the degree of inhibition will depend upon the relative concentration of surfactant and the inhibitory protein(s) and if the total active surfactant pool is reduced albumin may have a significant effect.

Although an abnormality of the surfactant system has been demonstrated in ARDS, its role in contributing to the abnormalities of pulmonary function remain unclear. ARDS is characterized by a reduction in lung volume and compliance, resulting in atelectasis and hypoxaemia secondary to an increase in shunt fraction. An impairment of surfactant function would certainly contribute to these abnormalities. It is attractive to consider that exogenous administration of surfactant could produce a significant improvement in respiratory function in ARDS. Current supportive therapy with positive pressure ventilation may expose the lungs to potentially damaging alveolar pressures and high inspired oxygen concentrations (Hickling, 1990) and the use of exogenous surfactant could prevent some of these adverse effects.

EXOGENOUS SURFACTANT PREPARATIONS

The first trials of replacement therapy in neonatal RDS revealed that pure DPPC was not effective (Chu et al., 1967) and highlighted the importance of the other phospholipid and protein components in promoting the formation of the surfactant monolayer within the lungs (Enhorning, 1977). Three sources of exogenous surfactant preparations have been developed: human, animal and synthetic (Table 11.1). Human surfactant, obtained by harvesting the amniotic fluid released during caesarean section, is highly efficacious in treating RDS (Hallman and Merrit, 1988). This material should be closest in composition to naturally-occurring lung surfactant and contains significant quantities of all three of the surfactant proteins. However, the logistical problems in obtaining adequate quantities and the theoretical risk of transmission of infections including HIV has restricted the use of this preparation.

Two methods have been employed to extract and purify animal surfactants. Calf lung surfactant extract (CLSE) is obtained by organic solvent extraction of cell free, whole lung bronchoalveolar lavage specimens. Alternatively, surfactant can be isolated by purification of a whole minced lung preparation (Curosurf, porcine) which can be supplemented by the addition of DPPC (Survanta, bovine). Both types of animal extract contain significant quantities of SP-B and SP-C but neither contains the most surface active protein, SP-A. As both human and animal surfactant preparations contain protein there is the potential risk of immunological sensitization. To date there has been no evidence of short-term adverse immunological effects in neonates who have received these preparations, although long-term effects cannot be ruled out (Merrit et al., 1988). However, the neonate is immunologically naive and the risk of immune-mediated adverse reactions may be of greater concern in adults.

Two synthetic preparations are available and consist of DPPC combined with agents to encourage surface adsorption. Artificial Lung Expanding Compound (ALEC, Britannia Pharmaceuticals, Crawley, UK) is a mixture of 70% DPPC and 30% DPPG derived from eggs which reduces mortality in RDS by approximately 30% (Ten Centre Study Group, 1987). When the mixture is applied to the airway, DPPG promotes the rapid adsorption of DPPC. It is postulated that repeated inflation–deflation cycles result in the extrusion of the DPPG component and the formation of a pure DPPC monolayer which is solid at 37°C, conferring great stability to the alveolus (Bangham et al., 1979). Exosurf (Wellcome Foundation, Crewe, UK) is a mixture of DPPC combined with hexadecanol and tyloxapol which act to encourage spreading. It has been demonstrated to be effective in RDS (Long et al., 1991) and some preliminary results suggest a beneficial effect in ARDS (Wiedmann et al., 1992).

Table 11.1 Exogenous surfactant preparations

Preparation	Source	Major constituents
Surfactant-HA	Human amniotic fluid	Phospholipids, neutral lipids and SP-A, -B and -C
CLSE	Calf lung washings	Phospholipids, neutral lipids and SP-B and -C
Survanta	Minced bovine lung extract modified with DPPC	Phospholipids, neutral lipids and SP-B and -C
Curosurf	Minced porcine lung extract	Phospholipids, neutral lipids and SP-B and -C
ALEC	Synthetic	Phosphatidylcholine (70%) and phosphatidylglycerol (30%)
Exosurf	Synthetic	Phosphatidylcholine (85%), Hexadecanol, Tyloxepol

Although the effects of overall mortality in RDS appear to be similar, the synthetic surfactants do not produce the same immediate improvement in lung function which often occurs after administration of the natural preparations (Horbar et al., 1993). This may reflect differing mechanisms of action, with the synthetic surfactants acting as a substrate stimulating endogenous surfactant synthesis. In future, the activity of synthetic surfactants may be enhanced by the addition of active proteins such as SP-A. Three separate genes for SP-A have been identified and current research is ongoing to allow the manufacture of this complex protein by biotechnology. Such a preparation would probably represent the ideal in terms of efficacy, availability, immunogenecity and risk of infection.

METHOD OF ADMINISTRATION

Surfactant can be administered either by direct installation into the lung or as an aerosol. The advantages of instillation include the ability to deliver a large quantity of surfactant rapidly with very little wastage. Aerosol delivery by nebulization is an inefficient method of drug delivery and may result in foaming and a reduction in the surface activity of the surfactant (Marks et al., 1983). Direct installation into the endotracheal tube has been employed in all the trials involving neonates and appears to be the optimal method in this patient group. Due to the greater distances involved in delivering the surfactant to the alveolar air–liquid interface, this may not be the ideal method in adults. In a recent study in adult sheep, installation of a modified bovine surfactant resulted in preferential distribution to the most injured areas, but nebulization produced the greatest improvement in lung function with the smallest amount of delivered drug (Lewis and McCaig, 1993). This apparent paradox may reflect the animal model used (whole lung lavage combined with localized acid installation) and may not be a true reflection of the heterogeneous appearance of ARDS. Both installation and nebulization have been shown to result in an improvement in lung function in ARDS and further trials are required in patients to assess the optimal method of delivery. Installation via a fibreoptic bronchoscope preceded by bronchoalveolar lavage to remove inhibitory proteins may prove to be an efficient method (Enhorning, 1989). Dry powder aerosols appear to be an efficient method of delivering bronchodilator drugs to the lungs and could be an effective method of delivering some of the synthetic surfactants (Bangham, personal communication).

The optimal dose is unknown and will depend upon the method of delivery. In neonatal practice doses of 100 mg/kg are usually employed. In the few case reports in ARDS, doses of between 50 mg/kg and 200 mg/kg have been instilled directly into the lungs. In the context of an estimated normal adult surfactant pool of between 5 and 15 mg/kg, these doses appear excessive and may reflect the effects of surfactant inhibition by proteins. The optimal timing of the treatment needs to be clarified. The reports to date have tended to be in moribund patients with severe lung injury. Exogenous therapy may be more effective if administered earlier in the natural history of the condition when the effects of alveolar capillary leak and protein inhibition may be minimized.

ANIMAL STUDIES

Surfactant therapy has been assessed in a number of animal models of acute lung injury. Repeated saline lung lavage not only produces a surfactant-deficient state but appears to cause a lung injury response which is characterized by a marked neutrophil influx, increased alveolar-capillary permeability and hyaline membrane formation. Not surprisingly, the lung injury induced by this model responds promptly to surfactant therapy (Berggren et al., 1986). Although this model may not reflect ARDS, it is useful for assessing such variables as different surfactant preparations, delivery techniques and modes of ventilation. Installation of hydrochloric acid into the lungs results in a severe lung injury which is improved by surfactant therapy (Kobayashi et al., 1988). Prolonged exposure to high concentrations of oxygen produces a free radical-mediated lung injury which has pathological similarities to ARDS. Surfactant treatment early in the course of the exposure reduces the injury (Matalon et al., 1987) but delayed therapy appears to be ineffective (Robertson, 1991). This may reflect an early surfactant abnormality due to direct free radical damage and dysfunction of type II cells which is responsive to replacement therapy. Late therapy may be ineffective secondary to protein inhibition.

Another animal model that has been the subject of studies is the lung injury that develops following subcutaneous exposure to *N*-nitroso-*N*-methylurethane (NNNMU). A progressive lung injury develops over 2–4 days which has some pathological similarities to ARDS. Surfactant abnormalities including a reduced pool of endogenous DPPC and an abnormal increase in the ratio of poorly functioning small aggregates to active large aggregates have been described (Lewis et al., 1990). Administration of either instilled or aerosolized surfactant resulted in improved lung function (Harris et al., 1989) although estimation of total pool size after therapy suggested that there was rapid metabolism or clearance of the exogenously administered surfactant (Lewis et al., 1990). Little is known of the fate of exogenously administered surfactant and more research is required.

Not all animal models of ARDS have shown favourable responses to surfactant therapy. One of the most extensively used models, intravenous oleic acid, does not appear to respond to artificial surfactant (Zelter et al., 1990) although it may have a protective effect if given before the onset of lung injury. Smoke inhalation causes a lung injury in part due to surfactant abnormalities but aerosolized artificial surfactant was ineffective in a recent study of rabbits (Feldbaum et al., 1993). The variable response to exogenous surfactant in animal models may reflect many factors such as the nature of the lung injury, its severity, the timing of therapy and the type of replacement therapy used (synthetic or natural). All these factors have important implications when considering therapy in clinical ARDS.

HUMAN STUDIES

The reported administration of surfactant to patients with ARDS has been limited to a few case studies and the preliminary results of a multicentre trial that is currently in progress (Wiedemann et al., 1992). Lachmann reported a dramatic improvement in lung function after direct tracheal installation of 300 mg/kg of a porcine surfactant in a 4 year old with sepsis induced ARDS (Lachmann, 1987). Richman and colleagues have described the response to 50 mg/kg of a similar porcine preparation (Curosurf) when delivered bronchoscopically to three patients with ARDS due to pancreatitis, aspiration and sepsis, respectively (Richman et al., 1989). There was an immediate improvement in oxygenation in all three patients but the effect lasted for less than 1 h in two of the subjects. Nosaka et al. (1990) have reported improvements in oxygenation and chest X-ray appearances in two patients who received considerably smaller doses (240 mg total) of a modified bovine preparation (surfactant-TA or survanta). In order to maintain the effect they gave repeated daily doses and were unable to demonstrate any evidence of an immunological response by antibody monitoring. Finally, bronchoalveolar lavage carried out before and after the administration of ALEC to four patients with severe ARDS resulted in no clinical improvement. PC levels 24 h later increased up to fourfold, and PG levels up to 34-fold. However, the ratio of PC to total phospholipids remained below the normal range and protein contamination was high (Haslam et al., 1994). These four different reports reveal a 50-fold range of surfactant doses. This may reflect the timing of the therapy in relation to the course of the disease. Delayed treatment in established ARDS may be ineffective unless very high doses are given, because of the effects of protein inhibition and alveolar flooding. Therapeutic formulations may also need to be modified according to the differing stages of ARDS.

The synthetic surfactant, Exosurf, is currently being assessed in a multicentre trial. Patients with sepsis-induced acute lung injury are being recruited at an early stage of their respiratory dysfunction. The surfactant is administered by a continuous aerosol and the results are being compared to a control group receiving saline. By studying less severely affected patients some of the problems of protein inhibition may be avoided. Preliminary results have suggested a 30% reduction in mortality although a significant improvement in gas exchange has not been demonstrated (Wiedemann et al., 1992). This may reflect a different mechanism of action compared to natural surfactants including stimulating endogenous synthesis or an effect on the host defence system. This trial is continuing and the results must be awaited before therapy can be recommended.

SURFACTANT AND OTHER RESPIRATORY DISEASES

Surfactant abnormalities may be important in the pathogenesis of a number of other respiratory conditions. In a study of HIV patients, BAL revealed an increase in protein:phospholipid ratio combined with a reduction in both DPPC and DPPG in those with active *Pneumocystis carinii* pneumonia (Escamilla et al., 1992). It is unclear whether these changes are the reason why this normally saprophytic organism becomes a pathogen or are secondary and underlie the severe pulmonary dysfunction commonly associated with the condition. The observation that gas exchange improves after surfactant therapy in rats with *Pneumocystis* pneumonia suggests the latter mechanism (Eijking et al., 1992). Surfactant function may be important in other types of pneumonia. Alterations in the lipid profile and a reduction in SP-A have been described in bacterial pneumonia (Baughman et al., 1993) while surfactant therapy has been reported to improve lung mechanics in mice with influenza pneumonia (Van Daal et al., 1992).

Lung transplantation appears to have adverse effects on the surfactant system where an increase in BAL protein concentration and small:large aggregate ratio occurs combined with a reduction in DPPC and SP-A concentrations (Veldhuizen et al., 1992). In a recent animal study, surfactant therapy improved gas exchange following experimental lung transplantation (Veldhuizen et al., 1993). Surfactant abnormalities may be an important cause of the pulmonary dysfunction which occurs following cardiopulmonary bypass (Macnaughton et al., 1992). Changes in the phospholipid content and surface activity have been described in BAL specimens obtained after bypass (Marcatili et al., 1990). However, a randomized, controlled study in 16 patients after cardiopulmonary bypass failed to show any improvement in lung function following the instillation of an artificial surfactant (Macnaughton and Evans, 1994). Moreover, there appeared to be a detrimental effect upon lung function which may have occurred secondary to uneven exogenous surfactant distribution.

Another area of current interest is the use of surfactant as a vehicle for drug delivery. Topical drug administration to the lungs by an aerosol may result in less than 10% of the dose reaching the airways. In addition, distribution depends upon a number of factors including particle size, breathing pattern, respiratory rate and airway calibre. The spreading ability of exogenous surfactant has the effect that its distribution is less influenced by these factors. A recent animal study has demonstrated improved distribution of pentamidine when a surfactant preparation (survanta) was used as a vehicle (Kharasch et al., 1991).

SUMMARY

The place of surfactant therapy in ARDS has not yet been established. Animal studies and some clinical reports suggest that there may be a role for this therapy although the results of prospective, randomized, controlled trials must be awaited. The data that are available suggest that single-dose therapy in those with established ARDS is unlikely to be of significant benefit due to the inhibitory effects of protein contamination of the alveolar compartment. Most benefit may occur when given early in the course of lung injury although, to avoid unnecessary treatment, better methods of predicting the course of lung injury are required. ARDS represents an arbitrary grouping together of a number of different conditions with the same clinical presentation. It is likely that the response to therapy will depend upon the underlying cause of lung injury. Thus, conditions which cause primary lung damage including acid aspiration, smoke inhalation, near drowning and pneumonia may be the most responsive to therapy. Many other questions remain to be answered. What is the optimal surfactant preparation: artificial or natural? Should it be delivered by instillation or as an aerosol? At what dose and how often? Finally, if this therapy is shown to be effective there will be significant financial implications. At current costs, the equivalent dose for a 1 kg neonate given to an adult would cost over £20 000.

REFERENCES

Ashbaugh, D.G., Bigelow, D.B., Petty, T.L., Levine, B.E. (1967) Acute respiratory distress in adults. *Lancet* **ii**: 319–323.

Avery, M.E., Mead, J. (1959) Surface properties in relation to atelectasis and hyaline membrane disease. *American Journal of Diseases of Children* **97**: 517–523.

Avery, M.E., Merritt, T.A. (1991) Surfactant replacement therapy. *New England Journal of Medicine* **324**: 910–911.

Bangham, A.D. (1991) Pattle's bubbles and Von Neergaard's lung. *Medical Science Research* **19**: 795–799.

Bangham, A.D., Morley, C.J., Phillips, M.C. (1979) The physical properties of an effective lung surfactant. *Biochimica et Biophysica Acta* **573**: 552–556.

Baughman, R.P., Sternberg, R.T., Hull, W. et al. (1993) Decreased surfactant protein A in patients with bacterial pneumonia. *American Review of Respiratory Diseases* **147**: 653–657.

Berggren, P., Lachmann, B., Curstedt, T. et al. (1986) Gas exchange and lung morphology after surfactant in experimental adult respiratory distress syndrome induced by repeated lung lavage. *Acta Anaesthesiologica Scandinavica* **30**: 321–328.

Chu, J., Clements, J.A., Cotton, E.K. et al. (1967) Neonatal pulmonary ischaemia: Clinical and physiological studies. *Paediatrics* **40**: 709–782.

Clemments, J.A. (1957) Surface tension of lung extracts. *Proceedings Experimental Biology and Medicine* **93**: 170–172.

Eijking, E.P., van Daal, G.J., Tenbrinck, R. et al. (1992) Improvement in pulmonary gas exchange after surfactant replacement in rats with *Pneumocystis carnii* pneumonia. *Advances in Experimental Medicine and Biology* **316**: 293–298.

Enhorning, G. (1977) Pulsating bubble technique for evaluating pulmonary surfactant. *Journal of Applied Physiology* **43**: 198–203.

Enhorning, G. (1989) Surfactant replacement in adult respiratory distress syndrome. *American Review of Respiratory Disease* **140**: 281–283.

Escamilla, R., Prevost, M.C., Hermant, C. et al. (1992) Surfactant analysis during *Pneumocystis carnii* pneumonia in HIV infected patients. *Chest* **101**: 1558–1562.

Feldbaum, D.M., Wormorth, D., Nieman, G.F. et al. (1993) Exosurf treatment following wood smoke inhalation. *Burns* **19**: 396–400.

Gregory, T., Longmore, W., Moxley, C. et al. (1991) Surfactant chemical composition and biophysical activity in acute respiratory distress syndrome. *Journal of Clinical Investigation* **65**: 1976–1981.

Gross, N. (1991) Altered surfactant subtypes in an experimental form of ARDS: radiation pneumonitis. *American Journal of Physiology* **260**: L302–310.

Hallman, M., Merritt, T.A. (1988) Human amniotic fluid surfactant: clinical trial experiences. In Shapiro, D.L., Notter, R.H. (eds) *Surfactant Replacement Therapy*, pp. 235–256. New York: Alan R. Liss.

Hallman, M., Spragg, R., Harrell, J.H. et al. (1982) Evidence of lung surfactant abnormality in respiratory failure. Study of bronchoalveolar lavage phospholipids, surface activity, phospholipase activity and plasma myoinositol. *Journal of Clinical Investigation* **70**: 673–683.

Harris, J.D., Jackson, F., Moxley, A.A., Longmore, W.J. (1989) Effect of exogenous surfactant instillation on experimental lung injury. *Journal of Applied Physiology* **66**: 1846–1851.

Haslam, P.L., Hughes, D.A., Macnaughton, P.D., Baker, C.S., Evans, T.W. (1994) Surfactant replacement therapy in ARDS. *Lancet* **343**: 1009–1011.

Hennes, H.M., Lee, M.B., Rimm, A.A. et al. (1991) Surfactant replacement therapy in respiratory distress syndrome: meta-analysis of clinical trials of single dose surfactant extracts. *American Journal of Diseases of Children* **145**: 102–104.

Hickling, K.G. (1990) Ventilatory management of ARDS: can it affect outcome? *Intensive Care Medicine* **16**: 219–226.

Hills, B.A. (1987) Bursting the alveolar bubble. *Anaesthesia* **42**: 467–469.

Holm, B.A., Notter, R., Siegle, J. et al. (1985) Pulmonary physiological and surfactant changes during injury and recovery from hyperoxia. *Journal of Applied Physiology* **59**: 1402–1409.

Holm, B.A., Keicher, L., Lui, M. et al. (1991) Inhibition of pulmonary surfactant function by phospholipases. *Journal of Applied Physiology* **71**: 317–321.

Horbar, J.D., Wright, L.L., Soll, R.F. et al. (1993) A multicentre randomized trial comparing two surfactants for the treatment of neonatal respiratory distress syndrome. *Journal of Paediatrics* **123**: 757–766.

Kharasch, V.S., Sweeney, T.D., Fredberg, J. et al. (1991) Pulmonary surfactant as a vehicle for intratracheal delivery of technetium sulfur colloid and pentamidine in hamster lungs. *American Review of Respiratory Diseases* **144**: 909–913.

Kobayashi, T., Ganzuka, M., Ueda, T. et al. (1988) Surfactant replacement in respiratory failure induced by aspiration of hydrochloric acid in rabbits. In Lachmann, B. (ed.) *Surfactant Replacement in Neonatal and Adult Respiratory Distress Syndrome* 245–257. Berlin: Springer Verlag.

Lachmann, B. (1987) The role of pulmonary surfactant in the pathogenesis and therapy of ARDS. In Vincent, J.L. (ed.) *Update in Intensive Care and Emergency Medicine* 123–124. Berlin: Springer Verlag.

Lewis, J.F., McCaig, L. (1993) Aerosolised versus instilled exogenous surfactant in a nonuniform pattern of lung injury. *American Review of Respiratory Diseases* **148**: 1187–1193.

Lewis, J.F., Ikegami, M., Jobe, A.H. (1990) Altered surfactant function and metabolism in rabbits with acute lung injury. *Journal of Applied Physiology* **69**: 2303–2310.

Long, W., Thompson, T., Sundell, H. et al. (1991) Effects of two rescue doses of a synthetic surfactant on mortality rate and survival without bronchpulmonary dysplasia in 700 to 1350 gram infants with respiratory distress syndrome. American Neonatal Study Group I. *Journal of Paediatrics* **118**: 595–605.

Macnaughton, P.D., Evans, T.W. (1992) Management of adult respiratory distress syndrome. *Lancet* **339**: 469–472.

Macnaughton, P.D., Evans, T.W. (1994) Artificial surfactant therapy after cardiopulmonary bypass. *Chest* **105**: 421–425.

Macnaughton, P.D., Braude, S., Hunter, D.N., Denison, D.M., Evans, T.W. (1992) Changes in lung function and pulmonary capillary permeability after cardiopulmonary bypass. *Critical Care Medicine* **20**: 1289–1294.

Matalon, S., Holm, B.A., Loewen, G.M. et al. (1987) Mitigation of hyperoxic injury by administration of exogenous surfactant. *Journal of Applied Physiology* **62**: 756–761.

Marcatili, S., Guarino, C., Giannattasio, A. et al. (1990) Alterations in endo-alveolar surfactant after surgery with extracorporeal circulation. *Respiration* **57**: 233–238.

Marks, L.B., Notter, R.H., Oberdorster, G. et al. (1983) Ultrasonic and jet aerosolization of phospholipids and the effects on surface activity. *Paediatric Research* **17**: 742–747.

Merrit, T.A., Strayer, D.S., Hallman, M. et al. (1988) Immunologic considerations regarding exogenous surfactants. In Shapiro, D.L., Notter, R.H. (eds) *Surfactant Replacement Therapy*, pp. 145–162. New York: Alan R. Liss.

Nosaka, S., Sakai, T., Yonekura, M. et al. (1990) Surfactant for adults with respiratory failure. *Lancet* **336**: 947–948.

Notter, R.H. (1989) Physical chemistry and physiological activity of pulmonary surfactants. In Shapiro, D.L., Notter, R.H. (eds) *Surfactant Replacement Therapy* 19–70. New York: Allen R. Liss.

Pattle, R.E. (1955) Properties, function and origin of the alveolar lining layer. *Nature* **175**: 1125–1126.

Petty, T.L., Silvers, G.W., Paul, G.W. et al. (1979) Abnormalities in lung elastic properties and surfactant function in adult respiratory distress syndrome. *Chest* **75**: 571–574.

Pison, U., Seeger, W., Buchhorn, R. et al. (1989) Surfactant abnormalities in patients with respiratory failure after multiple trauma. *American Review of Respiratory Diseases* **140**: 1033–1039.

Richman, P.S., Spragg, R.G., Robertson, B. et al. (1989) The adult respiratory distress syndrome: first trials with surfactant replacement. *European Respiratory Journal* **2**: 109s–111s.

Robertson, B. (1991) Surfactant inactivation and surfactant replacement in experimental models of ARDS. *Acta Anaesthesiologica Scandinavica* **35** (suppl. 95): 22–28.

Schlag, G., Redl, H.R. (1985) Morphology of the human lung after traumatic injury. In Zapol, W.M., Falke, K.J. (eds) *Lung Biology in Health and Disease, Vol. 24: Acute Respiratory Failure*, pp. 161–183. New York: Marcel Dekker.

Seeger, W., Lepper, H., Wolf, H.R.D. et al. (1985a) Alteration of alveolar surfactant function after exposure to oxidative stress and to oxygenated and native arachidonic acid in vitro. *Biochimica et Biophysica Acta* **835**: 58–67.

Seeger, W., Stohr, G., Wolf, H.R.D. et al. (1985b) Alteration of surfactant function due to protein leakage: special interaction with fibrin monomer. *Journal of Applied Physiology* **58**: 326–338.

Ten Centre Study Group. (1987) Ten centre trial of artificial surfactant (artificial lung expanding compound) in very premature babies. *British Medical Journal* **294**: 991–996.

Thomassen, M.J., Meeker, D., Antal, J.M. et al. (1992) Synthetic surfactant (Exosurf) inhibits endotoxin stimulated cytokine secretion by human alveolar macrophages *American Journal of Respiratory Cell and Molecular Biology* **7**: 257–260.

Van Daal, G.J., Bos, J.A., Eijking, E.P. et al. (1992) Surfactant replacement therapy improves pulmonary mechanics in end stage influenza A pneumonia in mice. *American Review of Respiratory Disease* **145**: 859–863.

Veldhuizen, R.A., Lee, J., Sandler, D. et al. (1992) Alterations in pulmonary surfactant composition and activity after experimental lung transplantation. *American Review of Respiratory Diseases* **148**: 208–215.

Veldhuizen, R., Mcdougall, K., Lewis, J., Novik, R., Possamayer, F. (1993) Surfactant supplementation in experimental lung transplantation. *American Review of Respiratory Disease* **147**: A261.

von Neergaard, K. (1929) Neue Auffasungen uber einen Grundbegriff der Atemmechanik die Retraktionskraft der Lunge, abhangig von der Oberflachenspannung in den Alveolen. Z, ges. exp. Med. **66**: 373–394. (Translated version: Arnold R., Hahn, H. (1976) The retractile force of the lungs, dependent on the surface tension in the alveoli. In Comroe, J.H. (ed.) *Pulmonary and Respiratory Physiology, Part 1*, pp. 214–234. Stroudsburg: Dowden, Hutchinson and Ross.)

Weaver, T.E., Whitsett, A.J. (1988) Structure and function of pulmonary surfactant proteins. *Seminars in Perinatology* **12**: 213–220.

Wiedemann, H., Baughmann, R., deBoisblanc, B. et al. (1992) A multicenter trial in human sepsis-induced ARDS of an aerosolized synthetic surfactant (Exosurf). *American Review of Respiratory Diseases* **145**: A184.

Wright, J.R., Clements, J.A. (1987) Metabolism and turnover of lung surfactant. *American Review of Respiratory Diseases* **135**: 426–444.

Yamada, T., Ikegami, M., Jobe, A.H. (1990) Effects of surfactant subfractions on preterm rabbit lung function. *Pediatric Research* **27**: 592–598.

Zelter, M., Escudier, B.J., Hoeffel, J.M., Murray, J.F. (1990) Effects of aerosolized artificial surfactant on repeated oleic acid injury in sheep. *American Review of Respiratory Diseases* **141**: 1014–1019.

Zimmerman, P.E., Voelker, D.R., McCormack, F.X. et al. (1992) 120-kD surface glycoprotein of pneumocystis carnii is a ligand for surfactant protein A. *Journal of Clinical Investigation* **89**: 143–149.

Index

Note: page numbers for illustrations and tables are in *italics*

Abruptio placentae, *58*, 59
Abscess drainage, 145
Academic Emergency Medicine, Society for, 15
'Accelerated starvation', 57
Acetaminophen, 94
Acetone, 86
2-Acetylaminofluorene, 225
Acetylcholine, 49–50, *49*
N-Acetylcysteine, *193*, 198
Acidosis
  nutrition, 145
  poisoning, 84
  pregnancy and childbirth, 68, 70, 72
  prehospital care, 27–8
Acids, 95, 268
Acinar cells, 213
Acral paraesthesiae, 60
Activated charcoal *see* Charcoal
Active Compression-Decompression (ACD), 24–5
Activins, *216*, 222
Acute fatty liver of pregnancy (AFLP), 69–72
Acute myocardial infarction (AMI), 31
Acute respiratory failure, 194
Acute respiratory distress syndrome (ARDS)
  antioxidant therapy, 175, 176, 188–9, 190, 194–5, 197, 198
  pregnancy, 68
  pulmonary vascular dysfunction, 41, 43–8, *42–3*, *45*
  surfactant, 256, 259–68
Adenosine, 30, 183, 196
Adenosine diphosphate, 176
Adenosine triphosphate, 180, *181*
Adipose tissue, 128, 129, 137
Adrenal gland, healing, 213
Adrenaline, 3, 24, 25, 26–7, 28
β-Adrenergic antagonists, 84, 96
Adult respiratory distress syndrome (ARDS) *see* Acute respiratory distress syndrome
Advanced cardiac life support (ACLS), 25, 26, 28, 31, 32
Advance directives, 113, 115–6
Advanced life support interventions, 2–6, 7, 8, 9, 10, 11
Advocacy, EMS, 16
Aerosols, surfactant, 263–4, 265, 266, 267, 268
Age, 113
Agitation, *87*
β_2-Agonists, 245
Air ambulance, 10
Air embolism, 66
Airway management, EMS, 8, 10, 15, 21–4
Alanine, 146, 162
Albumin
  antioxidant therapy, 186, 191, *192*, 197
  nutritional support, 147, *148*, 155
  pregnancy and childbirth, 70
  surfactants, 261
Alcohol, 72, 95, 212
Aldehydes, 179, 183, 188
Alkalosis, 27–8
Alkoxyl radical (RO), *177*, 184, 186, *187*
Allopurinol, *192*, 195–6
Alloxan, 186
ALT, 70
American Association of Poison Control Centers (AAPCC), 82

American Board of Emergency Medicine, 15
American Heart Association, 12, 21
Amino acids, 144, 146, 154, 151, *167*, 184
N-Amino-L-arginine, 196
Aminoglycosides, 243
21-Aminosteroids, 191
Amniotic fluid embolism (AFE), 65–9
Amphetamines, 86, *87*
Amphiregulin, 215, *216*, 217
Anabolic hormonal milieu, 146
Anaemia, 59, 228
Anaesthetics, 196
Analeptic agents, 84
Androgens, 213–4
Angiogenesis, 206, 210, 211, 221
Anoxia, 180
Anthropometric indices, 134–5, *135*
Antibiotics, 75, 145, *192*
Anticatalytic protection, 184, 185
Anticholinergic agents, 84, 85, 86, *87*
Anti-cholinesterase, 242
Anticonvulsants, pregnancy, 63–4, 65
Antidysrhythmic agents, 84
Antiemetics, 95, 118
Anti-endotoxin HA–1A, 102
Antihistamines, 84, *87*
Antioxidant therapy, 175–6, 190–8, *192–3*
  endogenous protection from free radicals and activated forms of oxygen, 184–6
  free radicals and activated oxygen species, 176- 80, *177*
    intensive care medicine, 186–90, *187*
  in vivo effects of free radicals and activated forms of oxygen, 183–4
  nutritional support, 144, 152, 169, *169*
  source of free radicals and activated forms of oxygen *in vivo*, 180–3, *181–2*
Anti-PAF, *193*
Antiproteinase, 184
Anti-receptors, *193*
APACHE (Audit scoring systems), 105–6, 107, 240
ARDS *see* Acute respiratory distress syndrome
Arginine, 144, 151, 154, 159–60, 169, *169*, 183
Arrhythmias, 30, 31
Arsenic, 84, 86
Arthralgia, *168*
Artificial Lung Expanding Compound (ALEC), 262, *263*
Ascorbic acid, 152, *169*, 178, 185, 186, *192*, 194–5
Aspiration, 22–3, 57, 91, 92, 266
  pneumonia, 66, 91
Aspirin, 46, 212
Assessment, nutrition, 147, *148*–9
AST, 70
Asthma, muscle dysfunction, 239, 245
Atelectasis, 261
Atenolol, 63
ATLS, 31, 32
ATP (adenosine triphosphate), 180, *181*
Atracurium, 244, 247
Atropine, 86, *87*
Autocrine secretion, 215, 249
Autonomy, 106, 111–2, 119
Autophosphorylation, 221, 229
Axonal neuropathy, 241–2, 244
Azotaemia, 147, 151

Bacterial pneumonia, 47
Barbiturates, 28, 84, 85, *87*
Basal energy expenditure (BEE), 147, 149
Bases, 95
Basic life support (BLS) provides, 4, 8, 9, 10
Belladonna, *87*
Beneficence, 119
Benzodiazepines, *87*, 118
β-Adrenergic antagonists, 84, 96
β_2-Agonists, 245
Beta stimulant tocolysis, 72–4, 75
Beta sympathomimetic agents, 72–4
Bicarbonate, 27
Bilirubin, pregnancy, 59, 70
Biochemical monitoring, *148*, 152–3
Bioimpedance analysis, 125, 133–4
Bland, Tony, 114

Bleomycin, 214
Blood pressure control, pregnancy, 62–3
Blood volume, pregnancy, 55, *56*
BMP (Bone morphogenetic proteins), *216*, 222, 223
Body cell mass, 129–30
Body composition, 125–6, *126*
  anthropometric indices, 134–5, *135*
  body composition models, 135–7, *136*
  bioimpedance methods, 133–4
  computed tomography, 128–9
  dilution methods, 130–3, *132*
  dual-energy X-ray absorptiometry, 127–8
  magnetic resonance imaging, 129
  neutron activation analysis (NAA), 126–7
  whole body counting, 129–30
Body mass, 134–5
Body volume, 134
Body weight, 134–5, *148*
Bombesin, 215
Bone, 126, 127–8, 137
Bone marrow transplantation (BMT), 109, 116, 156–7, *157*, 207
Bone morphogenetic proteins (BMPs), *216*, 222, 223
Bovine, surfactants, 262
Bowel irrigation, 90
Bradycardia, 84, *87*
Bradypnoea, 85
Bromide dilution, 133
Bronchoalveolar lavage (BAL)
  antioxidants, 188, 189
  surfactants, 259, 261, 262, 264, 266, 267
Bronchodilators, 264
Bronchopulmonary dysplasia, 256
Bronchoscope, 264
Buffer therapy, 27–8
Burn injury, 147, 149, 161
'Burn-out', 16
Burns, 84, 152, 161–5, *163–4*, *167*, 168, 175, 247

Caffeine, 84, *87*
Calcium
  antioxidant therapy, 180, 196
  body composition, 126
  EMS, 28, 30
  growth factors, 206, 231
  nutritional support, *148*, 161, 162, *164*,
  poisoning and overdose, 84, 96, 97
Calf lung surfactant extract (CLSE), 262, *263*
Calorimetry, 149, *149*
Camphor, 85
Cancer, 107, 206
Capnometry, 24, 25
Carbamate pesticides, *87*
Carbicarb, 28
Carbohydrates, 149, 159
Carbon, 126, 136
Carbon dioxide, 24, 130, 147, 149
Carbon monoxide, 85
Carbon tetrachloride, 213
Carcinogens, 184
Cardiac arrest, EMS, 7
Cardiac ischaemia *see* Ischaemia
Cardiac muscle cells, 207
Cardiac output, pregnancy, 55, 56, *56*
Cardiac surgery, 190
Cardiomegaly, 75
Cardiopulmonary bypass, 189, 195, 267
Cardiopulmonary resuscitation
  EMS, 2, 3–4, 5, 10, 12, 24–8
    open chest, 25–6
  pregnancy and childbirth, 57
  treatment limitation decisions, 104–5, 107, 112
Carpel tunnel syndrome, *168*
Cartilage, 137
Catabolic stress, 146, 147, 152, 156
Catalase, 185, 188, *193*, 197
Catalytic protection, radicals, 184, 185–6, 191, *192*, 194–5, 198
Catecholamaines, 145
Cathartics, 95–6
Caustic agents, 91, 95
Cefatzidime, *192*, 194, 195
Cell migration, 209
Cell proliferation, 209
Centoxin, 102
Central nervous system, 207, 214
Cephaeline, 91
Cerebral haemorrhage, *58*, 60, 62

Cerebral ischaemia, 191
Cerebral oedema, *58*, 62
Cerebral resuscitation, 28
Cervical spine, EMS, 22
Charcoal, 90, 91, 92, 93, 94–6, 97
Chemical model, body composition, 136
Chemical signalling, 214–5
Chemoattractant, 221
Chemotherapy, 207, 212, 228
Childbirth *see* Pregnancy
Children, 4, 22, 23, 27, 83
Chloral hydrate, *87*
Chloramines, 178, 185
Chlorine, 126, 136
Chlormethiazole, 64
Cholecystectomy, 161, 247
Cholecystokinin, 154
Cholestasis, 154
Cholinergic agents, 84, 86, *87*
Chondrocytes, 208
Chorioamnionitis, 73
Chronic lung disease, 47, 247
Circulatory shock, 41
Clara cells, 214
Clonazepam, 64
Clonidine, 86
Coagulation, 70, 175, 223
Coagulopathy, *58*, 62, 68, 69, 71–2, 75
Cocaine, 84, 85, 86, *87*, 96, 97
Coeliac disease, 219
Coenzyme Q10, 194
Colchicine, 86, 92
Collagen, 137, 210, 211, *222*
Collagenase, 210, 211
Colloid oncotic pressure, pregnancy, 55, 58
Colloid osmotic pressure, 75
Colony stimulating factors (CSFs), 206, 207, 227–8
Coma, 30, *87*
Combitube, 15, 22, 23
Communicable disease, EMS, 16
Complement, 175, 259
Computed tomography, 59–60, 65, 128–9, 137
Computers, EMS, 5, 9
Confused patients, 83, 113
Congestive heart failure, 1
Connective tissue, 208, 209, 211, 212, 245
Consciousness, poisoning, 85
Consensus, 113–4
Consent, 11–12
Convalescence, 145
Copper (II) 3,5 diisopropylsalicylic acid (CuDIPS), 197
Cor pulmonale, 67
Corneal injuries, 220
Coronary artery spasm, pregnancy, 68
Coronary disease, 1
Cortical blindness, *58*
Corticosteroids, 246
Cortisol, 145
Costs
  EMS, 2, 4, 6, 12, 16, 31–2
  nutritional support, 154
  surfactant, 268
  treatment limitation decisions, 102–4, 105, 106, 107, 108, 110
CPR *see* Cardiopulmonary resuscitation
Cranial nerves, poisoning, 85–6
Creatine kinase, 239, 246, *248*
Cripto, 215, *216*
Critical Illness Neurological Syndrome, 243, *248*
Critical illness neuropathy, 241–2, 244–5
Crohn's disease, 219, 227
Crypt cell, 212–3, 219
Culture, 111, 113
Curosurf, 262, *263*, 266
Cutaneous examination, poisoning, 86
Cutaneous injuries, 220
Cyanide, 85
Cyanosis, 86
Cyclo-oxygenase, 183, *192*, 196
  inhibitors, 46–7, 48, 50
Cysteine, 186
Cytochrome oxidase, 177, 180–1, *181*
Cytochrome P–450, 183
Cytokines
  antioxidant therapy, 175, 187
  growth factors, 214, 228
  nutritional support, 145
  pregnancy and childbirth, 74
  surfactant, 259

Cytomegalovirus, 109
Cytopathic virus, 213

D50W, 88, 89, 90
Dazoxiben, 45
Death, 118–9
Defecation, 86, *87*
Defibrillation, 2, 3, 4, 5, 8, 10, 11, 15, 28
Dehydroascorbate, 186
Delayed gamma activation, 126
Delirium, *87*
Demyelination, 241
Denervation, 241, 242, 243, 244
Deoxyribose, 184
Dermis, 137, 210
3-Desacetylvecuronium, 245
Desferrioxamine, *192*, 195
Desoxyhaemoglobin, 182
Deuterium labelling, 130
Dextrose
  nutritional support, 149–50, 151, 152, 153, 154, *155*
  poisoning and overdose, 88, 89, 90
Diabetes, 1, 88, 89, 102, 116
Diacylglycerol, 231
Diaphoresis, 86, *87*, 89
Diazepam, 64, 118
Diazoxide, 62, 63
Dienes, 188
Digoxin, 84, 86, 95
Dilution methods, 130–3, 136
Dimerization, 229
Dimethylsulfoxide (DMSO), 191, *192*
Dimethylthiourea, 191, *192*
Dinitrophenol, 85
Dipeptides, 169
Diphenhydramine, 86
Diphenoxylate, *87*
Disagreement, DNR, 114–5
Disseminated intravascular coagulation, 59, 66, 69
Disulfiram, 86
Diuretics, pregnancy, 74
DMTU, *192*
DNA synthesis, 210
DNR (Do not resuscitate), 104–6, 108, 111, 115
'Do not resuscitate' order (DNR), 104–6, 108, 111, 115
Documentation, treatment limitation decisions, 104, 115–9, *117*, 119
Dopamine, 62
Doxorubicin, 180
DPPG (phosphatidylglycerol), 257, 260, 262, *263*, 267
Drugs
  abuse, 86
  body composition, 136
  EMS, 2, 3, 6, 30–1
  muscle dysfunction, 238, 240, 243–5
  overdose, 28
  surfactants, 267–8
Dual-energy X-ray absorptiometry (DXA), 125, 127–8, 136, 137
Duodenal ulcers, 212, 219
Dynamic scoring systems, 108–9
Dyshaemoglobinaemia, 23
Dysphasia, 60
Dyspnoea, 73, 74, 107, 118
Dysrhythmias, poisoning, 84

Ebselen, 197
ECG (electrocardiogram), 5, 24
Echocardiography, 25, 74
Eclampsia, *58*, 60, 62, 63–5
Edrophonium, *87*
Edwin Smith surgical papyrus, 102
EEG (electro-encephalogram), 29
EGF *see* Epidermal growth factor
EGFR (epidermal growth factor receptor), 216, 218, 219
Eicosanoids, 45
Elastase, 184
Elastin, 137
Electrocardiogram, 5, 24
Electro-encephalogram, 29
Electrolytes, 145, 147, *148*, 151–2, *155*
Electro paramagnetic resonance (EPR) spectroscopy, 179, 189, 194
Elemental analysis, body composition, 135
Embryonal neoplasms, 221
Emergency medical services, 1–2, 16–17, 21
  airway management, 21–4

Emergency medical services (*cont.*)
cardiopulmonary resuscitation, 24–8
children, 4
drugs, 30–1
EMS management and deployment strategies, 8–11
ethics of research, futility and cost-containment, 11–13
National Association of Physicians, 7, 15
practice of medicine, 13
quality assessment, guidelines and reporting, 31–2
thrombolysis, 29
value of advanced life support interventions, 2–6
warning lights and sirens, 6–8
Emergency medical technicians (EMT), 3, 4, 14, 15
Emesis, 86, *87*, 90–2
Emetine, 91
Empowerment, 119
EMS *see* Emergency medical services
EMS-C (Emergency medical services for children), 4
Endocrine secretion, 214, 249
Endoscopy, 90
'Endothelial-derived relaxing factor' (EDRF), 183
Endothelin–1, 45
Endothelium
dependent relaxation, 48–9, *49*, 50
healing, 211, 221, 228
pregnancy, 57, 60
Endotoxaemia, 187, 194
Endotoxin, 74, 175, 187, 194, 228, 259
Endotracheal intubation
EMS, 2, 3, 4, 5, 21, 22, 23
pregnancy, 57, 64
poisoning, 92–3
surfactant, 263
treatment limitation decisions, 102
End-stage renal disease, 161, *167*
'Enduring' power of attorney, 112
Energy
nutritional support, 146, 147–51, *149*, 153, *155*, 169
stores, analysis, 136
Enteral nutrition, 144, 153–5, *155*
see also Nutritional support
Enteritis, *218*, 219
Enteroglucagon, 154
Enucleation, 213
Environmental poisoning, 83
Enzymes
antioxidant therapy, 182–3, *192–3*, 195–8
body composition, 137
Epidermal growth factor (EGF)
nutritional support, 144, 160, 168, *169*
tissue healing, 212, 215–20, *216–7*, 227, 229
Epidermis, 209–10
Epidural anaesthesia, 61–2
Epinephrine (Adrenaline), 3, 24,2 5, 26–7, 28
Epithelial cells, 207–8, 209–11, 212, 222, 223
EPO (erythropoietin), 207, *216*, 227, 229
Epoxides, 182
c-*erb*, 216–7
Erythromycin, 154
Erythropoietin, 207, *216*, 227, 229
Escherichia coli, 75
Ethane, 179, 183
Ethanol, 84, 85, 86, *87*, 88, 130
Ethchlorovinyl, 86
Ethclorvynol, *87*
Ethics, 2, 11–13, 102, 103, 105, 113
Ethylene glycol, 84
Euglycaemia, 90
European pharmacopoeia, 82
European Resuscitation Council (ERC), 32
Euthanasia, 105
Exosurf, 259, 262, *263*, 266
Extracellular domain, 229
Extracellular fluid, 126
Extracellular signal regulated kinase (ERK1), 231
Extracellular solids, 137
Extracellular water (ECW), 133, 136, 162, *167*

Fat
analysis, 125, 126, 127–8, 129

anthropometric indices, 134, *135*–6
body composition model, 136
dilution methods, 133
nutritional support, 144, 146, *148*, 150, 155, 159, 162
Fatty acids, 150, 169, *169*, 178, 179–80
Fenton reaction, 177, 178
Ferritin, 185
Fetal
development, 221
growth retardation, *58*, 59
squames, 68, 69
FGF (Fibroblast growth factor), *216*, 223, 229
Fibre, 154, 155, 169
Fibrin, 261
Fibrinogen, 59
Fibrinolysis, 223
Fibroblast growth factor, *216*, 223, 229
Fibroblasts, 208, 211, 221, 223, 228
Fibronectin, 210, 211, *222*
Fibrosis, 209
Ficke equation, 149
Firefighters, EMS, 3, 8, 9, 10–11, 16
Fish oil, 160
Flavonoids, 191, *192*, 194
Fluid status, 145, *148*
Fluid therapy, 60–1, 145
Focal liver infarction, *58*
Food and Drug Administration, US, 12
Free radicals *see* Antioxidant therapy
Frusemide, 62
Fulminant hepatic failure, 213
Furosemide, 3
Futility, treatment, 2, 11, 12, 109–10, 111

GABA agonists, 28
γ-radiation, 180
Gastric epithelia, 207
Gastric rupture, 92
Gastric ulcers, 219, 227
Gastrin, 154
Gastrointestinal tract
disease, 161
dysfunction, 158
haemorrhage, 70
healing, 211–3
nutritional support, *148*
poisoning, 86, *87*, 90–7
radiation syndrome, 212
Gastroparesis, 155
GDP (guanosine diphosphate), 231, *230*
Gene therapy, *193*
Genetic engineering, 197
Gestation *see* Pregnancy
Glasgow Coma Scale, 108
Glioma cells, 215
Glossitis, 147
Glucagon, 72
Gluconeogenesis, 146, 156
Glucose, 71, 89–91, 151, 152, *155*, *164*, *167*, 249
Glutamine (GLN)
muscle dysfunction, 247
nutritional support, 144, 146, 151, 152, 154, 155–9, *157–8*, *167*, 169, *169*
Glutathione (GSH), 157, 185, 188, 189, *193*, 198
peroxidase, 185, 188–9, 198
Glycaemia, 250
Glycogen, 136, 249
Glycogenolysis, 72
Glycoproteins, 228
Glycosaminoglycans (GAGs), 211
GM-CSF, *216*, 228, 229
Gram-negative sepsis, 102
Granulation tissue, 209, 210
Granulocyte colony stimulating factor (G-CSF), *216*, 228, 229
Granulocyte-macrophage CSF (GM-CSF), *216*, 228, 229
Granulocytes, 228
Grb-2, *230*, 231
Growth factors
body composition, 137
nutritional support, 144, 159, 160, 168–9, *169*
tissue healing, 206–7
signal transduction, 229–31, *230*
structure, function and application, 214–29, *216–8*, *220*, *222*, *224*–5
wound healing, 207–14, *208*

Growth factors (*cont.*)
see also Growth hormone, Insulin-like growth factor
Growth factor receptor bound protein 2 (Grb–2), *230*, 231
Growth hormone (GH)
muscle dysfunction, 247, 249, 250
nutritional support, 144, 159, 160, 161–8, *163–5*, *167–9*
GSH (glutathione), 157, 185, 188, 189, *193*, 198
GSSG reductase, 198
GTPase-activating protein (GAP), *230*, 231
Guanosine diphosphate, 231, *230*
Guedel airway, 22
Guidelines, EMS, 31–2
Guillain-Barre syndrome, 241, *248*
Gunshot wound (GSW), 7
Gut barrier function, 154, 157

H_2-receptor antagonists, 212
Haber-Weiss reaction, 178
Haematological malignancy, 109
Haematoma, 59–60
Haematopoiesis, 228
Haematopoietic growth factors, *216*, 227–9
Haemodynamics
ARDS, *42*
pregnancy, 55, *56*, 60–1, 67, 69, 74
Haemoglobin, *182*, 185
Haemolysis, *58*, 59, 75
Haemolytic uraemic syndrome, 65
Haemopoietic cells, 207
Haemorrhagic shock, 190
Haemosiderin, 185
Hair, 137
Hallucinogenic agents, 85
Harris-Benedict equation, 147, *148*
Head injury, 108
Healing by first intention, 209
Healing by second intention, 209
Health state, 116–8, *117*
Helicopters, 10
'HELLP', 59, 65, 70
Heme-base radicals, 179
Heparin, 69, 185, 223
Heparin-binding EGF, 215, *216*
Hepatectomy, 208, 213
Hepatic *see* Liver
Hepatitis, 70, 213
Hepatocyte growth factor (HGF), *216*, 223–6, *224–5*, 229
Hepatocytes, 208
Herbal medicine, 83
Heroin, 86, *87*, 96
Hexadecanol, 262, *263*
HGF (hepatocyte growth factor), *216*, 223–6, *224–5*, 229
Histamine, 175, 183, 212
Histidine, 184, 186
History, poisoning and overdose, 82–3, 97
HIV, 262, 267
HOCL *see* Hypochlorous acid
Homeopathic medicine, 83
Homicide, 83
'Hour glass' stomach, 212
Housebound lifestyle, 107
Human intestinal trefoil factor (hITF), 227
Human spasmolytic polypeptide (hSP), 226, 227
Hyaline membrane, 259, 264
Hyaluronic acid, 184
Hydralazine, 61, 63
Hydrocarbon, 85, 91, 95, 179, 183, 188
Hydrochloric acid, 265
Hydrocortisone, 239
Hydrodensitometry, 125
Hydrogen, 126, 127, 132
Hydrogen peroxide, 178, 179, 182, *182*, 184
endogenous protection from, 185
therapy, 191, *192–3*, 196
Hydroperoxide (ROOH), *177*, 179, 186
Hydroxyethyl starch, 195
Hydroxyl radical (OH), 176–7, *177*, 178–9, 182, *182*, 184, 185, 191
Hyperalimentation, 147
Hyperbilirubinaemia, 151
Hypercalcaemia, *168*
Hypercapnia, 24
Hypercarbia, 27, 64
Hyperglycaemia, 72, 89–90, 147, 149–50, 154, *168*
Hyperkalaemia, 28
Hypermagnesaemia, 96

Hypernatraemia, 27, 96
Hyperosmolarity, 27
Hyperoxia, 23
Hyperponea, 84
Hypertension, 42–5, *43–5*, 60, 62–3, 70, 84, *87*
Hyperthermia, poisoning, 84, 85, *87*
Hypertriglyceridemia, 150
Hypnosis, 118
Hypocalcaemia, 96
Hypocapnia, 24
Hypocarbia, 75
Hypochlorous acid (HOCL), 178, 179, 182, *182*, 184, 189
  antioxidant therapy, 191, 194
  endogenous protection, 185
Hypoglycaemia
  EMS, 6
  muscle dysfunction, 250
  nutritional support, 150, 168
  poisoning and overdose, 87–8, 89–90
  pregnancy and childbirth, 70, 71
Hypoglycaemic agents, 85
Hypokalaemia, 30, 72
Hypomagnesaemia, 30
Hypopnoea, 85, *87*
Hypotension
  antioxidant therapy, 183
  EMS, 27
  muscle dysfunction, 241
  poisoning, 84, 85, *87*
  treatment limitation decision, 107
Hypothermia, poisoning, 85, *87*
Hypovolaemia, 84
Hypovolaemic shock, 175
Hypoxaemia, 41, 46, 68, 261
Hypoxanthine, 180, 195
Hypoxia, 75, 85, 87–8

IFN-γ (interferon-gamma), 228
IGF *see* Insulin-like growth factor
IL *see* Interleukins
Immunity
  antioxidant therapy, 175, 194
  growth factors, 214
  nutritional support, 146, 152, 161, 166, *167*, *169*
  surfactant, 259, 262
Immunodeficiency, 158
Immunosuppression, 153, 184
Independence, 113
Indomethacin, 46
Infection
  antioxidant therapy, 175, 176, 184, 186, 195, 196, 198
  nutritional support, 145, 153–4, 155, 162, 164, *167*
  pregnancy, 73, 74
Inflammation, 206
Information, 112, 113
Inhibins, *216*, 222
Injury, EMS, 1, 5
Insulin
  muscle dysfunction, 247, 249, 250
  nutritional support, 146, 150, 160, 161, *167–8*
  poisoning and overdose, 88
  treatment limitation decisions, 102
Insulin-like growth factor (IGF)
  muscle dysfunction, 247, 249–50
  nutritional support, 144, 146, 152, 154, *157*, 160, 161, 162, *164*, 166–8, *167–9*
  tissue healing, *216*, 221, 229
Interferon-gamma, 228
Integrins, 196
Interleukins, 145, 206, *216*, 228, 229, 259
Intra-arterial pressure device, 25
Intracellular domain, 229
Intracellular water (ICW), 162, *167*
Intra-osseous injection, 4
Intravenous cannulation, 2
Intravenous (IV) fluid infusion, 4
Intubation *see* Endotracheal intubation
Invasive monitoring, pregnancy, 61–2, 63
Ion channels, 206
Iron
  antioxidants, 176–7, *177*, 178–9, 185, 190, 191, *192*, 195
  poisoning, 84, 86, 95, 96
Irradiation, 212
Ischaemia
  antioxidant therapy, 180, *181*, 188, 191, 194, 195, 198
  EMS, 30
  muscle dysfunction, 240–1

Ischaemia (*cont.*)
overdose, 88–9
pregnancy, 73
Isoniazid, 85
Isopropyl alcohol, 86
Isoproterenol, 213
Isotope dilution, 130–3, 136
ITF, *216*
Ito cells, 224, *224*, 226

Jaundice, 70
Joints, 137
Justice, 119

Keratinocyte growth factor (KGF), 223
Ketoacidosis, 30
α-Ketoglutarate (AKG), 156, *157*
Ketone bodies, 57, 72
Ketonuria, 72
Kidney, healing, 213
c-*kit*, *216*, 229
Klebsiella, 75

Labetalol, 63
Lacrimation, *87*
Lactate, 88, 89
Lactic acidosis, 27
Lactulose, 71
Laminin, 211
Laplace Law, 258
Laryngeal Mask Airway (LMA), 22–3
Latency associated protein (LAP), 222
Law, 111, 114–5
Lazaroids, 191, *192*
Lean, 125, 127–8, 146
Left ventricular failure, pregnancy, 68
Lethargy, *87*
Leukocyte adhesion molecules, 187
Leukocyte adhesion receptors, 196
Leukocytes, 180, 181–2, *182*, 186, 259
Leukotrienes, 45, 175, 183, 187, 196
Liability, EMS, 16
Lidocaine, 3
Limb circumference, 134
Lipids
antioxidant therapy, 175, 179–80, 183, 191
body composition, 128
nutritional support, 150, 153, 160, 169, *169*
surfactant, 257, *263*, 267
Lipolysis, 146, 161, 247, 249
Lipopolysaccharides, 228
Lipo-oxygenase, 183, 196
Lipoperoxidation, 176–80, *177*, 183, 186, 188, 194, 195
Lithium, 95, 96
Litigation, 119
Liver
healing, 213, 220
nutritional support, 147
pregnancy, *58*, 59–60, 70
transplantation, 72
Lividity, 12
Living wills, 113, 115–6
Losec, 212
Lungs
healing, 220
muscle dysfunction, 247
transplantation, 267
see also Pulmonary vasomotor dysfunction
Lysergic acid diethylamide, 85

α_2-Macroglobulin, 184
Macrophages, 181, 186, 228
Madin-Darby canine kidney (MDCK), 224
Magnesium
citrate, 95
EMS, 30–1
nutritional support, *148*, 151, 152, *155*, 161, 162, *164*, *167*
sulphate, 63–4, 72
Magnetic resonance imaging, 59–60, 65, 129, 137
Malabsorption, 154
Malignant cells, 215
Mallory Weiss tears, 92
Malnutrition, 144–5, 146, 147
muscle dysfunction, 238, 239, 246
Management and deployment, EMS, 2, 8–11, 13–15
Mannitol, 62, 191, *192*

Marketing, EMS, 9
MCF-7 human breast cancer cell line, 226
Mechanical ventilation
  muscle dysfunction, 238, 239, 241, 242, 243, 244, 245–6
  pregnancy, 64
  pulmonary vasomotor dysfunction, 41
  treatment limitation decisions, 114, 116, 118–9
Meclofenamate, 46
Meconium, 67, 68
MEK, *230*, 231
Mental status, 87–8, 90
Meprobamate, *87*
Mercuric chloride, 92
Mescaline, 85
Mesenchymal cells, 221
c-*met*, *225*
Metabolic state, 145
Metal chelators, 185
Metalloproteinases, 211, *222*
Methadone, *87*
Methaemoglobinaemia, 85
Methanol, 84, 86
Methemoglobin, 179
N-Methyl-L-arginine, 196
Methyldopa, 63
Methylene blue, 46, 47
Metoclopramide, 95
Micronutrients, 145, 146, 151–2
Microvillous atrophy, 219, *220*
Midazolam, 118
Migrainous auras, 60
Minerals, 136, *148*
Miosis, 86, *87*
Mitochondrial electron transport chain, 180–1, *181*
Mitochondrial enzymes, 188
Mitogen, 216, 220–1, 225
Mitogen Activated Protein Kinase (MAPK), *230*, 231
Mitosis, 210
Mitral stenosis, 73
Models, body composition, *126*, 135–7, *136*
Monoamine oxidase inhibitors, 84, *87*, 94
Monoclonal antibodies, 137
Monocytes, 221
Monomethylarginine (L-NMMA), 190, *193*, 196
Morals, 102, 113
Morbidity rates, 107
Morphine, 74, *87*
Mortality rates, 107
MPM II, 107
Mucosal defence barrier, gastrointestinal tract, 212
Mucositis, 219
Multiple organ dysfunction syndrome (MODS), 175
Multiple organ system failure, 242, 244, 250
Multiplication Stimulating Activity-MSA, 221
Muscle
  body composition, 128, 129, 137
  dysfunction, 238, 250
    acquired muscle disease, 238–41
    acquired peripheral nervous disease, 241–3
    amelioration of muscle wasting, 247–50, *248*
    neuromuscular disorders, 243–7
    nutritional support, 145, *148*, 156, 158
  healing, 208
  relaxants, 239, 243–5, 246, 247
  wasting, 158
Mutagenesis, 184
Mydriasis, 86, *87*
Myelin, 257, *258*
Myeloperoxidase (MPO), 178, 182, *182*, 189, 194
Myocardial
  infarction, 4–5, 6, 29, 31, 66, 207
  ischaemia, 73
  depression, 183
  dysfunction, 84
Myogenic stem cells, 208
Myoglobin, 185, 239–40
Myopathy, 238, 239, 240, 243, *248*

NADPH, 181–2
NADPH oxidase, 178, 181, 182, 196
Naloxone, 28
National Association of EMS Physicians (NAEMSP), 7, 15

National Institute of Health, US, 11–12
National Standards Conference on Emergency Cardiac Care, 12
Necrotizing myopathy, 243, *248*
Neomycin, 71
Neonate, surfactant, 259, 261–2, 263
Neoplastic growth, *168*
Neovascularization, 210
Nephrectomy, 213
Nephrogenesis, 224
Nephrotic syndrome, *58*
Neurological imaging, pregnancy, 65
Neuromuscular blocking drugs, 243
Neuromuscular disorders, 243–7
Neutron activation analysis (NAA), 125, 126–7, 135, 136, *136*
Neutropenia, 207, 228
Neutrophils, 264
NGF, *216*
Nicotinamide adenine dinucleotide phosphate, 181–2
  oxidase, 178, 181, 182, 196
Nicotine, 86
Nifedipine, 63
Nimodipine, 28
Nitric oxide
  antioxidant therapy, 183, *187*, 188, 196
  pulmonary vascular dysfunction, 46, 47, 48, 50
  synthetase, 183, 190, *193*, 196–7
N-Nitro-L-arginine, 46, 47–8, 196
Nitrogen
  body composition, 126–7, 130
  dioxide, 214
  growth hormone, 161, 162, 165–6, *163–5*, *167*
  muscle dysfunction, 238, 246, 247, 250
  nutritional support, 145, 146, 151, 152, 159, 168
    use of glutamine, 156, 157, *158*, 159
Nitrone, 194, *192*
Nitroprusside, 63
N-Nitroso-*N*-methylurethane (NNNMU), 265
NMDA antagonists, 28
Non-maleficence, 119
Non-steroid anti-inflammatory drugs (NSAIDS), *192- 3*, 196
NSAIDS, *192–3*, 196
Nucleic acids, 183, 184
Nucleotide, 156, 160
Nutritional assessment, 147, *148–9*
Nutritional status, 134
Nutritional support, 144–6, 169, *169*
  administration of growth factors, 160–9, *163–5*, *167–8*
  current practices, 146–55, *148–9*, *155*
  muscle dysfunction, 238
  pregnancy, 57
  use of specific nutrients, 155–60, *157–8*
Nystagmus, 86

'Oat cell', 215
Obstructive airways disease, 242, 245, 246
Obstructive lung disease, 161
Occupational poisoning, 83
Ocular movement, poisoning, 86
Oesophageal obturator airway (EOA), 21
Oestrogens, 214
Oleic acid, 265
Oliguria, 62
Ondansetron, 95
Open-chest CPR (OCCPR), 25–6
Opioids, 84, 85, 86, *87*, 118
Oregon 'experiment', 110
Organ donation, 109
Organ transplantation, 189, 190
Organophosphates, 84, 86, *87*
Organoselenium, *193*, 197–8
Ornithine a-ketoglutarate (OKG), 156, *157*
Orogastric lavage, 90, 92–3, 97
Orthopnoea, 73
Osteoblasts, 223
Osteocytes, 208
Osteogenetic protein–1, 223
Osteosarcoma, 215
Oval cells, 225, 226
Overdosed patient *see* Poisoned and overdosed patient
Oximetry, 23
Oxoferryl radical, 179, 182, *182*

Oxygen, 126, 130, 145
  see also Antioxidant therapy
Oxygen free radicals, 259, *260*, 261
Oxypurinol, *192*, 195

Paediatrics, 4, 22, 23, 27, 83
Pain, 113
Pancreatic acinar cells, 208
Pancreatic spasmolytic polypeptide (PSP), 226
Pancreatitis, 70, 150, 152, 175, 241, 266
Pancuronium, 244
Pancytopenias, 228
Panproctocolectomy, 136
Papanicolaou method, staining, 68–9
Paracetamol, 213
Paracrine secretion, 214–5, 227, 249
Paramedics, 1, 3, 4, 5, 6, 9, 13, 15
Paraquat, 180
Parasympathetic, 86
Parenchymal cells, 208
Parenteral nutrition, 144, 145, 247
  see also Nutritional support
Parietal, 212
Parotid gland, 213
PDGF (platelet-derived growth factor), 215, *216*, 220–1, 229
PEG catalase, *193*
Penicillin, 102
Pentamidine, 268
Pentane, 179, 183
Pentoxyfilline, *193*, 196
Peptic ulcers, 212, 219
Peptide growth factors *see* Growth factors
Peptides, 154, 155, 175, 215, 226–7
Perferryl ion, 177
Pericytes, 221
Peripheral motor polyneuropathy, 241
Peripheral nervous disease, 241–3
Peripheral neuropathy, 238
Peripheral vascular disease, 239
Peripheral vein access, nutritional support, *149*, 151
Peristalsis, *87*
Peritonitis, 175
Peroxyl radical (ROO), 177, *177*, 179, *187*
Peroxynitrite (ONOO), 183
Persistent vegetative state, 114
PET (Pre-eclamptic toxaemia), 57–65, *58*, 70
Phagocytosis, 175, 259
Pharyngo-Tracheal-Lumen Airways (PTLA), 21–2, 23
Phencyclidine, 85, 86
Phenothiazines, 85
Phenylbutazone, 196
Phenytoin, 64, 86
Phosgene, 85
Phosphatidylcholine (DPPC), 256–67, *258*, *263*
Phosphatidylglycerol (DPPG), 257, 260, 262, *263*, 266, 267
Phosphatidyl inositol (PI) 3-kinase, 206, 229, *230*, 231, 260
Phospholipase, 261
Phospholipase Cγ(PLCγ), 229, *230*, 231
Phospholipids
  body composition, 128
  surfactant, 257, 259, 261, 262, *263*, 266, 267
Phosphorus, 126, *148*, 151, 152, *155*, 161, 162, *163–4*, *167*
Phosphorylation, 221, 229
Physiotherapy, muscle dysfunction, 239
Physostigmine, *87*
Pilocarpine, *87*
Placental
  abruption, 66
  infarction, 58–9, *58*
Plasmin, 211, 223
Plasminogen, 210, 211, 226
  activator inhibitor (PAI-I), 211, *222*
Platelet activating factor (PAF), 45, 187, 196
Platelet-derived growth factor (PDGF), 215, *216*, 220–1, 229
Pleiotropic, 223
Pluripotential stem cells, 207, 221
Pneumatic anti-shock garment (PASG), 4
Pneumococcal pneumonia, 102, 109
Pneumocystis carinii, 259, 267
Pneumocytes, 214
Pneumomediastinum, 92

Pneumonectomy, 214
Pneumonia, 47, 48, 75, 107, 267, 268
Pneumonitis, 94, 260
Pneumothorax, 92, 256
POISINDEX, 82
Poisoned and overdosed patient, 82, 97, 213
  clinical evaluation, 82–6, *87*
  gastric emptying, 93–7
  gastrointestinal decontamination, 90–3
  treatment, 87–90
Polio, 102
Politics, EMS, 9,11
Polydipsia, 70
Polyethylene glycol, 97, 197
Polymorphonuclear neutrophiles (PMN), 178, 181–2, 186, *187*, 188, 189, 190
Polyoses, 184
Polypeptides, 215
Polyphenol, 185, 186
Polyribosone index, 247
Polysaccharides, 175
Polyunsaturated lipids, 183
Porcine, 262
Porphyrines, 176
Positive pressure ventilation, 102, 261
Post-partum, 65
Post-TPN syndrome, 219
Potassium
  body composition, 126, 129–30, 133
  EMS, 30
  nutritional support, 151, 152, *155*, 161, 162, *163–4*, *167*
  pregnancy and childbirth, 72
Power of attorney, 112
Pox virus growth factors, 215, *216*
pp60$^{c\text{-}src}$, 229
Practice of Medicine, EMS, 2, 13–15
Pre-arrest morbidity index, 107
Pre-eclampsia, 57–65, *58*
Pre-eclamptic toxaemia (PET), 57–65, *58*, 70
Pregnancy, 55, 76
  acute fatty liver of pregnancy, 69–72
  amniotic fluid embolism, 65–9
  biological changes, 55
  medical care, 55–7, *56*
  pulmonary injury complicating pyelonephritis, 72–6
  pulmonary oedema due to tocolytic therapy, 72–4
  severe pre-eclampsia and eclampsia, 57–65, *58*
Prehospital care *see* Emergency medical services
Primary union, healing, 209
Procarcinogens, 183
Procollagenase, 184
Proelastase, 184
Prompt gamma activation, 126, 127
Propofol, 118
Propoxyphene, *87*
Prostacyclin, 46, 48, 50
Prostaglandin, 28, 44–5, *44–5*, 46, 69, 183
Prostaglandin E1, 44–5, *44*, *45*
Prostanoids, 175, 187, 196
Prostatic acinar cells, 208
Protease, 180, 184, 195, 222, *222*, 223
Protein
  antioxidant therapy, 183, 184
  body composition, 125, 126, 128, 129–30, 134, *135*
    models, 136, 137
  bone morphogenetic proteins, *216*, 222, 223
  kinase C, *230*, 231
  muscle dysfunction, 249–50
  nutritional support, 144–6, *148*, *149*, 152, 153, 154, *155*, 156, 169
    administration, 147–51
    growth factors, 161, 162, *167*
  phosphorylation, 206
  surfactant, 257, 260, *260*, 262, 264, 266, 268
  tyrosine kinase (PTKs), *225*, 229, *230*
α_1-Proteinase inhibitor, 184
Proteinuria, 57, 70
Proteoglycans, 211
Proteolysis, 146
Proton-pump inhibitors, 212
Protoplasm, 126
pS2, *216*, 226, 227
Pseudo-diabetes insipidus, 70
Psilocybin, 85
Psychology, pregnancy, 56

Pulmonary capillary wedge pressure, pregnancy, 55, *56*, 61
Pulmonary, healing, 213
Pulmonary hypertension, 41–50, *42–5*, *47*, *49*, 67
Pulmonary oedema
  pregnancy, 55, 74–6
    amniotic fluid embolism, 66, 67, 68, 69
    pre-eclampsia and eclampsia, 58, *58*, 61, 62, 63
    tocolytic therapy, 72–4
  surfactant physiology, 259, *260*
  vasomotor dysfunction, 41
Pulmonary thromboembolism, 67
Pulmonary vasomotor dysfunction, 41–2, *42*, 50
  endothelium-dependent relaxation, 48–9, *49*
  hypertension, mechanisms of, 44–5, *44–5*
  hypertension, nature of, 42–4, *43*
  vasodilator release, 46–8, *47*
Pulse oximeters, 23
Pyelonephritis, 72–6
Pyloric mucosa, 212
Pyloric stenosis, 212
Pyrexia, 75

Quality assessment, EMS, 31–2
Quality of life measures, 106, 109, 112, 113

Race, 111
Radiation, 180
Radiation pneumonitis, 260
Radiosulfate, 133
Raf, *230*, 231
Ras, *230*, 231
Rat intestinal trefoil factor (rITF), 227
Rat spasmolytic polypeptide (rSP), 226–7
Reactive gliosis, 207
Recombinant DNA techniques, 206
Recombinant human erythropoietin (rhEPO), 228
Re-epithelialization, 212
Refeeding syndrome, 151
Regeneration, healing, *208*, 209
Regional poison centres, 82
Rehabilitation, muscle dysfunction, 238–9, 246
Relatives, 112, 113–5, 118–9
Religion, 111, 113–4, 115
Remodelling, 209
Renal
  ammoniagenesis, 156
  disease, 161, *167*
  failure
    growth factors, 207, 228
    muscle dysfunction, 239–40, 241, 244, 247
    nutritional support, 161, *167*
    pregnancy and childbirth, *58*, 70
    treatment limitation decisions, 107
  secretion, 72
  tubule cells, 208
Repair, healing, 209
Reporting, EMS, 31–2
Research, EMS, 11–13
Respiration, 177–8, 180–1, *181*
Respiratory
  burst, 186, *187*, 196
  distress, 74–5, 219
  distress syndrome (RDS), 256–7, 262–3
  failure, 194, 241, 242
  muscle, nutritional support, 165–6, *165*, *167*
  see also Acute respiratory distress syndrome
Restitution, 212
Resuscitation
  cerebral, 28
  see also Cardiopulmonary resuscitation
Retinal detachment, *58*
Retinol binding protein, 147
Reye's syndrome, 69
Rhabdomyolysis, 239–40, 241, 246
rhEGF, *218*, 219, *220*
Rigor mortis, 12
Risk benefit, 106–10, 116
  ratio, 144
Ritodrine, 72
RNA, 160, 226–7
Rous sarcoma virus, 229

Salbutamol, 72, 244
Salicylates, 84, 85, 86, 88, 95, 97
Salivary glands, 213
Salivation, 86, *87*
SAPS II, 107
'Sarcoma growth factor', 215
Satellite cells, 208
Scar tissue, 209
Scatter factor, *216*, 223–6, *224–5*, 229
SCF (Stem cell factor), 109, *216*, 229
Scombroid intoxication, 86
Scopolamine, *87*
Scoring system, 107–9
Secondary union, healing, 209
Sedation, 118
Sedative-hypnotics, 84, 85, *87*
Seizures, 6, 30, 63, 64, 65
Selectins, 196
Selenium, 152
Sensory polyneuropathy, 241
Sepsis
  antioxidants, 188, 194
  body composition, 134, *135*, 136
  muscle dysfunction, 240, 241, 242, 244, 247, 248, 249
  nutritional support, 162, 166
  pregnancy and childbirth, 74–5
  pulmonary vasomotor dysfunction, 41
  surfactant, 266
Septic shock
  free radicals, 175, 183, 186, 187, 188
    antioxidant therapy, 194, 196, 198
  pregnancy and childbirth, 66
Septicaemia, muscle dysfunction, 241
Serotonin, 175
Sex glands, 213–4
SH2 (Src homology 2), 229
Short bowel syndrome, 159
Siderophores, *192*, 195
Simian sarcoma virus, 221
Singlet oxygen, 178, 179, 182, *182*
Sinus tachycardia, 73
Skeletal muscle, 137, *148*, 156, 208
Skin, *148*, 209–11
  grafts, 223
Skinfold anthropometry, 125, 134, 135, *136*
SLUDGE, *87*
Smoke, 265, 268
Smooth muscle cells, 208
Social isolation, 113
Society, 110
SOD (superoxide dismutase), 180, 185, *193*, 197, 188
Sodium, 72–3, 126, 133, 161, 162, *167*
  nitroprusside, 49
Soft tissue, 137
Somatomedin C, 221
Sorbitol, 95, 96, 155
SP, *216*
SP-A protein, 257, 259, 262, 263, *263*, 267
SP-B protein, 257, 262, *263*
SP-C protein, 257, 262, *263*
Sphingomyelin, 128, 260
Spin trapping agents, 189, 194
Spinal immobilization, 3
Src family, 229
Standards, EMS, 32
Stature, 134
Status eclampticus, 60, 64
Stem cell factor (SCF), 109, *216*, 229
Stem cell regulation, 228–9
Steroids, muscle dysfunction, 239, 245–6
Stoichiometric protection, radicals, 184, 185, 186, 191, 194, *192*, 198
Stratified squamous cells, 207
Stroke, 1
Stromelysin, 211
Stupor, *87*
Subcutaneous tissue, 210
Submaxillary gland, 213
Sudden Death Syndrome, 3
Suicide, 83, 111
Sulfhydryl, 184
Superoxide anion, 178, 180, 181, 182, *182*, *187*, 188, *193*, 195
Superoxide dismutase (SOD), 180, 185, 188, *193*, 197
Supine hypotension syndrome, 56
Supraventricular re-entry tachycardia, 3, 30
Surface tension *see* Surfactant
Surfactant, lung injury, 220, 256, 268
  abnormality in acute lung injury, 259–61, *260*

animal studies, 264–5
exogenous surfactant preparations, 261–3, *263*
history, 256–7
human studies, 265–6
method of administration, 263–4
structure and physiology, 257–9, *258*
surfactant and other respiratory diseases, 267–8
Surfactant-HA, *263*
Surgery, poisoning, 90
Surrogacy, 112–3
Survanta, 262, *263*, 268
SVTs (Supraventricular re-entry tachycardia), 30
Swan-Ganz catheter, 62
Sympathomimetic agents, 72–4, 75, 84, 85, 86, *87*, 213
Syrup of Ipecac, 90–2, 93, 97
Systemic inflammatory response syndrome (SIRS), 175, 176

Tachycardia, 3, 73, 74, 84, *87*, 89
Tachypnoea, 84
Tagamet, 212
Teeth, 137
Teichopsia, 60
Terbutaline, 72, 239
Terminal illness, EMS, 12
Tetany, 30
Tetracycline toxicity, 69, 71
TGF-α, 212, 215, 216–7, *216*, 219–20
TGF-β, *216*, 221–3, *222*
Thallium, 86
Theophylline, 84, 85, 86, *87*, 95, 96, 97
Thermogenesis, 137
Thiobarbituric acid reactive substances (TBARS), 188
Thiol compounds, 186
Thiyl radicals (RS), 186
Thrombocytopenia, *58*, 59, 71, 75
Thrombolysis, EMS, 29
Thrombolytics, 4–5, 6
Thrombotic thrombocytopoenic purpura, 65
Thromboxane, 45
Thyroid
dyshormonogenesis, 213
follicular cells, 208
stimulating hormone, 213
Tissue, 125, 127, 128–9, 145
see also Growth factors
Tissue inhibitor of metalloproteinase (TIMP), 211, *222*
TLO (Treatment limitation order), 104, 105–10, 113
TNF-α (tumour necrosis factor), 48, *49*, 228
Tocolytic therapy, 72–4, 75
Tocopheryl radical, 186
Torsades des pointes, 31
Total body fat (TBF), 135, *136*
Total body nitrogen (TBN), 126, 127
Total body protein (TBP), 126, 127, 137
Total body water (TBW), 130–2, *131*, 133, 134
Total parenteral nutrition (TPN), 217
Tracheal intubation *see* Endotracheal intubation
Tracheostomy, 119
Transferrin, 147, 185
Transforming growth factor alpha (TGF-α), 212, 215, 216–7, *216*, 219–20
Transforming growth factor-βs, *216*, 221–3, *222*
Transition metals, 176–7, *177*, 185, 195
Transmembrane domain, 229
Transoesophageal echocardiography, 25
Trauma
antioxidant therapy, 175, 186
body composition, 134, *135*, 136
centres, 1
EMS, 4
muscle dysfunction, 240
nutritional support, 147, 161, 164
pulmonary vasomotor dysfunction, 41
surfactant, 260, 261
Traumatic shock, 194, 195
Treatment limitation decisions, 102–4, 105–6, 119
assessment and measurement of risk-benefit, 106–7
autonomy, 111–2

Treatment limitation decisions (*cont.*)
  consensus, 113–4
  disagreements, 114–5
  'do not resuscitate' orders, 104–5
  individual risk-benefit, 107–110
  risks and benefits to society, 110
  surrogacy, 112–3
  withdrawing or withholding treatment, 115–9, *117*
'Treatment limitation order' (TLO), 104, 105–10, 113
Trefoil growth factor family, *216*
Trefoil peptides, 226–7
Tremor, 89
Tricyclic antidepressants, 84, 85, *87*
Triglyceride, 128, *148*, 150, 152, 154, 160, 162, *169*
Tritiated water dilution method, 135
Tritium dilution methods, 130–3
Trunk circumference, 134
Tryptophan, 184, 186
  dioxygenase, 187
TSH (thyroid stimulating hormone), 213
Tube feeding 114
Tubular necrosis, 62
Tumour angiogenesis, 223
Tumour cells, 221
Tumour necrosis factor (TNF), 145, 187–8, 228, 259
Tumour necrosis factor-α, 48, *49*, 187–8, 228
Tyloxapol, 262, *263*
Tyrosine kinases, 206, 221
Tyrosine phosphorylation, 229

UACL, 227
Ubiquinone, 181, *181*
Ulcer Associated Cell Lineage (UACL), 227
Ulcerative colitis, 219
Ulcers, 212, 219–20, 223, 226, 227
Urea dilution, 130
Urea generation, 161, 162, *167*
Uric acid, 185, 186, 191, *192*
Urination, 86, *87*
URO-EGF, 216, *216*, 217, 218–9
β-Urogastrone, 216, 217
'Utstein' style reporting, 32
UV radiation, 180

Vascular endothelial cells, 208
Vascular endothelial growth factor (VEGF), *216*, 221
Vasoconstriction, 44–8, 50
Vasodilators, 44–5, 46–8, *47*, 50, 61
Vasospasm, 30
Vecuronium, 244, 247
VEGF (vascular endothelial growth factor), *216*, 221
Ventilation
  muscle dysfunction, 238
  poisoning, 84
Ventricular fibrillation, 3
Verapamil, 30
Visual disturbances, 89
Vitamin C, 152, *169*, 178, 185, 186, *192*, 194–5
Vitamin E, 152, *169*, 185–6, 188, 189, *192*, 194–5
Vitamin K, 71

Warning lights and sirens (WL and S), 2, 6–8, 11
Water, body, 125, 128, 134–5, *135*, 136
Weight change, 134–5, *135*, *148*
Whole body counting, 129–30, 133
Whole bowel irrigation, 96–7
Withdrawing treatment, 103, 111–9, *117*
Withholding treatment, 103, 111–9, *117*
Wolff-Parkinson-White syndrome, 30
Wound healing, growth factors, 207–9, *208*
  gastrointestinal tract, 211–3
  liver, 213
  nutritional support, 145, 146, 152, 161, 162, *167*, 168
  other tissues, 213–4
  skin, 209–11
  see also Growth factors

Xanthine
  dehydrogenase, 180, 195
  oxidase, 178, 180–1, 182, 188, 189, *192*, 195, 196
Xenobiotics, 180, 213
X-radiation, 180

Zantac, 212
Zinc, 146, 147, 152, *155*